# NEW YORK

# JOURNAL OF PHARMACY,

PUBLISHED BY AUTHORITY OF

**THE COLLEGE OF PHARMACY OF THE CITY OF NEW YORK,**

EDITED BY

BENJAMIN W. McCREADY, M. D.

PROFESSOR OF MATERIA MEDICA AND PHARMACY IN THE COLLEGE OF PHARMACY,

ASSISTED BY A PUBLISHING COMMITTEE, CONSISTING OF

JOHN H. CURRIE, THOMAS B. MERRICK, EUGENE DUPUY,
JOHN MEAKIM, GEORGE D. COGGESHALL.

VOLUME II.

New York:
CHARLES SHIELDS, PRINTER,
CORNER OF PLATT AND GOLD STREETS,

1853.

# CONTENTS.

## INDEX OF AUTHORS.

# NEW YORK JOURNAL OF PHARMACY.

JANUARY, 1853.


## ON THE PURIFICATION OF SAL-AMMONIAC.

BY HENRY WURTZ.

Many chemists must have become aware that the loaves of sal-ammoniac which occur in commerce almost invariably contain iron in some form of combination. It is the separation of this iron which is particularly to be brought under consideration in this paper. The occurrence of this contamination is not noticed by Gmelin, but I find that Pereira in his materia medica, mentions it, apparently entertaining the opinion, however, that the iron is contained exclusively in the brownish yellow layers which usually appear in a section of one of the loaves. He remarks,* "For several years past I have been accustomed to demonstrate in the Lecture-room that a solution of these yellow bands in water gives no traces of iron on the addition of ferrocyanide of potassium, until a few drops of nitric acid be added when a copious blue precipitate is formed; and I therefore inferred that this yellow matter was a double chloride of iron and ammonium. My opinion has been fully confirmed by the experiments of Dr. G. H. Jackson."

In the examination of several specimens of commercial sal-ammoniac, however, I have myself found the quantity of protochloride of iron in the transparent colorless portions of the mass to be apparently equal to that in the yellow portions. Neither the colorless nor the yellow portions give any reaction with yellow prussiate of potash or with sulphocyanide of patas-

* Pereira's Materia Medica, 1, 446.

sium, or any precipitate upon heating with ammonia; but strong solutions of each are equally blackened by sulphide of ammonium, and after boiling with a drop of nitric acid give quite considerable and apparently equal flocky brown precipitates of hydrated sesquioxide of iron upon heating with ammonia, and apparently about the same blue coloration with prussiate of potash, and red with sulphocyanide of potassium. The yellow substance in the colored bands I am disposed to regard as some organic matter. The iron is evidently all present in the form of protochloride, which has sublimed together with the vapor of the sal-ammoniac in the process of manufacture. In fact, judging *a priori* from the well known reducing properties of sal-ammoniac, when aided by heat, the presence of sesquichloride of iron, which, from its yellow color, and easy volatility previous to examination, would naturally be supposed present in the yellow portions, seems improbable. The reaction between sal-ammoniac sesquichloride of iron, when heated together would probably be something like the following:

$$3\ Fe^2\ Cl^3 + NH^4\ Cl = 6\ Fe\ Cl + 4\ H\ Cl + N.$$

The sesquichloride of iron being thus converted into protochloride.

Gmelin* who does not notice the presence of iron, states that commercial sal-ammoniac may be purified both by resublimation and recrystallization. To test this, two experiments were made. First, a quantity of crude sal-ammoniac was slowly and carefully sublimed in a glass tube. An aqueous solution of the sublimate which, it is worthy of observation, had a slightly brown color, and an empyreumatic smell, when tested with prussiate of potash and sulphide of ammonium, still gave most unmistakeable indications of the presence of protochloride of iron. Next, some of the crude sal-ammoniac was crystallized from water—the crystals rinsed with distilled water and dried by strong pressure between folds of filtering paper. A solu-

* Handbuch der Chemie, 1, 887.

tion of these crystals still gave a coloration, though faint, with sulphide of ammonium. By two or more recrystallizations every trace of iron might, in all probability, be separated, but at the expense of a large loss of material.

While an instructor in the Chemical School, connected with Yale College, at New Haven, I became acquainted with a method of separating the iron from ferriferous sal-ammoniac, devised, I believe, by Mr. Wm. H. Brewer, a former student in that institution, and in common use in the analytical department for the preparation of pure sal-ammoniac solution, for use in analysis, which leaves nothing whatever to be desired in point of economy, perfection and facility of execution; and as Mr. Brewer has never, to my knowledge, published his process, I have concluded, in view of the importance of the matter and the fact that I have myself verified the accuracy of the process by repeated trials, to make it public.

Brewer's process was founded upon the hypothesis, confirmed as above by Pereira and myself, that the iron is in the form of protochloride, and consists simply of a conversion of this protocholride into sesquichloride by passing a few bubbles of *chlorine* gas through a nearly saturated hot solution of crude sal-ammoniac and the subsequent decomposition of the sesquichloride of iron by ammonia. The solution is then kept hot on the sand bath for a short time or until the precipitate separates in flocks and then quickly filtered while hot. On cooling the sal-ammoniac crystallizes out absolutely pure.

When passing the chlorine gas into the liquid, special care must be taken to keep the liquid hot and not to prolong the action sufficiently to allow the formation of the well known dangerously explosive compound $NHCl^2$* usually called chloride of nitrogen. It is evident that the sal-ammoniac obtained

* The discovery by Adolphe Wurtz, of the detonating compound formed by the action of chlorine upon ethylamine, and called by him "*l'ethylamine bichlorée.*" (*Memoire sur les ammoniaques composées, par M. Ad. Wurtz, p.* 33) leaves us hardly any alternative, if we consider the perfect analogy between the two cases, than to assign the above formula to the *soi-disant* chloride of nitrogen.

cannot contain any free chlorine, all the chlorine introduced being converted into chlorohydric acid, which combines with the excess of ammonia, or according to the long known reaction.

$$4\ NH^3 + 3\ Cl = 3\ NH^4\ Cl + N.$$

---

## PILLS OF IODIDE OF IRON.

BY JOHN LOINES.

The intensely styptic taste of the solution of iodide of iron as well as the unpleasant stain it imparts to the teeth and lips is often felt to be a serious inconvenience in the use of this valuable remedy, and has given rise to considerable inquiry by the medical practitioner for some more palatable mode of administering the iodide. Such, however, is the nature of this compound, that it is scarcely to be expected that any form of preparation will supersede the salt with gum or the combination of saccharine matter in various proportions. Meantime it has been proposed, in order to conceal the taste of the officinal solution, to enclose it in capsules or, by the addition of suitable substances, to make of it a mass capable of being formed into pills. It has even been thought advisable to evaporate the solution till it should acquire a suitable consistence for this purpose. To the capsules the expense will probably be urged as an objection by some, while their liability to leak, unless made with more than ordinary care, will be found a constant source of complaint. On the other hand, although it is easy enough, by the addition of gum, to make a mass that can be rolled into pills, the bulk of this adjuvant in connection with that of the sugar already employed renders the dose inconveniently large. It was in view of these objections that the writer, about a year ago, devised the plan of making a very concentrated syrup of the iodide of iron, which may be readily made into pills, two or three of which contain the ordinary dose o that medicine, and having made use of them in his own case for a considerable time, with advantage, he would respectfully recommend them to the favorable notice of physicians and pharmaceutists. The formula he employs is the following viz:

Take of iodine (dry)................................1 oz.
fine iron wire, cut in pieces.....................3 ʒ.
Sugar in powder...........................2¼ oz.
Water....................................1½ fl. oz.

Measure 2½ fluid ounces of water into a three or four ounce phial, and mark upon it the height at which the liquid stands, then pour out the water and introduce the sugar in its stead. Proceed, with the other ingredients, to make the solution of iodide of iron in the same manner as in the formula of the U. S. P. taking care to use a flask or matruss of the capacity of only 3 or 4 ounces in order to avoid waste of the materials. The filter employed should also be very small (from one to two inches in depth) and its apex must be protected by a small cap of muslin without which a rent is almost certain to occur; or, a small piece of fine linen or muslin might be substituted for the double filter thus formed. Having filtered the liquid into the sugar, shake the phial containing them, and suspend it in a vessel of hot water until perfect solution takes place. If the product measures less than 2½ fluid ounces, add simple syrup to make up the deficiency.

This concentrated syrup is four times the strength of the officinal solution and should contain, by calculation, twenty-nine grains of the dry iodide in every fluid drachm. As some loss is, however, unavoidable the proportion is actually rather less.

To prepare the pills, two fluid drachms of the concentrated syrup are to be triturated in a mortar, with 3 drachms of powdered gum arabic, and the mixture set aside for several hours, during which time it acquires the consistence of very stiff paste, but needs the addition of a little more gum, which should be worked in by hand, to make it into pills. When brought to the proper consistence it is to be divided into 60 pills, each of which may be assumed to contain the equivalent of 8 minims of the officinal solution of iodide of iron. They do not become hard by keeping; some have been kept a year and then beaten anew into a mass and made again into pills. Neither does any perceptible alteration appear in their color, taste or smell.

New York, 12 mo. 21, 1852,

---

## ON A NEW CRYSTALLINE BODY FROM HELLEBORUS NIGER.

BY MR. WILLIAM BASTICK.

The natural order Ranunculaceæ contains a number of plants of great activity on the animal economy; and most of these employed as medicinal agents have been thoroughly examined by Chemists, by whom their active principles have been separated beyond doubt. It has been found, as is well known, that these active principles are organic bases of extreme virulence, and possess the properties of the plants from which they are derived, in a highly concentrated form. Black hellebore root has been several times examined for the purpose of ascertaining what were its active constituents, and more especially to learn whether, like other members of this family, it contained an organic base. Vauquelin ascribed its activity to the presence of an acrid oil, and Gmelin to a soft resin which exists in it. The most recent and complete examination of black hellebore root is that of MM. Feneulle and Capron;* whose researches were principally directed to prove the absence or presence of an alkaloid in this root. However, they came to the conclusion that no such body existed in it, and that its activity

* *Journal de Pharmacie*, vol. vii., p. 503.

was due to a combination of a fatty oil with a volatile acid, which they separated from it. Doubting the truth of their conclusions, and réasoning from analogy, I was led to believe that by the improved methods of research, of the present day, an organic base might be extracted from it; I therefore employed a method which experience has shown will eliminate an alkaloid from any substance, if any such alkaloid, soluble in ether, exist therein, and which is as follows:—

The black hellebore root was finely bruised and maccrated with alcohol, containing $^{1}$th part of strong sulphuric acid. After three days the tincture was filtered from the root, and supersaturated with calcined magnesia. The liquid was then filtered and sufficient sulphuric acid added to it to render it slightly acid. It was again filtered to remove the sulphate of magnesia formed. The filtrate was now mixed with twice its volume of distilled water, and the mixture evaporated to expel the alcohol, and to reduce considerably the bulk of the solution. To remove the soft resin which was separated by replacing the alcoholic menstruum with water, filtration was resorted to. The concentrated fluid was then carefully saturated with carbonate of potash, but nothing was precipitated. A large excess of that carbonate was now added, and the solution agitated for some time with four times its volume of ether, and afterwards set aside so that the ethereal part of the liquid might separate from the watery portion. When this separation had taken place, the ethereal portion was removed from the bottle by means of a pipette, and exposed to spontaneous evaporation in a capsule. Had an organic base been present in the root, it would have been found in the ethereal solution; but this solution was entirely free from any reaction on litmus paper. Thus far my experiments corroborate those of MM. Feneulle and Capron, as to the non-existence in black hellebore root of any body, having the more distinct characteristics of an alkaloid, but no farther. For I found in the ethereal solution by its evaporation, a well-defined *crystalline* organic body, to what I propose giving the name of *helleborine*, although that name has been already given to the soft resin by Gmelin, and undeservedly so, as I think: because it possesses no peculiarities either physical or chemical. This new body readily separates by evaporation from its watery, alcoholic, and ethereal solutions, in white translucent crystals. It is slightly soluble in water, more soluble in ether, and readily soluble in alcohol. It dissolves more freely in these liquids when they are heated. It is bitter to the taste, and produces on the tongue a tingling sensation like the root. Strong sulphuric acid decomposes it, and gives with it a reddish-brown solution which, when diluted with water, affords a brown precipitate. Concentrated nitric acid dissolves it, but does not oxidize it until the solution has been exposed to heat. After it had been thus oxidized, the usual tests shewed that oxalic acid was not one of the products. This substance is not volatile, and when heated is decomposed, and leaves a carbonaceous residuum, but does not inflame. It is as previously indicated, entirely without reaction on litmus paper, and does not combine with or saturate acids or alkalies. A dilute solution of caustic potash appears to produce no change in it, as is also the case with dilute mineral acids. It is not precipitated from its solutions by acetate of lead, bichloride of mercury, or iodide of potassium. When heated in a dry state with fused caustic potash in a tube, ammonia is evolved, which shows that it is a nitrogenous body. It therefore closely resembles piperine in many of its properties, which is classed amongst the alkaloids, although like helleborine it is devoid of alkaline reaction. But whether it possesses an elementary constitution similar to that of piperine, or the alkaloids in general, remains to be determined by ultimate analysis.

Having so far endeavored to learn its characters, I proceeded to ascertain if this new body could not be extracted from black hellebore root by a more simple process. I treated the bruised root with alcohol to form a strong tincture. The filtered tincture was diluted with water, and heated for some time to expel the alcohol. The aqueous solution was then filtered to remove the separated resin, and afterwards further evaporated, when some helleborine crystallized out of the solution, but in a less pure condition than by the former process, consequently I treated the solution with carbonate of potash in excess, and agitated it with three or four times its volume of ether, which extracted the helleborine almost in a state of purity. This substance may be further purified by solution in alcohol and re-crystallization.

It is probable from this latter process that helleborine exists in an uncombined state in the root, and that it is the soft resin contained therein which chiefly interferes with its recognition and extraction, by a simple solvent as a crystalline substance. There is also a free acid in black hellebore root, which it is necessary to neutralize with a base before the helleborine is extracted from its aqueous solution with ether, as it contaminates the product. This is not gallic acid, which is said to exist in this root, according to the analysis of MM. Feneulle and Capron, as it did not give a black precipitate with a persalt of iron, but a brown gelatinous one; it also afforded white precipitates with acetate of lead and with nitrate of silver. Neither is it the volatile acid found by them, as it is not expelled by long boiling from its solutions. It seems to resemble closely the aconitic acid found in another member of the natural order Ranunculaceæ, especially when it is remembered, that like that acid, it is soluble when free in alcohol, ether and water.

It may be mentioned, that in consequence of the insolubility in ether of the coloring-matter extracted by alcohol from black hellebore root, it is scarcely necessarry to use animal charcoal to decolorize the helleborine, as its ethereal solution is colorless in the above process, and this substance crystallizes thereout with care nearly in the same condition.—*Pharmaceutical Journal and Transactions*, *Dec.*, 1852.

# ON TANNATE OF ALUMINA.

BY WILLIAM PROCTER, JR.

The London Medical Gazette contains an article on the medical application of Tannate of Alumina, in which it is stated that Mr. Rogers Harrison had prepared a combination of alumina and tannic acid which "was of a dirty yellowish color, and in crystals about the size of those of coarse sugar, and readily soluble in hot water." It had been used successfully for inflammation of the urethral passages in the form of injection, two to ten grains of the salt, according to circumstances, dissolved in sufficient distilled water.

Having recently received a prescription for ten grains of this salt dissolved in two fluid ounces of water, and being unable in any of a number of chemical works at my command, to find any account of the salt, I undertook to make it, but could not succeed in obtaining a soluble compound of tannic acid and alumina that answered to the description of that of Mr. Harrison, all of them being insoluble or nearly so in water, and entirely amorphous.

1st. An equivalent of tannic acid was triturated with one of alumina in the pulpy hydrated condition; combination ensued, and an insoluble or slightly soluble compound resulted. The same result occurred when two and three equivalents of alumina were employed. When agitated with water after standing in a pulpy state for several weeks, and the water filtered off, the latter gave no evidence of tannic acid or a soluble tannate.

2nd. A solution of alum in water was prepared, containing 37 grains to the fluid ounce, which quantity contains four grains of anhydrous alumina. A solution of tannic acid in water was then made, containing 16 grains to the fluid ounce. The alumina and tannic acid existed nearly in the proportion of their equivalents in these solutions.

Equal measures were mixed together without any precipitation, showing that free tannic acid is unable to displace alumina from its combination with sulphuric acid, notwithstanding the insolubility of the aluminous tannate, even when they are boiled.

3rd. When, however, ammonia is carefully added to a fluid ounce of the tannic acid solution until it is saturated, and an equal measure of the solution of alum is added, an immediate bulky gelatinous precipitate occurs, similar in appearance to the magma in No. 1. When washed and dried it weighed 13 grains. The washings had a slight astringent taste, and afforded a slight inky blue precipitate with ter-chloride of iron.

4th. As tannic acid is considered by Liebig to be tribasic, three parts of solution of alum was added to one of solution of tannic acid, with sufficient excess of ammonia to liberate all the alumina. On filtering out the precipitate, the clear liquid yielded no precipitate with ammonia, but was precipitated bluish-black by ter-chloride of iron; showing that in the presence of enough alumina to form a tribasic salt, a part of the tannic acid remains in solution probably as tannate of ammonia.

5th. The liquid filtered from No. 3, with the washings, was evaporated to a small bulk, and on standing, dirty yellowish colored crystals in small quantity were deposited. The mother liquid poured off and evaporated gave other mamillary crystals admixed with dark matter. The first crystals had the well known triangular facets of alum, and when tested by solution in hot water, yielded a bluish-black precipitate with ter-chloride of iron. When powdered and boiled in repeated portions of alcohol, nearly all the color is removed, and they give but a trace of color with the ter-chloride, whilst the alcohol when evaporated yielded a yellowish, non-crystalline residue, which reacted as tannic acid with the ter-salts of iron, and was not precipitated by an excess of ammonia. The crystals, after treatment by alcohol, yielded, when dissolved in water, a white insoluble precipitate with chloride of barium, and a gelatinous precipitate with ammonia and were alum. The residue from the mother liquid contained sulphate of ammonia, tannin and some undecomposed alum.

From these results it appears that tannate of alumina formed by direct combination, is an amorphous salt, nearly insoluble in water. That the same salt is precipitated from alum on the addition of tannate of ammonia, and, finally, that it is probable that the tannate of alumina of Mr. Harrison is a mixture of tannic acid and alum, derived either from the evaporation of a mixture of alum and tannic acid, or from the washings of tannate of alumina, as treated in No. 5.—*American Journal of Pharmacy, January*, 1853.

---

## ON CHLOROFORM.

BY WILLIAM HUSKISSON, JR.

A process appeared some time since, by Dr. Gregory, on the purification of chloroform by means of sulphuric acid; a short time after its publication, an article was added by Professor Christison, (*in the absence of Dr. Gregory,*) stating that chloroform, purified by sulphuric acid, had speedily undergone decomposition—had become loaded with chlorine, and thus rendered quite unfit for use—and that the manufacturer had failed, in almost every instance, in obtaining a permanent article. Since that period, no process for the preparation or the purification of chloroform has been published, except in the pharmacopœia; it has been left entirely to the discretion of the manufacturer. Recently, at a meeting of the Pharmaceutical Society, Dr. Pereira exhibited a specimen of chloroform, which had not only undergone change, but had become of a pink color.

Having prepared chloroform on a large scale, and having had considerable experience in the changes it undergoes when purified by sulphuric acid, the following is the only process by which I have always obtained a permanent article; and one which I have never found, under any circumstance, undergo change or decomposition. I take 130 lbs. of chloride of lime and 7 lbs. of common lime, put them into a capacious still, with sufficient water to make a thin paste; when well stirred together, I then add more water with 25 lbs. of rectified spirit; (*taking care that the still shall not be more than half full*,) dilute it down—load it; apply a gentle heat and commence distillation; separate what comes over from the supernatant liquor, and wash it several times with distilled water; *put the washings and supernatant liquor again into the still, with one half the above quantities, and proceed as before;* then introduce the chloroform thus obtained into an ordinary still, with four or five times its weight of distilled water, with a small quantity of lime; apply heat, and let the chloroform bubble through the water, and pass over; separate the chloroform from the water that comes over with it, by means of a separatory funnel, and agitate it with a little highly dried carbonate of potash, to entirely abstract from it a small portion of water it generally contains.

With regard to the product, there is considerable uncertainty, owing to the great difference in the quality of the chloride of lime employed; it is necessary that the chloride should be rendered alkaline by means of lime, otherwise formic acid is not so readily produced; it also prevents, in a great measure, the action being so violent when the ingredients are mixed; and the chloroform that passes over is rarely contaminated with chlorine, which is frequently the case when the lime is omitted. I have occasionally added a weak solution of chlorine instead of water, and a larger quantity of lime: but neither by this, nor by any of the other processes I have tried, have I obtained a result so uniform or satisfactory, as by the foregoing. The chloroform, when thus carefully prepared, answers to the following tests: It is exceedingly bright and transparent in any moderate temperature, possessing a highly penetrating aromatic odor; when dropped upon the hand it rapidly evaporates, leaving no faint unpleasant odor behind.

It is not affected by litmus or turmeric paper; when dropped into water the greater part immediately sinks, leaving a little floating on the surface, which, after a time, sinks also, imparting a sweetish taste to the water. It has a specific gravity of 1,500, which is the best test of its strength; when agitated with sulphuric acid, the acid becomes colored yellow, the chloroform loses its fine odor and undergoes decomposition, which takes place still more rapidly if allowed to remain in contact with the acid, giving off a gas somewhat resembling hydrochloric. If it contains the smallest amount of alcohol or spirits of wine, on the addition of a little bichromate of potash, and a few drops of sulphuric acid, the green oxide of chromium is formed, which floats on the surface, and, if allowed to evaporate spontaneously, the aldehyd which is formed thereby can be easily recognized. It is miscible with alcohol; if rather more than 13 parts of chloroform and 6 parts alcohol, (.835 S. G.,) be mixed, they will unite and give a specific gravity of about 1,200, and if more chloroform be added, they will separate. When it contains the smallest amount of water, it will become clouded with every variation of temperature.

It is quite evident that the carbonizing or charring of the volatile oil by concentrated sulphuric acid, which is said to have caused nausea, &c., in peculiarly sensitive persons (*even when agitated with the purest sulphuric acid*,) has caused decomposition of the chloroform as well as of the oil. It occurred to me, that the sulphuric acid converted the chloroform into formic acid by affording it sufficient oxygen, and the free chlorine combined with hydrogen, thus forming hydrochloric gas. When chloroform has been treated with sulphuric acid, it is usually agitated with oxide of manganese, which decomposes any free sulphurous acid that might be present.

Another remarkable phenomenon in decomposed chloroform is the formation of a number of crystals round the upper surface of the chloroform, and after the lapse of a few weeks, its becoming a delicate pink color, which is sometimes fugitive, owing, no doubt, to a salt of manganese, most probably a sulphate; and this opinion is strengthened by the fact of its being observable in the following preparation:

When acetic acid is obtained by decomposing acetate of soda by sulphuric acid, the sulphurous acid that is formed passes over with the acetic acid; to remove this mineral acid, it was usual to add oxide of manganese; after a short time, the acetic acid that has been thus deprived of its sulphurous acid will frequently become pink, and deposit pink crystals; also in the preparation of chlorate of potash, if the heat applied to the mixture be too great, and the mixture boils over, the mother liquors will frequently be of a rich pink color. From these results I think we may safely infer, that it is a salt of manganese, like the mineral chameleon, which gives rise to the formation of crystals in, and to the changing color of chloroform, when subjected to Dr. Gregory's process.

I have tested and examined large quantities of Edinburgh and Dublin chloroform, but have never met with any to supersede, or even equal in its general characters, that prepared from the spirit obtained from the best London distillers; I regret that many scientific journals should have stated that the Edinburgh manufacturers have devoted more care and attention to its preparation, and have produced the best chloroform. The fact is, while the London manufacturers were using every effort to cover the actual expenses of materials, &c., to say nothing of profit, owing to the great difference in the duty on spirit or whiskey in England, and Scotland, and Ireland, (*chloroform is admitted free of duty into England;*) they, in the latter countries, manufactured at a profit, and we at a loss; and the result was, after repeated attempts, the London makers were compelled to give way to their Scotch friends, though not in quality but in price.—*Annals of Pharmacy, Jan.* 1852.

# ON THE EMPLOYMENT OF COLLODION IN PHOTOGRAPHY.

BY MR. BINGHAM.

Photography has made rapid progress during the last two years, especially in the methods of operating on paper and glass. We cannot but accord to M. Niepce the merit of having contributed to the perfecting of this art by his beautiful discovery of the process of albumen on glass. The admirable proofs obtained by M. Martens by this means have a beauty of design, a clearness and fineness of detail which leave nothing to be desired. Nevertheless, we cannot conceal the serious inconvenience which this process presents. The length of exposure in the camera obscura necessary for obtaining an image compels us to limit its application to landscapes and architecture and renounce its employment in portraiture.

I am about to give the details of a process on glass by means of collodion; this process rivals in beauty the albuminised plate, and even surpasses the daguerreotype in sensibility to the light.

In a pamphlet on photography, which I published in London in January, 1850, I mentioned the employment of collodion in photography, and communicated the secret of this discovery to the most distinguised photographers of London: but it it is only very recently that all its advantages have been appreciated. The process is very simple ; it consists solely in the substitution of a layer of collodion for the albumen of M. Niepce.

No operator accustomed to the manipulations of albumen on glass can fail to succeed with collodion, and to arrive at the best results.

To obtain an image, two or three different methods should be followed, which I will now point out. We shall divide the manipulations into four distinct operations :—

1. The preparation of the collodion.
2. The application of the collodion on the plate.
3. The development of the image.
4. The fixation.

## 1. PREPARATION OF THE COLLODION.

The collodion is prepared by dissolving gun-cotton in ether; it is necessary that the gun-cotton and ether employed for this preparation should be perfectly pure, that is to say, that they should not contain the smallest trace of sulphuric or nitric acid.

The collodion is more or less fluid, according to the proportions of gun-cotton and ether which are employed. It is only required to be so liquid that, on being poured on to a glass-plate, it shall flow, and be easily spread over the surface. When it is too thick, pure ether is added to it, until the degree of fluidity proper for operating is obtained. A few experiments will suffice for arriving at this. When the collodion is too thick, it is difficult to obtain a uniform surface; when it is too fluid its sensibility appears to be very slight.

The collodion is poured into a six-ounce phial, containing fifty-three grains of iodide of ammonium and two grains of fluoride of potassium, with four or five drops of distilled water. The iodide of ammonium should not be entirely dissolved in the water; that is to say, the proportion of water should not be sufficient for making a perfect solution. It is sufficient for the salt to be almost dissolved; the solution is completed by the addition of the collodion.

It is important to pay attention to these details, and for this reason; if too much water is put into the mixture, the layer of collodion will not take well to the plate, and is liable to be detached in the nitrate of silver bath. Agitate the flask once or twice, and allow it to stand until the liquor has become clear and limpid: its color will be of a pale yellow, but if by chance the ether or the collodion retain a trace of acid there will, in that case, be a decomposition of the iodide of ammonia, and the iodine, in being disengaged, will give to the liquid a deep red color.

This method is the most expeditious, but it also presents rather more difficulty than that with the iodised collodion which I now describe.

Into a six-ounce phial introduce twelve grains of iodide of potassium and seven or eight grains of iodide of silver; add a few drops of water, but not more than sufficient for dissolving the iodide of potassium; then fill the phial with collodion of the requisite degree of fluidity, agitate once or twice, and leave the mixture to repose for two or three days, until it has become perfectly transparent; it should be almost white, it is ordinarily rather yellow.

2. PREPARATION OF THE PLATE FOR RECEIVING THE IMAGE.

Fix the glass plate on a piece of gutta percha: this substance readily adheres to glass when it is heated; pour on a few drops of ammonia mixed with tripoli, and rub the glass with cotton, describing small circles, as is done with daguerreotype plates; then, with another pledget of cotton, remove the tripoli left on the glass; pour on a second mixture of tripoli and alcohol, and rub as with the first mixture: a few particles of tripoli and fibres of cotton may remain on the glass: to remove these pour on a little pure alcohol, make a very compact pledget, so that the fibres of cotton may not project, and rub the plate with the greatest care; finally rub for the last time with a new dry pledget. It is ascertained that it is fit to be employed when, on breathing on it, the moisture condenses uniformly over the whole surface. Always holding the plate by its handle of gutta percha, gently pour the collodion on it, and incline it from side to side, in order that the liquid may run into the corners; then pour the excess of liquid, by one of the corners, into the phial. The plate will then appear to be covered with very fine groves, all perpendicular in the direction of the flowing; by inclining it in another direction, the grooves will be obliterated, and the layers will become thin and uniform. Then, before the collodion has time to dry, the plate is introduced into a bath of nitrate of silver, the prepared surface being held downwards.

This bath should contain forty grains of nitrate of silver to each ounce of distilled water. The surface of the plate will not be wetted immediately ; a certain time is required for the ether to become mixed with the water; the plate is therefore allowed to remain in the bath at least half a minute without allowing it to touch the bottom of the vessel, and supporting it by the aid of a silver or platinum hook.

As soon as it is perceived that the plate is covered with a whitish uniform layer, and that the water has flowed well over its surface, it is removed and placed immediately in the frame of the camera obscura; it must be used within ten or fifteen minutes—the sooner the better.

DEVELOPMENT OF THE IMAGE.

Place the glass on a support, and quickly pour on the surface a solution composed of two parts of pyrogallic acid, sixty parts of glacial acetic acid, and five hundred parts of water. If the exposure in the camera obscura has not been sufficient, a few drops of nitrate of silver may be added, but ordinarily this is not necessary.

As soon as the image is perfectly developed, which takes about two minutes, it is washed with a current of water, and then it is fixed by pouring on a saturated solution of hyposulphite of soda. The layer of iodide of silver disappears, and the image is perceived, which sometimes is positive; it is then washed in a large quantity of water to remove all the hyposulphite; the plate is then dried either over a lamp or spontaneously in the air; before drying the layer is very tender; afterwards it becomes hard and adheres to the glass like albumen.

By means of this process, it would be easy, if desired, to obtain at once a positive image of great beauty, and possessing much more force and purity than those of the daguerreotype, and not having, like the latter, the inconvenience of a reflection which prevents them from being seen except in a certain position. To obtain this result, the exposure of the camera obscura should be much shorter than for a negative proof; but it is also necessary to allow this image, which we desire to make into a positive, to remain in a solution of pyrogallic acid, with one or two drops of nitrate of silver.

Then the luminous parts are formed of white layers having the same character as the crystalline layers formed by the mercury in the daguerreotype process.

When the positive image is quite developed, it is fixed by the same means as the negative.

I must add, in conclusion, that the time generally necessary for obtaining a good negative in the shade with an ordinary German object-glass is from two to three seconds, or less than half the time requisite for obtaining the same result with the daguerreotype.—*Comptes Rendus*, No. 19, May 11, 1852.

---

## THE COMPOUNDS OF IODINE WITH QUININE AND MORPHINE.

BY F. W. WINCKLER.

*Iodide of Quinine.*—When iodide of potassium and sulphate of quinine are dissolved in boiling water, in equivalent proportions, regular crystals (free from iodine) of sulphate of quinine are formed. A similar result is obtained when, instead of sulphate of quinine any other salt of quinine formed with an oxy-acid is used. The hydracids give a contrary result. A mixture of hydrochlorate of quinine and iodide of potassium, in equivalent proportions, precipitates a small quantity of iodide of quinine in a resinous state. To the complete decomposition of the hydrochlorate of quinine, Winckler has found that four equivalents of iodide of potassium are necessary. The compound then produced consists of two equivalents of quinine, with one equivalent of iodine, or 126 parts of iodine and 328 parts of quinine. This combination has, when dried, the properties of a resin. When cold, after being thoroughly dried, it is easily powdered without being electric, as the pure quinine is when rubbed. It is white, without smell, permanent in the air, and possesses a very bitter taste. It dissolves considerably in water, almost in any quantity of spirit and also in ether. All these solutions are clear, colorless, and leave behind, when evaporated, the iodide of quinine in the form of a transparent resin. By chlorine and concentrated sulphuric and nitric acids, this salt is immediately decomposed with the separation of its iodine. Its combustion on platina foil is with difficulty effected, and the residuum, after combustion, contains no trace of potash. The analysis of this salt gave—

| | Found. | Calculated. |
|---|---|---|
| Quinine, - - - | 71,58 - - - - - - | 72,166 |
| Iodine, - - - | 28,42 - - - - - - | 27,834 |
| | 100,00 | 100,000 |

*Iodide of Morphine.*—This salt consists of one equivalent of morphine and one of iodine. It is to be obtained by dissolving 120 parts by weight of dry acetate of morphine in 960 parts of cold distilled water, and filtering the solution. Add previously to filtration a few drops of acetic acid, if any of the morphine remains undissolved. Decompose the filtered solution with a solution containing sixty parts of iodide of potassium. The iodide of morphine crystallizes out of this liquid after some time in very fine crystals, and may be obtained in still finer crystals if the mixed solutions are warmed in a water-bath, and then slowly cooled. It thus separates in transparent, shining, colorless, four-sided prisms, which cannot be distinguished by their appearance from sulphate of quinine. Iodide of morphine dissolves slightly in cold water, but readily in hot water, and easily in alcohol. Its solutions have a bitter taste. The analysis of this salt gave—

| | Found. | Calculated. |
|---|---|---|
| Morphine, - - - | 71,4 - - - - - - | 71,24 |
| Iodine, - - - - | 28,6 - - - - - - | 28,76 |
| | 100,0 | 100,00 |

*Jahrbuch fur Prakt. Pharm.*

## ELDER FLOWER OINTMENT AND OIL.

BY SEPTIMUS PIESSE.

In the London Pharmacopœia the flowers are directed to be boiled with the lard, in making unguentum sambuci. By this process the odor of the flowers is entirely destroyed, and the ointment acquires an empyreumatic smell from the action of the heat upon the flowers. To obviate this result, and to make an ointment possessing the pleasant odor of elder flowers, I beg to suggest to the readers of the "Annals," the following process, which I have found effectual.

Melt the lard at the lowest possible temperature at which it assumes the fluid form, and introduce into it as many flowers as the melted lard will cover. Macerate them at the above temperature for twelve hours, and then strain off the lard through a piece of linen, without the least pressure. By this means an ointment will be made, when the lard is cold, which represents that which the College really intends it should be.

The oil of elder flowers requires no heat for its preparation, and is prepared precisely as the ointment, with the exception of the heat; as the only object of its use is to obtain the menstruum in a fluid form, and besides, its employment on any other ground is objectionable, especially as it volatizes the odorons principle of the flowers.—*Annals Pharmacy*, *Aug.* 1852.

---

## ON THE BOUQUET OF WINE.

BY DR. F. L. WINCKLER.

In his recent experiments on the vegetation of plants, Winckler has arrived at very satisfactory results explanatory of the specific odor peculiar to the various sorts of wine produced in different districts, which is known by the expression of "*blume*," or "*bouquet.*"

If about half a pint of any sort of grape wine be evaporated in a porcelain vessel by means of steam, until not only all the spirit of wine, but also the œnanthic ether, and, in general, all parts volatile at this temperature (80° R.) are evaporated, a thickish liquid of more or less dark color, and of a peculiar, pleasant, acidulo-vinous odor remains behind, from which, after it has become cold, a greater or lesser quantity of tartar separates. By diluting this liquid with water, so that the weight of the solution is about a quarter of a pound, and subjecting the solution, with an equal weight of fresh burnt lime, to distillation, there is obtained, even during the slacking or hydrating of the lime a very agreeable and intensely smelling distillate, which, like ammonia, is a strong base, and forms with acids neutral salts, possessing in a high degree the odor corresponding to the so-called "bouquet" of the employed wine.

This fact suggested the idea that this compound may be in a similar manner contained in the wine itself, and the supposition was fully corroborated by experiments.

If the residuary lime of the evaporated wine be treated with water after the conclusion of the distillation, the solution filtered, and the filtrate distilled with a small quantity of moderately strong sulphuric acid, a new volatile acid of a highly specific, almost balsamic odor is obtained, which being neutralized by the necessary quantity of the first-obtained nitrogenous base, yields a neutral volatile salt, which possesses the peculiar odor ("bouquet") of the employed wine in the highest degree. There is, therefore, no doubt that this compound is not only contained as such in the wine, and constitutes the "bouquet," but that it is the nitrogenous compound which determines the chemical constitution, the durability, and all those changes to which it is subject by keeping.

Although for the present only six different sorts of red and white grape wine from various districts of the Grand Duchy have been examined, yet the results are so uniform and decisive, that there exists no reason to doubt their correctness. The contrast was very striking on comparing the "bouquets" of a fine red Oberingelheim wine, of 1846, with a very excellent sort of white Bergstraszer, of 1846, and with one of the worst qualities of 1851, from the latter district. The first two sorts yielded quite a different bouquet, of a very pleasant odor, whilst the latter betrayed but too distinctly the year and quality by its unpleasant earthy smell.

Beer also contains a considerable proportion of nitrogen, which can be obtained from it in the same way as from the wine. It is this component from which beer obtains its importance as a nutrient.

The anthor has, moreover, found, that the coloring matter of wine, and chiefly that of red wine, is closely connected with this nitrogenous compound; that most, and perhaps all, fresh vegetable juices contains nitrogen, and undergo during the process of vegetation, changes which are analogous to the fermentation of wine; that the fragancy of the vine-flowers, and very likely also the odors of most flowers and leaves are dependent on similar compounds, which are characteristic, and of a peculiar chemical composition in each genus of plants.—*London Pharm. Journ.*, from *Jahrbuch f. prakt. Pharmacie*, Bd. xxv., Hft. 1, p. 7.

---

## ON THE ENEMIES OF THE MEDICINAL LEECH.

BY DR. EBRARD.

Every year France imports leeches to the value of nearly three million of francs, from Sardinia, Italy, and Spain, and even these countries obtain them elsewhere. In England and in America the high price of leeches almost precludes the use of them among the lower classes.

These circumstances naturally lead one to imagine, that any person who could succeed in propagating leeches in confinement, would realize an immense fortune. Numerous trials have been made with this view, a few have not been entirely unsuccessful; but in no case that I am aware of, have the results equalled the expectations of the experimentalists.

Nevertheless, in several cases where reproduction was attempted, the first apparent results were most satisfactory; for in some pieces of water which had been properly stocked with them, and presented favorable conditions of soil, aspect, and vegetation, there appeared each year, in the months of May and September, large quantities of young leeches moving on the surface of the water. But after the lapse of a few years, with scarcely any exceptions, there remained only those which were placed in the water, and those just hatched.

What then had become of the young leeches which were seen in each of the preceding years? Had they perished from want of food, or had they suffered from an epidemic disease? Had they emigrated? Without doubt, in certain cases, the disappearance of the leeches might be attributed to the depopulation of the ponds, but more frequently it was caused by their various enemies. Animals having their freedom are not exposed to many diseases, and if they sometimes perish from want of nourishment, they more commonly are the victims of other animals. The leech forms no exception to this general rule.

Which then are the enemies of the leech? A memoir by M. Hedrich, of Dresden, the work of M. Huzard, on the breeding of leeches; that of M. Martin, the monograph by M. Moquin, and the report made to the Academy of Medicine by Professor Soubeiran, contain some information on this question, but the information is incomplete, and insufficient for the guidance of those persons having pieces of water stocked with leeches. Therefore, I have thought it useful to publish my own notions and experience on this subject, in addition to those already made known by others. Such is the object of this notice, in which I propose, first, to describe the enemies of the leeches, known and unknown; secondly, to point out a means of diminishing, if not of preventing, their ravages.

*Quadrupeds.*—Pigs devour leeches. On the edge of a pond,

in which I had some considerable number of leeches, I observed that the pigs were turning over the ground, from which the water had just receded, or sometimes it was covered by a few centimètres of liquid. A great portion of this ground was without the least vegetable production; for what, therefore, could these animals be seeking, unless it were for aquatic animals buried in the mud? On the same day, I threw some leeches to the pigs, who devoured them with that greediness which is poverbial with these animals.

The otter, the hedgehog, and the mole have been mentioned by leech-gatherers, as being enemies of the leech.

M. Joseph Martin has found leeches in the stomachs of rats and water shrew-mice. These animals are most prejudicial, as they destroy the cocoons which the leeches deposit in the holes formed by them.

*Birds.*—" A cultivator in Sologne," says Paymaurin, " having realized 30,000 francs in four years by commerce in leeches, tried to breed them in a small pond. He put in more than 200,000, when several flocks of ducks took possession of the pond, and depopulated it in twenty-four hours."

This fact is at the least exaggerated; for had the pond been covered for several days by millions of ducks, these birds could not have caused so considerable a loss, as leeches remain in large numbers buried in the earth. However it may be, I consider it as certain that ducks are very fond of leeches. At a farm of Dombe's where I had been called in, the leeches which had been applied to a sick person were crawling before the door of the house on some muddy soil. The ducks seized them with avidity and swallowed them, after having washed and shaken them in an adjacent pool.

It is probable that teal, ducks, and other palmipedes (I except the domestic goose) are enemies to the leech. This supposition is equally applicable to the heron and other wading birds. A young bittern or pouch, which I reared in 1850, much preferred fish or frogs to leeches, but ate the later when deprived of other food. Geese have never eaten the leeches I have offered them, neither do they eat frogs and water-lizards.

The fowl is also an enemy of the leech. I was occupied in cleaning a jar containing leeches before a window from which the crumbs from the table were usually thrown into the yard. A number of chickens came under the window and I threw them some leeches, which they quickly swallowed, and notwithstanding the fears of the farmer's wife, continued in good health.

*Reptiles and Batrachia.*—From birds I pass to reptiles and batraceians, and my attention will be first directed to the water-adder, the head of which is so often seen above the water of ponds. It eats leeches, although they are not a favorite food with it. One of these pretty reptiles, which I kept under a wire-gauze cover, swallowed a frog or a salamander every three or four days; but it would not take leeches until after a week's fasting. But although it devours frogs and salamanders, which serve as nourishment to the leech, yet the water-adder must be considered as an injurious animal.

I had seen terrestial toads swallow worms, and I therefore imagined they would do the same with other kind of anniledes. But one of these animals, which I confined with some leeches, died without having touched one of them.* Should I have concluded from this fact that toads do not eat leeches? Not at all. The loss of liberty is with some animals the cause of so much sorrow, that they will allow themselves to die of hunger. I had recourse to another means of testing this fact. I watched for the appearance of a toad, who had domiciled himself in a hole in the house, and then threw him a leech; it instantly disappeared.

Doubtless there exists a great similitude of confirmation and habits between the terrestrial and aquatic toad; it might, therefore be imagined that the latter would also eat the leech. My experiments have given me proof to the contrary. Several aquatic toads, which I placed in a glass jar, seized with avid-

*Leeches attach themselves to toads without biting them.

ity some earth-worms, but would never touch the leeches which I offered them. Ten toads which I opened contained only non-aquatic insects.

Aquatic toads, salamanders, and frogs, are bitten by leeches, who feed on their blood;* they have, therefore, been recommended as useful in leech ponds. But if these anniledes were devoured by water-lizards or frogs, it would be introducing the wolf into the sheep-fold. From thence to my experiments on batrachia. I have stated all relating to the toad, and I will now state the facts I have obtained relative to the water-lizards and frogs.

Some water-lizards which I kept in a jar, having become sufficiently tame to take worms out of my fingers, fled instantly to the opposite side of the jar when I offered them some young leeches. A leech-gatherer assured me he had seen a frog swallow a leech. This circumstance is not improbable, as the frog is very carnivorous; the frog, as is known, is caught by means of a fish hook baited with the skin of another frog. Nevertheless, several frogs, which I had kept without food for some days, would never touch leeches, either when in the water or on its surface; they on the contrary, seized on worms of the same size, which I had placed with the leeches. Twelve frogs, taken out of a swamp stocked with leeches, were found to contain, when opened, only beetles, spiders, and flies. Although aquatic toads, salamanders, and frogs, are not enemies of the leech, yet I have made known my experiments relative to them, as my silence respecting them might have appeared to be the result of an omission.

*Crustaceæ.*—M. Demarquette, of Douai, informed me that the animal which caused the greatest ravages among leeches was known in that country by the name of *scorpion*. At Bresse this name is given to the fresh-water shrimp. Wishing to convince myself if this was the animal alluded to by M. Demarquette, I plunged a small leech into a stream where

*The contrary has been said relative to toads, but I am certain of the fact above stated.

these crustaceæ were numerous; it was instantly surrounded on all sides, and when I withdrew it from the water its body was covered with wounds.

In the middle of April, 1850, Professor Soubeiran, erected a reservoir for leeches in the central Pharmacie of the hospitals of Paris, with the view of studying the reproduction of these animals. At the end of the year, on examining the contents of the reservoir, he only found about a hundred fillets, but instead of them he found a large quantity of the *oniscus aquaticus.* M. Soubeiran, jun., suspecting that these crustaceæ were enemies of the leech, placed a number of them in a jar with leeches; they soon attached themselves to the bodies of the latter, who tried without effect to get rid of them, but ultimately become their victims.

The *oniscus aquaticus* are very numerous in the ponds in the neighborhood of Paris. M. Soubeiran thinks that this circumstance explains an observation frequently made by dealers in leeches. "Frequently," they say, "they have seen in their ponds the young leeches produced by the adults which they had placed there, but in all cases after a short time this hope of a new generation completely disappeared.

As will be perceived, this opinion of M. Soubeiran's much resembles that entertained by myself, and which induced me to write this memoir.

The *oniscus aquaticus* of Linnæus only differs from other lice in the form of its tail. The body is flat, composed of eight rings, including the tail. The head is broader than it is long. The seven crustaceous laminæ which cover the body are almost equal, but the eighth, which forms the tail, is larger, rounded, and terminates above in a blunt point; it is furnished on each side with forked appendages attached to its extremity, and terminating in four long bristles. The *oniscus aquaticus* has seven pairs of claws.

It is probable that those aquatic lice, which are of the same size and of the same habit as the *oniscus aquaticus*, such as the *branchia*, also devour the leech. The *branchia* has a long body, and is yellow and tranparent. Its head is furnished with two immoderately long horns, forked at the points. The eyes are very large, black, and *fixed on a moveable neck.* The tail is terminated by two fins furnished with long feathered webs.—*Journal de Pharmacie.*

# VARIA—EDITORIAL.

In cities, the offices of the apothecary and the physician are entirely distinct; but, unfortunately, there is more than one point of contact between them. The apothecary, apart from his legitimate business, in selecting and compounding medicines, is presumed to have some knowledge of their applications, and is called upon to prescribe in cases of disease; the physician is sometimes tempted to add to his legitimate fee the profit upon the medicines which he orders. The apothecary may do harm by assuming the responsibilities of an art of which he is ignorant; the physician avails himself of the skill and knowledge of the apothecary in the preparation of the medicines which he furnishes to his patients, and then deprives the latter of the reward which is justly due to him; nay, the physician, indirectly perhaps, encourages a belief in the patient, that the apothecary is not to be relied upon, unless under the supervision of his superior knowledge and sagacity. These are not the only evils which result from this interference; but they are the most marked and prominent, and they lie at the root of the others. In the code of Ethics, promulgated by the American Pharmaceutical Association, which was re-published in our last number, the right ground is taken on this subject. "All such professional amalgamation" is denounced; in conducting their business, apothecaries "should avoid prescribing for diseases, when practicable, referring applicants, for medical advice, to the physician. On the other hand, the practice of some physicians (in places where good apothecaries are numerous) of obtaining medicines at low prices from the latter, and selling them to their patients, is not only unjust and unprofessional, but deserving the censure of all high minded medical men." Now we do not, of course, believe that the general recognition of the justice of an abstract ethical principle, will cause its mandates to be invariably respected. The love of gain is not always to be restrained by such a feeble barrier. But in endeavoring to correct an evil, it is something to have it recognised as an evil. There are many who, without giving much attention to the matter, do what they find convenient and profitable, who, if they believed it to be wrong and unprofessional, and knew that it was generally regarded as so, would scrupulously avoid it. The apothecaries have led the way. They have distinctly denounced on their part all interference with the physician, all prescribing at the counter, except in necessary and unavoidable cases. Will not the physicians follow? Will they not, too, recognise "the practice of some physicians (in places where good apothecaries are numerous) of obtaining medicines at low prices from the latter, and selling them to their patients," as "not only unjust and unprofessional, but deserving the censure of all high minded medical men?"

---

PARTHENIUM INTEGRIFOLIUM.—Dr. Mason Houlton has lately employed the parthenium integrifolium, or prairie dock, with perfect success in intermitting fever. The parthenium grows abundantly in the open prairies of the western and south western states. The flowering tops are the parts employed; they are intensely bitter, having somewhat a quinine flavor. Dr. H. has employed the infusion and finds that two ounces of the parthenium thus employed are equivalent, in therapeutic effects, to twenty grains of the disulphate of quinine. The new remedy bids fair to form a valuable accession to our indigenous materia medica; but numerous and careful experiments must be made before its value can be regarded as ascertained. Many vegetable bitters possess considerable power in the treatment of intermitting fever, but the immense superiority of quinine seems to be connected with the influence it exercises on the nervous system, rather than with its bitterness.

---

LINIMENT OF HYDRIODATE OF AMMONIA.—The following formula, which was furnished by Mr. George D. Coggeshall, has been extensively used as a quack remedy. It forms a nearly colorless liniment, containing an excess of Ammonia, is slightly stimulating, and exerts the specific effect of the iodine compounds.

℞ Iodine gr. xv.
Alcohol ℥vij.

Dissolve and add—

Oil of Rosemary,
Oil of Lavender, of each ʒi.
Camphor ʒij.
Water of Ammonia ℥i.

Mix.

Half an ounce of tincture of iodine might be conveniently substituted for the iodine in substance, diminishing the quantity of alcohol to 6½ ounces.

Hand Books of Natural Philosophy and Astronomy, by Dionysius Lardner, D. C. L., &c.—Second Course.—Heat, Magnetism, Common Electricity, Voltaic Electricity.—*Illustrated by upwards of two hundred Engravings on wood.*—Philadelphia: Blanchard & Lea, 1853.—Duo. pp. 451.

The merit of Dr. Lardner, as a popular teacher of science, is well known. He has great clearness of expression, great variety and fertility in illustration, and remarkable readiness in showing the applications of science to the arts, and to the purposes of every day life. His books are not too learned, but can be readily understood by those who have received merely a good elementary education, and he has a happy method of drawing attention to the more important propositions, which greatly facilitates the progress of the learner. The present volume treats of subjects with which the pharmaceutist is constantly conversant, and with which it is necessary for him to be thoroughly acquainted, and he will nowhere find them more lucidly or agreeably treated of.

---

Manual of Physiology, by William Senhouse Kirkes, M. D., Licentiate of the Royal College of Physicians, &c. assisted by James Paget, F. R. S. &c.—Second American, from the Second London Edition.—*With one hundred and sixty-five Illustrations.*—Philadelphia: Blanchard & Lea, 1853.—Duo. pp. 568.

Kirkes' and Pagets' manual is a book of established reputation. Those who are interested in the study of Physiology, and to whom is it not a matter of interest, will find in it all of importance that is known upon the subject set forth concisely and clearly.

---

Biographical Sketch of J. Kearney Rodgers, M. D. &c., by Edward Delafield, M. D.—Read before the New York Academy of Medicine, on Wednesday, Oct. 6, 1852, and Published under its Authority.

The late Dr. John Kearney Rodgers must have been well known to many of our readers. The kindness of his heart, and the urbanity of his manners, rendered him beloved wherever he was known, while his great skill as a surgeon extended his reputation far beyond the bounds of his personal friends, or the city of his birth. The memoir of Dr. Delafield, the testimony of a friendship of thirty-seven years duration, gives a simple but admirable account of his life, while, from such a man, the motive which suggested the memoir is the highest testimonial to the uprightness and amiability of its subject.

NEW YORK

# JOURNAL OF PHARMACY.

FEBRUARY, 1853.

## VESICATING OIL.

BY E. DUPUY.

The solubility of cantharidin in chloroform, as shown by the experiments of Professor W. Procter, suggested to me the idea of using that vehicle in combination with a fixed oil to obtain a vesicating agent, freed from the disagreeable concomitants of the ordinary fly blister, and retaining the cantharidin in a soluble state. I proceeded thus:

Powdered Cantharides, one part.
Chloroform, } of each (by weight) one and a half parts.
Castor Oil, }

To the powder was added the mixture of chloroform and oil in a close vessel; the ingredients were transferred after some hours, to a glass apparatus and the liquid displaced in the usual way. It amounted to about two-thirds of the original bulk of the liquid employed. A few drops of the vesicating oil applied to the arm of an adult produced a perfect blister in eight hours. Its easy application on any given surface may be of value as a vesicating or epispastic. I would suggest the use of oil silk over the application of it to the skin; by retaining the moisture of the skin it will favor the action of the oil.

# ON THE MEAT BISCUIT OF GAIL BORDEN,*

BY B. W. M'CREADY, M. D.

The preservation of animal food, by which the surplus products of one section of country can be made available for the use of another, and by which, too, it can be made serviceable in long journeys by land or sea when other supplies cannot be obtained, is an object of the highest importance. The employees of the Hudson's Bay Company convert their meat into what is called pemican. The muscular parts of the animal are cut into thin strips, thoroughly dried, reduced to powder, and mixed in proper proportion with melted fat. This answers perfectly the purposes for which it was intended. All the nutriment of the meat is preserved, it is compact, easily transported, and keeps for a long time, particularly in high latitudes. There are objections, however, to the process, which prevent it being used on a large scale.

In curing meat by salting it, the salt acts mainly by abstracting moisture from the meat. When fresh beef is covered with dry salt, the salt soon becomes moist, and is finally dissolved. The water is supplied by the beef; the latter is reduced in bulk, it becomes dryer and corrugated. The same process goes on when meat is placed in strong brine, and the abstraction of moisture continues for a considerable time, until the greatest possible amount is withdrawn, and the meat becomes dense and hard. Unfortunately, the moisture does not consist of simple water, it contains, dissolved in it, various salts, of which potash is the principal base, and forms what has been termed the juice of the flesh. Now, in the living animal, these salts play an important part in the wonderful process

* This article was prepared for a different purpose, but as the subject was an important one, and has been noticed at length in some of the foreign Pharmaceutical Journals, it is inserted here.

which constitute nutrition. During life, together, with the other materials of the body, they are exposed to constant waste, and need to be constantly replaced. Salt meat, deprived of these necessary ingredients, which are to some extent replaced by the salt itself, does not contain all the elements which are necessary to perfect nutrition; consequently, those fed on it exclusively for any length of time, become ill, they are affected with scurvy.

Mr. Gail Borden, of Galveston, Texas, residing in a land where cattle are numerous, and meat exceedingly cheap, has attempted another method of rendering the abundance of his adopted state serviceable in supplying the wants of other countries, in that respect, less favorably situated. In doing this, Mr. Borden has hit upon a preparation, which, though it may not be all its more sanguine friends claim, is still exceedingly useful, and merits, perhaps, the encomium which Professor Lindley, in his lecture on the results of the Great Exhibition of 1851, in London, assigns to it, as being the most important of the many wonderful things which were there exposed for the admiration of the English public.

In the preparation of the Meat Biscuit, according to the specification of the patent, meat from animals in good condition, and fresh from the slaughter-house, is divided into small pieces by means of a cutting machine, and is then boiled in a large quantity of water for sixteen hours. The soup thus made is passed through strainers of wire-cloth, and then evaporated by steam heat in a pan or tub, or by means of the vacuum-pan, to the consistence of thick treacle. Previous to, and during this process, all the fat which rises to the surface is removed. With the extract thus obtained, good flour is incorporated, until the whole attains a consistence proper for rolling into a thin layer, which is then cut up by a common biscuit machine. The biscuit are then baked in a slow oven until they are thoroughly crisp and dry. The quantity of flour employed, according to Mr. Borden, is about three parts by weight to two parts of the syrup, and eleven pounds of beef produce one pound of extract. The biscuit are afterwards ground to a coarse powder, and packed away into air-tight casks or tin cases.

In this process, it will be observed, that in the first place, all the fat is removed; in the second place, as neither fibrin nor albumen are, to any extent, soluble in boiling water, they likewise will be separated by the wire gauze through which the decoction is strained. The extract can contain then only the flocculi of coagulated albumen, which escape through the meshes of the strainers, together with a minute portion of the albumen, which, according to Dr. Bence Jones, is altered by the continued boiling, being rendered soluble, and converted into what Dr. Jones terms albuminose, the gelatine, the principles kreatine, kreatinine, and inosinic acid, which in a comparatively recent period, have been discovered to exist in flesh, and the various salts which form an important ingredient of its juice.

In the part which flesh, taken as food, plays in nutrition, it is now generally admitted, that the fat serves as respiratory food, the carbon and hydrogen of which it is composed, combining with oxygen in the course of the circulation, and becoming converted into carbonic acid and water and thus maintaining the animal temperature. What escapes oxidation is either stored away directly as fat, for the future use of the system, or passes out of it with the various excretions. The fibrin and albumen serve mainly to nourish the muscles, imparting by their decomposition strength and activity to the body and maintaining the activity of the heart and of the various other muscles of organic life.

It cannot consequently be admitted that the meat biscuit, or any similar preparation, contains the whole nutriment of the flesh from which it is made; on the contrary, the fibrin, the albumen, and the fat, which, in reality constitute its most nutritive portions are removed, and for all purposes of nutrition, lost. What, then, are its advantages, and what purpose does it really serve in the human economy?

"Fresh meat when incinerated," says Liebig, "leaves three and one-half per cent. of the weight of the dried flesh as salts. Meat, exhausted by boiling, leaves hardly one per cent. Ten pounds of fresh meat yield in all, 42.93 grms. (two and a half oz. avoirdupois, or 662.8 grains); but when these ten pounds are exhausted by lixiviation and boiling, 544.7 grains of the 662.8 enter the soup, and there remains in the meat only 118 grains. The fresh meat contains in its ash upwards of 40 per cent. of potash, the exhausted flesh only 4.78 per cent. of that alkali." It is on the presence of these salts, we believe, that the restorative effects of soup and of extracts of flesh mainly depend. They are essential ingredients of the body, and are necessary in the minute chemical changes of which vital activity is the product; they are constantly passing away with the excretions, and required to be constantly renewed; and in the form of aliment under consideration, they are presented to us in a condition and in proportions best suited for immediate assimilation.

Liebig attributes much of the effect of extract of flesh to the kreatinine, a nitrogenous compound, somewhat analogous to theine in its composition, and which exists in the juice of the flesh in exceedingly minute quantity. There is no proof, however, that kreatinine produces any such effect, and it is more probable that this substance is merely one of that series of bodies, the result of the decomposition of the tissues, which, commencing with muscle and nerve, terminates with urea.

In his biscuit, Mr. Borden unites wheaten flour in large proportion, with the extract of meat. He thus replaces the animal fibrin and albumen by the gluten of the wheat, while the starch, as respiratory or heat-producing food, takes the place of animal fat; the whole forming an economical, portable, and nutritious food, which can be preserved for an indefinite length of time. Biscuit, which had been in the Arctic ocean with the Grinnell expedition, and another portion, which had made the voyage to Australia and back, was perfectly unaltered, and when cooked, formed as palatable a soup as could be made directly from fresh meat.

The real merits of Mr. Borden's preparation can then be very briefly summed up. It affords a cheap and nutritious aliment, perfectly suited to the wants of convalescent patients and in hospital practice, must be invaluable.

On long voyages, it affords a nutriment, abounding in those substances, the want of which renders the continued use of salt provisions so unwholesome. It will probably be found beneficial in the treatment of scurvy, and will do much to prevent its occurrence.

Under similar circumstances, it affords a change of diet, which could not otherwise be obtained, unless at a greatly increased expense. Its cheapness renders its use for ordinary consumption in families a matter of economy.

Finally, it is compact, portable, and may be preserved unaltered for a great length of time.

---

## UPON THE DECOLORIZING POWER OF CARBON AND OTHER BODIES.

Filhol states, that many substances, besides carbon, have the power of decolorizing liquids. Sulphur, arsenic, and metallic iron, reduced from its sesquioxide by hydrogen gas, possess this quality. Indeed, the number of substances which possess decolorizing power appears to be quite large, and this property would seem to be a purely physical one, depending more upon the state of division of a body, than upon its chemical properties. Also, a substance which extracts from a liquid, one coloring matter, has frequently no action upon another. Filhol, gives the following table, showing the quantities of tincture of litmus, and of solution of indigo-sulphate of soda, respectively decolorized by equal quantities of various substances:—

| | Tincture of Litmus. | Indigo-sulphate of Soda. |
|---|---|---|
| Charcoal - - - - - - | 100 | 100 |
| Hydrated peroxyd of iron - | 129 | 2 |
| Alumina - - - - - - | 116 | 10 |
| Phosphate of lime - - | 109 | 2 |
| Iron reduced by hydrogen - | 95 | 100 |
| Precipitated sulphur - - | 27 | 0 |
| Black oxide of manganese - - | 89 | 14 |
| Indigo - - - - - - | 80 | 14 |
| Oxide of zinc - - - - - | 80 | 7 |
| Stannic acid - - - - - | 70 | 0 |
| Antimonic acid - - - | 67 | 2 |
| Chromate of lead - - - | 70 | 2 |
| Litharge - - - - - - | 67 | 4 |
| Sulphate of antimony - | 59 | 0 |
| Sulphate of lead - - - | 50 | 14 |
| Black oxide of copper - - | 27 | 0 |
| Calomel - - - - - - | 22 | 0 |
| Precipitated sulphate of baryta | 50 | 0 |
| " sulphide of lead | 130 | 17 |

(*Comptes rendus*, xxxiv, 247.)

I have, myself, observed also that precipitated carbonate of baryta and oxalate of lime, also calcined magnesia have, to a very considerable degree, the power of abstracting an organic coloring matter from the "Croton water," with which New York city is supplied. The color of this water is usually sufficiently deep, to be easily perceptible in a stratum two or three feet thick.

H. W.

# UPON THE OPERATION OF CARBON AS A DECOLORIZER.

Guthe, of Andreasberg, has taken the first prize offered for the year 1850–51 by the *Hagen Buchholzs'chen* Institution, for answer to the following question. "How far are charcoals, both animal and vegetable, applicable as decolorizers, without loss of the substance which is to be decolorized?" His experiments were made with blood-charcoal, bone-charcoal, and different wood-charcoals. His first experiments were made with the coloring matter of crude morphine. It was found to be insoluble in water, but easily soluble in alcohol and diluted acids. The author has given a table showing the quantities of the different coals respectively required to remove one part of this coloring matter from the solutions in alcohol and very dilute acids, from which it appears that the acid solutions require a little less of each kind of coal for decolorization, than the alcoholic solutions. The acids used were acetic and sulphuric diluted with 100, and muriatic alcohol with 300 parts of water.

| | Alcohol. | Acids. |
|---|---|---|
| Charcoal from fresh blood | 6 | 5 |
| " " dry blood | 8 | 7 |
| Pure ignited bone charcoal | 9½ | 8 |
| " moist bone charcoal | 1½ | 1¼ |
| Crude bone charcoal | 14 | 12 |
| Charcoal from Cream of Tartar | 22 | 20 |
| Linden and mahogany charcoal | 42 | 40 |
| Alder wood charcoal | 48 | 45 |
| Ash " " | 60 | 56 |
| Fir-tree " " | 64 | 60 |
| Chestnut tree wood charchal | 65 | 61 |
| Elder and apple tree charcoal | 67 | 64 |
| Beech " | 80 | 76 |
| Pear-tree " | 84 | 82 |
| Oak " | 90 | 84 |

He found that to precipitate one part of morphine itself from its neutral solutions in acetic, muriatic acid, and sulphuric acids, required four parts of charcoal from fresh blood, six parts of that from dry blood, and seven parts of purified ignited bone charcoal. The morphine thus precipitated was found to be difficultly and incompletely taken up again by boiling alcohol from purified bone charcoal, but easily from the crude. With regard to vegetable coals, the author opines that they cannot be applied profitably to the decolorization of morphine. It is necessary after the decolorization of solution of morphia by crude bone charcoal, to filter off immediately, in order to avoid greater loss.

Guthe divides animal charcoals into three different kinds, according to their properties. 1. The reignited purified blood and bone charcoals, which decompose the salts of the alkaloids while decolorizing them, and absorb a proportionate quantity of the alkaloid. 2. Crude bone charcoal, which, by the action of the carbonate of lime, which it contains, precipitates, but without absording morphine from its muriate and sulphate, but not from its acetate. 3. Purified bone charcoal, freed from lime by muriatic acid and water, but not reignited, which separates morphine from none of its solutions. The most advantageous way of decolorizing morphine appears to be, to operate upon its neutral acetic acid solution with crude bone charcoal. 100 parts of opium, treated with water, required 700 parts of crude bone charcoal for decolorization, and 6 per cent. of morphine was obtained. When moist, purified charcoal was used, the yield was increased to 8.66 per cent., and by treating the opuim with dilute acetic acid and crude bone charcoal, 8.66 per cent. was also obtained.

*Quinine and Cinchonine.*—A mother liquor obtained in the manufacture of quinine was precipitated by ammonia, in a state resembling chinoidine; the precipitate dissolved in alcohol, and treated with crude bone charcoal, yielded 70 per cent. of pure quinine; one part of pure quinine is completely absorbed from its acetic acid solution by six parts of charcoal, from fresh blood. A solution of crude quinine cannot be completely decolorized by charcoal, but its use is nevertheless, so far advantageous, that the quinine crystallizes afterwards more easily. Cinchonine in solution behaves towards charcoal like quinine, but is completely decolorized, 130 parts of moist bone charcoal being required for 100 parts of bark.

*Santonine.*—Good results were obtained in the decolorization of santonine by crude bone charcoal.

Finally, Guthe's result may be summed up as follows:—

1. Vegetable charcoals are not profitably applicable in any case for decolorizing, on account of the large mass required, and the abstraction of the substance to be decolorized from the solution.

2. In all cases, in which the presence of lime is not hurtful, crude bone charcaal is the most advantageous decolorizer.

3. In cases in which lime must not be present, bone charcoal, which has been treated with muriatic acid, and washed with water, but not reignited, is the proper agent.

(*Archiv der Pharm.*, 2 R. lxix., 121.)

---

## UPON THE GREEN COLOR OF PLANTS AND THE RED COLOR OF BLOOD.

Verdeil has announced that the substance called *chlorophylle*, and hitherto considered as a definite chemical compound, is a mixture of a colorless crystallizable fat, with a coloring matter which Verdeil has not obtained in a perfectly pure state, but which he thinks has a great analogy with the coloring matter of blood. By the addition of a small quantity of milk of lime to an alcoholic solution of chlorophylle, he precipitated all the coloring matter, leaving behind a colorless solution of the fat. The coloring matter was separated from the lime by means of chlorohydric acid and ether, and obtained by evaporation of the etherial solution. This coloring matter, like that of blood, contains according, to Verdeil, a large quantity of iron. (*Comptes Rendus*, xxxiii, 689.)

In connection with the above may be taken the statement of the Prince of Lalur-Horstmar, in one of his recent memoirs, that the presence of iron in the soil has an influence upon the coloring matter of plants. It occurs to me, however, as somewhat remarkable, that Verdeil's content of iron in chlorophylle should have been overlooked by one and all of the previous investigators of chlorophylle, namely—Vauquelin, Pelletier and Caventou, Prout, Macaire-Princep, Preisser, Mulder, and above all, by Berzelius. With this exception, however, Verdeil seems to have promulgated little or nothing that is new in his paper. Berzelius, in fact, in his memoirs upon chlorophylle, (*Annalen der Pharm.* 27, 296,) seems to have shown, quite distinctly, that this was a combination of a coloring matter with a fatty or waxlike substance.

H. W.

---

## ON THE CHEMICAL COMPOSITION OF QUINIDINE.

BY H. G. LEERS.

Quinidine, discovered several years ago by Winckler,* in a bark resembling Huamalies cinchona, and also in Maracaibo cinchona, has never yet been subjected to an accurate analysis, although this base appears to be daily acquiring a greater importance in relation to quinine.

In consequence of the government of Bolivia having monopolized the exportation, and by this means raised the price of

---

* Buchner's ***Repert. d. Pharm.*** [2] xlviii. [See also a paper in the ***Pharmaceutical Journal***, vol. vii., p. 527.]

*Calisaya cinchona* (the principal material for the manufacture of quinine), a cheaper bark is now imported, under the name Bogota cinchona,* which contains chiefly quinidine, and but a small proportion of quinine.†

From this Bogota cinchona, large quantities of quinidine are now prepared for admixture with quinine. The proportion of alkaloids in this bark was in two experiments, 2.61 and 2.66 per cent. It appeared, therefore, of great interest to obtain a more exact knowledge of the chemical relations of this substance, which, in the crude state in which the author received it from Mr. Zimmer, was beautifully white and distinctly crystalized, but still not perfectly pure. It contained an uncrystalizable, yellowish green resinous substance, together with quinine (according to the test with chlorine water and ammonia), and very probably also a third substance, containing a larger portion of carbon.

The following operations were performed in the laboratory of Prof. Will:—

In order to obtain the base in a perfectly pure state, the rough quinidine was dissolved in alcohol of 90 per cent., and the solution allowed to evaporate spontaneously in the air, when a greenish-yellowish resinous substance soon appeared on the walls of the vessel. The most beautifully formed crystals were then selected, washed with alcohol, and re-dissolved in spirit of wine, when the same greenish-yellow substance was deposited. The re-crystalization having been performed five or six times, until the yellow substance was no longer perceived, and the proportion of carbon in the base not yet prov-

---

* The bark here called *Bogota cinchona* is usually known in England as a Carthagena bark; and to distinguish it from common hard Carthagena bark, it is sometimes called *fibrous Carthagena bark*. Coquetta bark is one sort of this bark.—[Ed. *Pharm. Journ.*]

† In order to ascertain whether Bogota cinchona, like other cinchona barks, contained kinic acid, some finely powdered Bogota bark was boiled with hydrate of lime, and the obtained kinate of lime submitted, along with peroxide of manganese and sulphuric acid, to distillation, by which was obtained a liquid containing kinone.

ing uniform, the crystals obtained after five or six times repeated re-crystalization were finely powdered and shaken with ether, until all reaction of quinine disappeared, and the proportion of carbon remained constant.

If quinidine be dissolved in spirit of wine of 90 per cent., and the solution left to spontaneous evaporation, it forms colorless, hard prisms, shining like glass, with edge angles of 86° and 94°; the planes of the prisms are strongly striped, these stripes being also observable on the planes of truncation of the more obtuse edges of the prism; and in the direction of the latter planes the crystals admit of perfect cleavage. The crystals are terminated by shining planes, which converge at 114° 30', and are applied on the more aeute edges of the prism.

The rather hard crystals are easily rubbed to a snow-white powder, which becomes electrical by friction. If the crystals be heated in a platinum crucible over the flame of spirit of wine, they at first retain their brilliancy and form, and fuse without decomposition, and without yielding water, at 175° C., and form a clear, wine-yellow liquid, which, when cold, solidifies into a greyish-white crystaline mass. If the heat be increased above 175°, the wine-yellow fluid ignites, burns with a red, vividly flaring, strongly sooty flame, evolving at the same time an odor of kinoyl and of oil of bitter almonds, and leaves behind a voluminous easily combustible charcoal. The taste of quinidine is not so intensely bitter as that of quinine.

In order to determine its solubility, quinidine was rubbed down with water of 17° C. and shaken. 36.1 grammes of the solution left after evaporation of 0.014 grms. of quinidine dried at 100°; one part of quinidine, therefore was soluble in 2580 parts of water at 17°.

42.7 grms. of pure quinidine dissolved in water at 100°, and treated as before, left 0.023 grms. of quinidine =1 part to 1858 parts of water at 100° C.

The solubility in ether was determined by shaking finely powdered pure quinidine with ether of 0.728 spec. grav. at

17°; 19.4 grms. of this solution, by evaporation yielded 0.137 grms. of quinidine dried at 100°, or 100 parts of the solution contain 0.70 of quinidine. According to Winckler, 100 parts of ether dissolve 0.6923 parts of quinidine. One part of quinidine dissolves in 12 parts of alcohol of 0.835 spec. grav. at 17°.

*Analysis of Quinidine.*—1. *Crude quinidine* finely powdered and dried at 110° until it lost nothing, yielded:—

| | I. | II. |
|---|---|---|
| Carbon | 77.34 | 77.02 |
| Hydrogen | 7.86 | 7.90 |

2. *Pure quinidine*, obtained by being four or five times recrystalized from alcohol, finely triturated and shaken five or six times with ether, till chlorine water and ammonia produced no reaction of quinine, was washed with water and dried at 110°, till the weight remained constant. The results were:—

| | I. | II. | III. | IV. | V. | VI. | VII. |
|---|---|---|---|---|---|---|---|
| Carbon | 76.88 | 76.82 | 76.79 | 76.40 | 76.55 | 76.49 | — |
| Hydrogen | 7.70 | 7.76 | 7.77 | 7.73 | 7.70 | 7.81 | — |
| Nitrogen | — | — | — | — | — | — | 9.99 |

With reference to the analysis of the salts of quinidine, and the determination of the atomic weight of the base from the proportion of platinum in the platinum double salt, the following formula is calculated for quinidine:—

$C_{36} H_{22} N_2 O_2$.

| | | Calculated. | | Average of the Experiments. |
|---|---|---|---|---|
| 36 equiv. | Carbon | 216 | 76.59 | 76.66 |
| 22 " | Hydrogen | 22 | 7.80 | 7.74 |
| 2 " | Nitrogen | 28 | 9.93 | 9.99 |
| 2 " | Oxygen | 16 | 5.68 | — |
| 1 " | Quinidine... = | 282 | 100.00 | |

If quinidine be subjected with hydrate of potash and a small quantity of water to distillation, a yellow oleaginous substance is obtained, which reacts as an alkali, and possesses all the properties of quinoline. Repeatedly washed with distilled water, it yielded a beautifully yellow, oily liquid, from which muriatic acid and chloride of platinum threw down an orange yellow precipitate, which, after having been perfectly exhausted by cold water, was dissolved in hot water. When cold, the platinum salt precipitated from the solution in the form of small orange-red needles. Dried at 110°, 0.695 grms. of the platinum salt yielded, after being burnt, 0.204 grms. of platinum = 39.35 per cent. If the formula for quinoline, $C_{18}$ $H_7$ N, be correct, that of the platinum salt of quinoline would be $C_{18}$ $H_7$ N, H $C_4$ Pt $Cl_2$, and the salt would contain 29.47 per cent. of platinum.

Finely powdered quinidine dissolves in chlorine water without any particular phenomenon; quinine and cinchonine have the same relation to chlorine water. But if ammonia be added to these solutions, the cinchonine falls down from the cinchonine solution of a white color, the quinine solution becomes green like grass, and the quinidine solution remains unaltered. The reaction upon quinine becomes still more sensible by ether, if the substance to be tested for quinine be first finely powdered, then shaken with ether, and to the ether chlorine water and ammonia be added, the least trace of quinine may be detected by the liquid becoming green. By this test, the absence or presence of quinine could very easily be detected in the preparation of the quinidine salts.

*Salts of Quinidine.*—Most of these salts are much more readily soluble in water than the salts of quinine. In spirit of wine, they dissolve very easily, in ether scarcely at all. There are acid and neutral salts of quinidine, of which there are but few which are not distinctly crystallizable; some furnish beautiful large crystals with a vitreous brilliancy. The aqueous solutions of the quinidine salts yield with potash, soda, and ammonia, the mono and the bicarbonates of the alkalies, white pulverulent precipitates, which crystallize after long standing, and are insoluble in an excess of the precipitant.

Phosphate of soda, bichloride of mercury, and nitrate of silver, yield white precipitates. Chloride of gold gives a light yellow, chloride of platinum an orange yellow, and chloride of palladium a brown precipitate. Sulphocyanide of ammonium yields a white and tannic acid, a dirty yellow color, with the salts of quinidine.

*Neutral Sulphate of Quinidine.*—This salt was prepared by dissolving quinidine in diluted sulphuric acid, till the latter was neutralized. The neutral solution having been evaporated in the water-bath, yielded by cooling long, silky, shining, acicular crystals, arranged in star-like groups, of sulphate of quinidine, the watery solution of which was neutral. In order to establish the solubility of this salt, the crystals were rubbed down with water of 17°, and then some time shaken. The perfectly saturated solution was afterwards filtered, 43.1 grms. of the filtrate were evaporated to dryness, and the residue dried at 110°, the result was 0.325 grms. of sulphate of quinidine. It required, therefore, 130 parts of water at 17° to dissolve one part of the sulphate.

33.5 grms. of a solution saturated at 100°, yielded, after being evaporated and dried at 100°, 1.904 grms. of the salt= one part of the salt in 16 parts of water. Sulphate of quinidine dissolves very readily in alcohol, but is almost insoluble in ether. Analysis of 100 parts :—

| | Found. | | | | | |
|---|---|---|---|---|---|---|
| | I. | II. | III. | IV. | Average. | Calculated. |
| Carbon | 64.70 | 64.79 | — | — | 64.75 | 65.25 |
| Hydrogen | 8.18 | 6.91 | — | — | 7.05 | 6.95 |
| Sulphuric acid | — | — | 11.99 | 12.02 | 12.01 | 12.08 |

Corresponding formula :—

$$C_{36}\,H_{22}\,N_2,\,O_2,\,SO_3\,HQ.$$

*Acid Sulphate of Quinidine.*—The salt was obtained by adding to the neutral sulphate as much acid as it already contained.

The clear, very acid, and strongly opalizing solution was evaporated in the water-bath, and then placed under the air-pump, over sulphuric, acid. After the solution had arrived at the consistency of a syrup, and had assumed an intensely brown color, a crystalline mass of rather thick asbestos-like needles, of a slight yellow color, was formed. These crystals, after being removed from the mother-liquor, were washed with a mixture of alcohol and ether, and pressed between folds of filtering-paper, which did not deprive them ef their yellowish color. The proportion of sulphuric acid in the salt varied considerably several times, which arose very likely from the presence of some neutral sulphate, and for this reason no analysis is given.

*Neutral Hydrochlorate of Quinidine.*—Pure quinidine was finely powdered and mixed with water, then as much muriatic acid added by drops with the addition of heat, till the whole of the quinidine was dissolved, and the solution was neutral to test paper. By the spontaneous evaporation of the solution, the muriate of quinidine was obtained in the form of large rhombic prisms of a vitreous lustre. The mother-liquor yielded no crystals, even after having been evaporated to the consistency of a syrup and left standing for several weeks in the dry air. The solubility was determined by rubbing down the crystallized salt with water of 17°, and shaking, till the latter took up no more salt. Of the filtered liquid 7.067 grms. were evaporated, and the residue dried at 100° weighed 0.252 = 1 part of the salt, therefore, required 27 parts of water. Alcohol dissolved the salt very easily, ether scarcely at all. Analysis showed in 100 parts:—

| | Found. | | | | Calculated. |
|---|---|---|---|---|---|
| | I. | II. | III. | IV. | |
| Carbon | 64.57 | 64.11 | — | — | 64.19 |
| Hydrogen | 7.28 | 7.06 | — | — | 7.13 |
| Chlorine | — | — | 9.95 | 10.16 | 10.54 |

Corresponding formula:—

$$C_{36} H_{22} N_2, 2 H Cl_2, 2 HO.$$

*Acid Hydrochlorate of Quinidine.*—To the last salt as much muriatic acid as it already contained was added, and the solution, left to evaporate spontaneously, yielded beautiful, large, slightly yellowish crystals, which are monoklinometric and have the appearance of rhombic prisms.

Perfectly dried over sulphuric acid at 100° the acid muriate of quinidine lost 5.8 per cent. of water. It is easily soluble both in water and spirit of wine. In 100 parts were:—

| | Found. | | | Calculated. |
|---|---|---|---|---|
| | I. | II. | III. | |
| Carbon | 58.30 | — | — | 57.93 |
| Hydrogen | 7.12 | — | — | 6.97 |
| Chlorine | — | 18.96 | 19.00 | 18.99 |

Corresponding formula:—

$$C_{36} H_{22} N_2 O_2, 2H Cl+2 HO.$$

*Platinum-Chloride of Quinidine.*—The most beautiful crystals of the muriate of quinidine were dissolved in water, the solution diluted, acidulated with muriatic acid and chloride of platinum added as long as a precipitate was obtained. The orange-yellow precipitate was then placed on a filter and washed with acidulated water till chloride of platinum was no longer detected in the washings. The precipitate dried at 100°, was burnt, and gave the following results. In 100 parts were:—

| | Found. | | | Average of experiments | calculated. |
|---|---|---|---|---|---|
| | I. | II. | III. | | |
| Platinum | 27.05 | 27.17 | 27.13 | 27.11 | 27.04 |

These numbers correspond to the formula:—

$$C_{36} H_{22} N_2 O_2\ 2\ H\ Cl, Pl\ Cl\ 2+4\ HO.$$

*Mercury-chloride of Quinidine.*—Pure quinidine was dissolved by the aid of heat in alcohol of 85 per cent., acidulated with muriatic acid and an equal weight of bichloride of mercury dissolved in ether, added to the solution. When the mixture had become cold the murcury-chloride of quinidine was obtained in the form of small, scaly, pearly crystals, which dissolved with great difficulty in water. The crystals were placed on a filter, thoroughly washed and pressed between folds of filtering-paper; when dried over sulphuric acid they lost no water at 100°. In 100 parts were:—

| | Found. | | | | | Calculated. |
|---|---|---|---|---|---|---|
| | I. | II. | III. | IV. | V. | |
| Carbon | 34.77 | — | — | — | — | 34.52 |
| Hydrogen | 4.01 | — | — | — | — | 3.83 |
| Quicksilver | — | 31.98 | 31.91 | — | — | 31.97 |
| Chlorine | — | — | — | 22.60 | 22.31 | 22.63 |

Corresponding formula:—

$$C_{36} H_{22} N_2 O_2, 2 H Cl, 2 Hg Cl.$$

*Nitrate of Quinidine.*—If pure quinidine be dissolved by the aid of heat in moderately diluted nitric acid until the solution is neutral to test-paper, and the strongly opalizing mixture evaporated over sulphuric acid, the nitrate of quinidine crystallizes after some time in beautiful, large, warty crusts, resembling enamel. If the mother-liquor be allowed further to evaporate, a hemispherical white mass, resembling wax, forms on the surface, whilst the liquor becomes slightly green. This salt readily dissolves in water.

*Chlorate of Quinidine.*—By the mutual decomposition of neutral sulphate of quinidine and chlorate of potash, this salt was obtained in a perfectly pure state after having been re-crystallized from alcohol of 90 per cent. It forms long, white, silky prisms grouped in tufts. By a gentle heat it fuses into a transparent mass, but explodes very violently at a higher temperature.

*Hyposulphite of Quinidine.*—It was obtained by the mutual decomposition of neutral sulphate of quinidine and hyposulphite of soda. When the solution cools, the hyposulphite of quinidine crystallizes in thin, long, asbestos-like needles. In water this salt dissolves with some difficulty, but is very soluble in ether.

*Fluate of Quinidine.*—Pure quinidine in fine powder was suspended in water and placed in an apparatus for the development of fluoric acid; after some time, the quinidine contained in the water entirely dissolved, and a clear, intensely acid, slightly opalizing liquid was obtained. The solution was left to spontaneous evaporation, and yielded a mass of fluate of quinidine, consisting of white, silk-like, crystalline needles, which dissolved with great readiness in water. Upon the addition of chloride of calcium a precipitate was formed, which was insoluble in acetic acid.

*Acetate of Quinidine.*—This compound is obtained by dissolving by the aid of heat finely powdered quinidine in diluted acetic acid. When cold the acetate of quinidine appears in the form of thin, long, silky needles, which do not easily dissolve in cold water. When dried, the salt easily loses part of its acid. On removing the first crystals and allowing the mother-liquor to evaporate spontaneously, a salt crystallizes from it, consisting of a mass of semi-globularly grouped, small pointed needles, having an appearance of porcelain. This salt is by far more soluble in water than that above mentioned.

*Oxalate of Quinidine.*—If an alcoholic solution of oxalic acid be added to an alcoholic solution of quinidine with the application of heat, till the liquid is neutral to test-paper, the oxalate of quinidine crystallizes from the solution after the latter has become cold, in the form of long, white, silky needles, which dissolve with great difficulty in water. From the spontaneously evaporated mother-liquor a salt in the shape of warty crusts with an opaque white appearance, crystallizes, which dissolves with less difficulty in water.

*Tartrate of Quinidine.*—With tartaric acid quinidine forms two compounds, which appear to possess great resemblance to the oxalates. On saturating tartaric acid with quinidine, at a boiling heat, a salt separates, when the solution cools, in the shape of small, pearly needles, which dissolve, but with greater difficulty in water. The solution of neutral tartrate of quinidine having been allowed to evaporate spontaneously, yielded beautiful vitreous needles, and by the further evaporation of the mother-liquor, small, semi-globular, white, opaque, shining crusts of small needles appeared.

*Citrate of Quinidine* was obtained by saturating pure quinidine with pure citric acid at a boiling heat. From the cold neutral solution of the citrate of quinidine, small, but slightly glittering needles crystallized, which did not easily dissolve in water.

*Formate of Quinidine*, obtained by saturating the pure aqueous formic acid with quinidine. The salt forms long, beautiful, silky needles, readily dissolving in water.

*Butyrate of Quinidine.*—Aqueous butyric acid was saturated with an alcoholic solution of quinidine. The salt crystallized from the neutral solution in large, warty crusts resembling porcelain. It was very soluble, and smelt strongly of butyric acid.

*Valerianate of Quinidine.*—Aqueous valerianic acid being saturated with an alcoholic solution of quinidine, and the neutral solution left to spontaneous evaporation, the salt soon appeared in the shape of warty crusts, in the centre of which was a lighter body of a radiating structure. The salt smelt strongly of valerianic acid. The solution of the valerianate of quinidine having been evaporated in the water-bath, the liquid assumed a brown color, emitting a penetrating odor of valerianic acid, whilst at the same time oily drops were evolved.

*Kinate of Quinidine.*—Pure kinic acid dissolved in water, was saturated whilst heated with quinidine. The spontaneously evaporated neutral solution yielded a white, milky mass of small needles, soluble both in water and spirit of wine.

*Hippurate of Quinidine.*—Pure hippuric acid, dissolved in spirit of wine, was saturated with quinidine under the application of heat. The hippurate of quinidine crystallized from the cold neutral solution in long, silky crystals, which had the appearance and shape of fern-leaves. It dissolves readily in water and in spirit of wine.

In comparing the formula for quinidine with those for quinine and cinchonine, the following relations are established:—

| | |
|---|---|
| Quinidine | $C_{36} H_{22} N_2 O_2$. |
| Quinine | $C_{38} H_{22} N_2 O_4$ (Laurent).<br>$C_{20} H_{12} N O_2$ (Liebig). |
| Cinchonine | $C_{38} H_{22} N_2 O_2$ (Laurent).<br>$C_{20} H_{12} N O_4$ (Liebig). |

According to this quinidine differs from cinchonine by a lesser proportion of two atoms of carbon, whilst the equivalents of the other elements are the same. An homologous relation between these bases, which appears so very probable, cannot, therefore, be established.—*Ann. der Chem. u. Pharm., Mai,* 1852, *in London Pharm. Journal.*

---

## ON FLUID EXTRACT OF RHUBARB AND SENNA.

BY WILLIAM PROCTER, JR.

Notwithstanding that two preparations of Rhubarb and Senna are already known, it is believed that the new one now proposed, possesses sufficient claims to gain for it the favorable opinion of physicians and patients, in many cases where a cathartic is needed, simply as such, or in connection with other medicines. It is well known that senna has little, if any, tonic influence on the alimentary surfaces; that an overdose has a depleting effect, often inconvenient, and that griping is a frequent attendant on its exhibition. On the other hand, it is equally understood, that rhubarb is remarkable for being a sort of therapeutical paradox, in so far as it possesses both a purgative and an astringent property, the latter coming into play *after* the former has manifested itself, and thus repairing, as it were, its effects. It is also well known, that this astringent or tonic action, is so strongly marked, that it is necessary, in most cases, to combine it with some other cathartic to overcome or modify this peculiarity, when a simple cathartic is needed. By the union of these two drugs in the concentrated form presented by a fluid extract, and in a due proportion, a resulting cathartic action is obtained which is safe, unattended by unpleasant symptoms, and not followed by constipation when the dose has been properly graduated. It has been ascertained that the association of alkalies and alkaline salts with rhubarb and senna, has a tendency to prevent their unpleasant griping effects, and in the case of senna, to increase its activity. The introduction of the bicarbonate of potassa is with this view, and the aromatics from their carminative properties also aid. The following is the formula:—

| | |
|---|---|
| Take of Senna, in coarse powder, | twelve ounces, (troy) |
| Rhubarb, in coarse powder, | four ounces, |
| Bicarbonate of potassa, | half an ounce, |
| Sugar, | eight ounces, |
| Tincture of ginger, | a fluid ounce, |
| Oil of cloves, | eight minims, |
| Oil of aniseed, | sixteen minims, |

Water and alcohol, of each a sufficient quantity.

Mix the senna and rhubarb, (by grinding them together is a convenient way,) pour upon them two pints of diluted alcohol (U. S. P.), allow them to macerate twenty-four hours, and introduce the mixture into a percolator furnished below with a stopcock or cork to regulate the flow. A mixture of one part of alcohol and three of water should now be poured on above, so as to keep a constant but slow displacement of the absorbed menstruum, until one gallon of tincture has passed. Evaporate this in a water bath to eleven fluid ounces, dissolve in it the sugar and bicarbonate, and after straining, add the tincture of ginger, holding the oils in solution, and mix. When done the whole should measure a pint.

*Remarks.*—If the percolation has been properly conducted, the ingredients will have been sufficiently exhausted when six pints of fluid have passed. As by far the larger portion of the soluble matter passes in the first two pints, it is well to set these aside and evaporate them separately to six fluid ounces, subsequently adding it to the other liquid when it has been reduced to five fluid ounces. As the cathartic principles of senna and rhubarb are very susceptible to injury from heat, especially in contact with the air, the propriety of using the best available means for conducting the evaporation need not be urged.

When the evaporation is conducted in open vessels, some advantage is gained by adding the sugar to the tincture, and continuing the process until it measurs fifteen fluid ounces. The sugar protects the extractive matter from oxidation, and more completely suspends or dissolves the resinous part of the rhubarb contained in the tincture. The bicarbonate should not be added to the extract while it is above 140° Fahr., and should be reduced to powder previously.

It may be objected to this formula that we already have fluid extracts of rhubarb and of senna of the same ratio of strength, and that when physicians need such an association, they can mix them. In answer, it may be stated that the cases where a simple cathartic is needed, are so numerous that this preparation will be found useful to the physician, and a good medicine for travelers and others who resort to this kind of purgative habitually.--*American Journal of Pharmacy, Jan. 1st,* '53.

---

## PREPARATION OF SANTONINE WITHOUT THE EMPLOYMENT OF ALCOHOL.

BY J. LECOCQ, OF SAINT-QUENTIN.

To obtain santonine, we take one part of semen-contra of Aleppo reduced to coarse powder, and boil it with ten parts of water, and after boiling for a quarter of an hour, a sufficient quantity of slaked lime is added to it to render the liquor slightly alkaline; it is again boiled for ten minutes, then strained through a cloth, and the residue pressed. If it is not considered sufficiently exhausted, which may be ascertained by its leaving in the mouth the hot and pungent taste of semen-contra, it is boiled again with five quarts of water and a little slaked lime; it is strained, and the residue submitted to pressure. The united liquors are evaporated until they do not weigh more than the semen employed; they are then put into a stone-ware pot, allowed to cool, and are then treated with an excess of hydrochloric acid. A fatty and resinous matter instantly separates, in thick flakes, which float, and santonine is precipitated as an impalpable powder; it is strained through a fine cloth; the santonine passes with the liquor, and the resinous matters remain on the cloth. This substance, which contains only very little santonine, is rejected; after a day's repose, the impure santonine is deposited at the bottom of the vessel.

It is washed with distilled water, and purified by combining it *de novo* with lime. For that purpose, it is put into a porcelain capsule, with about two quarts of distilled water; it is boiled. A certain quantity (50 to 60 grammes) of quick lime reduced to powder, is then added to it, and the combination is operated in a short time.* The liquor is filtered and decolorized with animal charcoal, and then treated with hydro-chloric acid; the santonine is immediately precipitated; it is collected on a paper filter, washed with distilled water until the washing water does not redden litmus paper, and dried in a stove sheltered from the light.

Thus obtained, santonine occurs in pearly white bracteæ, of great billiancy, and promptly becomes colored by light. It is therefore essential to keep it in a black glass flask and well corked.—*Repertoire de Pharmacie, Oct.*, 1852.—*M. Chemist, Nov.*, 1852.

---

* It is important for the success of the operation not to add an excess of lime in combining the impure santonine with this base, for the bibasic salt of santonine is very sparingly soluble in water; it is better to leave a slight excess of santonine which will remain on the filter and which may be treated *de novo* with lime.

## ON THE HEMOSTATIC EFFCTS OF THE EAU PAGLIARI.

BY PROFESSOR SEDILLOT.

The formula for the preparation of the styptic water invented by Signor Pagliari, an apothecary at Rome, and which has attained a high celebrity on the Continent, is thus given by Professor Sedillot, to whom it was transmitted by the inventor:—

Take of benzoin, eight ounces; sulphate of alumina and potassa, one pound; water, ten pounds. Boiled together in a glazed earthen vessel for six hours, constantly stirring the resinous mass, and supplying the loss by evaporation by successive additions of hot water, so as not to interrupt the ebullition. Finally, filter the liquid, and preserve it in well-stopped glass vessels. The portion of benzoin which remains undissolved will be found to have lost its odor and inflammability.

The hemostatic water thus obtained is limpid, resembles champagne in color, has a slightly styptic taste, and a sweet aromatic odor. It leaves, on evaporation, a transparent deposit, which adheres to the sides of the vessel.

The following are the conclusions deduced by M. Sedillot from his experience of this and other styptics:—

1. There are fluids which instantaneously coagulate the blood, and convert it into a thick, homogeneous and consistent clot.

2. The eau Pagliari enjoys this remarkable property, and does not exercise any injurious action on the tissues with which it comes into contact.

3. Theory, experience, and clinical observation equally concur in demonstrating its efficacy as a styptic.

4. The object of compression, in the application of hemostatic liquids, is to permit the coagulation of the blood, as well as the adhesion of the clot to the mouths of the wounded vessels.

5. In all cases in which recourse cannot, without serious in-

convenience, be had to ligature, as well as in those in which the alteration of the blood prevents its coagulation, and renders hemorrhage dangerous, the eau Pagliari may be advantageously employed, and deserves to be classed among the valuable resources of our art.—*Gazette Medicale de Strasbourg, May*, 1851.

---

# VARIA—EDITORIAL.

## DR. STEWART'S LETTER UPON ADULTERATED DRUGS.

To G. B. Guthrie, M. D.

Dear Sir:— 77 N. Eutaw St., Baltimore, *Jan. 4th*, 1853.

Only a few days have elapsed since my attention was called to your letter in the New York Journal of Pharmacy, for December, 1852, or it should have met with a prompter response. I thank you for it, especially in view of the publication of my report, and the kind manner in which you have reviewed my little speech in the convention. The fact is, I was not aware that it would be published, or I might have been reminded that I had lost my individuality on the point referred to. You will remember that when we met in 1852, you told me that "my letter to our friend Coggeshall," (expressing the same opinions to the New York Convention of 1851, which I reiterated in 1852, in the Philadelphia Convention), "was pretty freely discussed." You also expressed a wish to delay your report until after the next annual convention, in order to a further discussion and settlement of these few mooted points. But in my letter to Mr. G. D. Coggeshall, I also pledged myself to submit my opinion to the majority, in order to establish a uniform system of examination at all the ports. Then, as soon as you told me that the New York Convention had not adopted my resolution, I at once said to you, "I will, in my report, adopt the views of the Convention, and sustain them as soon as they are sanctioned by the Honorable Secretary of the Treasury." You will remember that I was anxious that these should obtain the sanction of another National Convention before submitting your report to the Honorable Secretary.

Well, the Convention assembled, and we very naturally went over the subject *de novo;* I, taking the position of my letter to my friend Coggeshall one year before, 1851 is then consistent with 1852, and neither are opposed to your report, as it was suspended in order to a second discussion of the whole matter.

There is no defect in the law as it *now* stands. There is no hesitation about the exclusion of the *products of fraud;* the foreign merchant can no longer flood our market with refuse and adulterated drugs. But the attempt is now made to so construe the law, that it shall *also prevent fraud at home.* Now, I am not inconsistent, if, with the same breath, I oppose this effort *as calculated to break down a good law*, (that now does its whole duty, and nothing but its duty,) while I sincerely wish to accomplish this second object, and pledge myself to sustain you in its accomplishment by the most feasible means that can be adopted by the most intelligent portion of our citizens (*on this subject*), viz., the National Pharmaceutical Association. I do not feel that I have bemeaned myself in thus losing my individuality, and sustaining in my report, the system of examination adopted by the convention in 1851. See American Journal of Pharmacy, vol. xviii, pp. 24, 25. Moreover, I may with propriety use the very arguments which I had intended to give importance to *my own* plan, and if asked for my *private* (individual) opinion, I may say, that I would prefer to admit all articles "that are good of the kind," and no others, thus protecting all the states from adulterations by *irresponsible*, nameless *foreigners, in other countries.* Then, let each state protect itself against *responsible* citizens of our own country, who adulterate good medicines, flour, coffee, tea, spices, or any other necessary article.

It is useless for any one state to make such a law, unless the general government protects us from foreign fraud, and *since* the general government has offered the protection from abroad, we find our United States National Medical Convention is really engaged in arranging a home protection. I have been appointed to attend that Convention by our state faculty for several years, and at the request of their committee, gave them the plan annexed. Now, by way of illustration, suppose we construe the law so that it shall include *all* inferior varieties of Peruvian bark, not admitting any that are good of the kind, (most bastard barks contain tonic and valuable principles, Maracaibo, for instance). What is the consequence? "The most respectable druggists are at once supplied with powdered Peruvian bark, made of the refuse bark of the quinidine manufacturer, entirely destitute of all tonic principles; yet it can be declared to be "real, genuineTabla Calisaya," and it is: but the quinine has been extracted. I ask you, would you not prefer the Maracaibo, if you were the patient? The fact is that the supply of the *pure*, true, quinine bark is not sufficient, and even in France they are seeking a substitute. And moreover, for 23 years, I know, that some varieties, not at all characterized by quinine, are actually preferred *when given in powder*, to the yellow Calisaya or quinine bark. A most reliable man, and a contributor to the Journal of Pharmacy, told me, that when an apprentice in one of the most respectable and most extensive wholesale drug-stores in the United States, (15 years since.) "He really did not know that there was any true red bark, as all they sold was made by coloring the pale bark with red ochre."

This house monopolized all the trade with one or two of our Western States.

Nevertheless, this was more potent than the leached bark that is now supplied to our patients, although it be real Calisaya Tabla, and this is no fancy sketch; a few weeks since, on the same day I received two samples of bark for analysis, one from a first class prescription store, perhaps the oldest and most central in Baltimore, with a note from the Pharmacien, which I have here annexed.

This proved to be, not only the refuse leached bark above referred to, but also the magma of carbonate of lime, &c., that results in the manufacture of quinine, showing that it was not supplied by the quinine manufacturer, but taken with other refuse, without his participation, otherwise he would have kept the magma separate from the refuse bark.

The other sample was from an importing merchant of our city, who wished to know the value of a bastard quill bark, that could be obtained in South America, perhaps at 10 or 12 cents per pound, and it yielded more than two per cent. of alkaloids, cinchonine, &c.

Now, as it contained no quinine, his inducement to import it must depend on the value of "bark for powder," and the government will lose all the duty on his importation, *if it is prevented*, by the supply of refuse bark from quinine manufactories. Moreover, the two per cent. of tonic principles is double the proportion in officinal bark, [true loxa or crown bark contains 39 grains of alkaloids per pound, (Gœbel.) The above contains 154 grains per pound.]

Another argument for the appointment of an independent state officer in every state, is the encouragement of science, and especially Toxicology and medical jurisprudence. Professors of chemistry and others have united in sending me the contents of a stomach from another state, (pronounced to contain arsenic without the shadow of a reason.) And why should the time of the chemist be employed by other states, and he expected to leave his business and home to attend court without any pay. Where will you find a lawyer, or a man of any other profession who will spend two weeks in performing an analysis; in macerating stomachs and their contents, then be haled to court, criticised by lawyers, and receive as a compensation, the satisfaction of knowing that on the evidence of chemical tests, one poor wretched woman was hung? This is literally the truth with regard to two of our best chemists in Baltimore. They were denied by the court any compensation, although it sealed their services with death.

There should be, in every state, at least one chemist to whom the poor as well as the rich could apply when poison or adulteration was suspected. His salary should be $2000 per annum, and whenever an adulteration was detected, the vender should be fined $100, unless he could prove that he purchased it in the same condition. One such exposure of a drug grinder would make him harmless, and there are few merchants who would pay the fine rather than inform. I have in my possession a sample of cream of Tartar adulterated largely with alum. The proportion of Indian meal that is used to adulterate mustard and ginger, would, I suppose, stagger the credulity of the most credulous. It is well known that sulphate of copper and other noxious drugs have been used to make white bread out of bad flour, and it would be difficult to find one keg of saltpetre containing a tithe of its weight of nitrate of potash in some manufactories; but the poor are generally the only sufferers in these cases; and we are apt to think that they deserve the blame for seeking cheap articles; every good government should really protect the poor and the ignorant above all others.

By this plan of mine, the fines would pay the government more than the salary of the officer, and if they did not, the amount could be raised by compelling all who sell or practice medicine to take out a license, *except graduates of Pharmacy, or those possessing diplomas*, and double the licence for every secret nostrum vender. This would be found a two edged sword for the protection of the poor by the suppression of empiricism, quackery, and fraud, and the encouragement of science.

Respectfully,

*Baltimore, Jan. 4th*, 1853. DAVID STEWART, M. D.

---

*Copy of Note referred to above.*

*November 29th*, 1852.

DEAR SIR:—

I herewith send you a parcel of Peruvian bark, which I have reason to believe does not represent its label, "Cinchona flava, powdered Calisaya bark." I bought it in the city of ——, some time since, as the best of its species, from a house, the name of which is a guarantee to all Pharmaceutists, and am forced to believe that it was an oversight on their part, or criminal substitution and adulteration on the part of the powderer. The price paid for the article was $2.70 per pound. Should it prove of sufficient interest to command a few moments of your valuable time, the subscriber will be happy to acknowledge the favor, in common with all the apothecaries, who feel a solicitude that such drugs only as are pure and genuine, shall be dispensed to the public:— Very Respectfully, &c.,

To DR. D. STEWART, Eutaw-st. A. S——s..

---

NEW METHOD OF EMPLOYING IODINE.—M. Hannon recommends that when iodine is to be employed externally, instead of using it in the form of ointment, it should be sprinkled in substance between two layers of cotton batting, and kept applied directly on the part by means of a bandage. The iodine volatilized by the heat of the part permeates the cotton-wool, and acts directly upon the skin. It is best to cover the outer layer of batting with a piece of oiled-silk or sheet gutta percha, to prevent the vapor from discoloring the dress. This mode of employing iodine is convenient, cleanly, and efficacious. The quantity used at one time must be very small; ten grains applied over a chronic glandular enlargement, produced in a stout young man so much irritation that he was compelled in a short time to remove the epithem.

---

COLLODION.—Ordinary collodion when applied over a surface of any extent, is apt to crack or break. M. Robert Latour proposes to correct this defect by the following formula:

| | |
|---|---|
| Collodion, - - - - | 30 grammes. |
| Castor Oil, - - - - | 50 centigrammes. |
| Soft Turpentine, - - - | 50 centigrammes. |
| | Mix. |

M. Guernsaut who has employed the collodion thus prepared, finds that it is pliable, gives less pain on application than ordinary collodion, dries quickly, and adhers well. It has been used in cases of erysipelas, cutaneous eruptions, &c. Collodion has been recommended as giving immediate relief in chilblains.

**Hospital Sulphate of Quinine.**—Under this title an English apothecary, Mr. Edward Herring, recommends a preparation consisting of disulphate of quinine only partially purified. It differs from the ordinary disulphate chiefly in its color, which is brownish. As the final purification of quinine is attended with considerable trouble, and some loss from animal charcoal, the new preparation can be afforded at a cheaper rate. The principal objection to its employment is the increased facility it would afford for adulteration.

---

**Glycerin Ointment.**—The bland and unirritating character of pure glycerin, its permanence, when exposed to the atmosphere, the completeness with which it shields the parts covered by it, rendered it susceptible of many important applications. The following formula for the preparation of a Glycerin ointment, is published by Mr. John H. Ecky, in the last number of the American Journal of Pharmacy. Mr. E. has found it particularly useful in cases of chapped and excoriated hands, &c :

| | | |
|---|---|---|
| Spermaceti, | - - - - | ℥ ss. |
| White Wax, | - - - - | ʒ i. |
| Oil of Almonds, | - - - | fl ℥ ij. |
| Glycerin, | - - - - | fl ℥ i. |

Melt and incorporate the wax and spermaceti with the oil of almonds at a moderate heat; put these into a wedgewood mortar, add the glycerin, and rub until *well mixed and cold.*

---

M. Dizé whose name is associated with that of Le Blanc, in the discovery of the method of manufacturing carbonate of soda from common salt, has lately died at Paris, at the advanced age of eighty-eight years. For fourteen years under the republic and the empire, M. D. was pharmacien en chef of the armies of France. The history of the discovery on which his reputation mainly rests, perhaps the most valuable which modern science has given to the arts, is sufficiently curious. We condense the following account of it from the eulogium pronounced upon Dizé by M. Frederic Dubois before the Academie Nationale de Medicine. Le Blanc, a surgeon of Paris, and an attentive auditor of the chemical lectures which were delivered at the college of France, first conceived the idea of obtaining soda by the decomposition of chloride of sodium. Applying to Darcet he was by him referred to his pupil Dizé. The first experiments made at the Collage of France were unsuccessful, and Darcet was inclined to report unfavorably, and give up the attempt. Le Blanc was not so easily discouraged. New experiments were instituted. Finally Dizé noticed in one of Le Blanc's experiments that the fusion of a mixture of sulphuret of sodium, carbonate of lime and charcoal, produced a soda much less sulphuretted than that of any of the numerous preceding trials. Dizé communicating this observation to Darcet, the latter recommended him to place the mixture in a crucible, and to elevate the temperature until the whole was in a state of perfect fusion. The experimenter followed his advice, and for the first time obtained crystals of carbonate of soda. This discovery, which saved France alone twenty millions of francs per annum, never proved of any direct advantage to the discoverers. The Duke of Orleans having furnished the means, a large manufactory was established at Saint Denis; but, on the arrest and execution of that prince, this was, with the rest of his property, sequestrated. Le Blanc and Dizé made numerous attempts, under the successive governments of the period, to obtain indemnification, but without success. Disappointed and destitute, Le Blanc finally committed suicide; while the talents and information of Dizé opened to him in other pursuits a long and honorable career.

---

MATERIA MEDICA, OR PHARMACOLOGY AND THERAPEUTICS. BY WILLIAM TULLY, M.D. VOL. I., No. I. NOVEMBER, 1852. SPRINGFIELD: George W. Wilson's power presses. 8vo., pp. 64.

We have received this publication at so late a period, that we must defer an extended notice of it until our next number.

---

THE ESCULAPIAN, DEVOTED TO POPULAR MEDICAL LITERATURE. C. D. GRISWOLD, M.D., 108 Nassau-street.

There is much in many departments of medicine that would be useful and interesting to the public at large. Matters relating to hygiene, diet, the causes and the hereditary nature of many diseases, the history of epidemics, the laws of contagion, &c., can be understood without any very profound knowledge of anatomy or physiology. Confining himself to topics, of which the public are able to judge, Dr. Griswold will afford valuable information, while the diffusion of real knowledge will operate as the best antidote to charlatanism. His journal is well printed on good paper. The subscription price, $1 per annum, is exceedingly cheap. We cordially wish him success in his enterprise.

NEW YORK

# JOURNAL OF PHARMACY.

MARCH, 1853.

## GERMAN AND AMERICAN PHARMACY.

BY FREDERICK F. MAYER.

SOME months since, I published in the *New York Journal of Pharmacy*, a notice of the etherial solution of Sesquichloride of Iron, and the rebuff I then received from another contributor, nearly disheartened me from any further communication; but I am again encouraged to contribute something more from the information gathered during forty years experience, and hope that my new countrymen will extend to me the indulgence that I found in the land of my birth.

If the philosopher of old Greece could say for himself that "the wiser a man becomes, the more he is aware of his own ignorance," the same thing will be acknowledged by other honest men who have a sincere desire for their own improvement, and, of course, by physicians and pharmaceutists, in whose profession every year is bringing forward new facts, such as not only cannot be arranged under existing systems, but such as require new arrangements and modified theories.

To promote and to forward any science, such as pharmacy, it is useful to learn its conditions, such as they have existed in other countries, and at earlier periods of their development, by which our view is extended, and becomes objective. Something of this kind I should like to undertake myself, and by placing my older experience parallel with my later, give occasion for further comparison, and reciprocal acknowledgment.

Not that I would here, where all the conditions are still new and strange to me, attempt to speak didactically,—I would only attempt to draw a parallel between the state of pharmacy in two countries which are daily drawn into closer intercourse with each other, and between which an attentive spectator cannot fail to find many interesting points of difference. Such a parallel, if well drawn, cannot fail to be interesting, and by it many of the differences would be defined, explained, and finally reconciled.

To perform this task, I would propose to go through with the preparations, which in a marked degree differ from those used in the United States. But before doing this I would say some few words regarding the education of a German pharmaceutist, and the relation which he bears to the state and to the physician.

The following, then, is the regular course of education of the German apothecary. In the fourteenth or fifteenth year of his age, he commences an apprenticeship of three or four years, after having by an examination tested his knowledge of the Latin, and, in some cases, of the Greek language, and of the elements of mathematics, physics, and natural history.

At the expiration of his apprenticeship, the future pharmaceutist has again to prove, by an examination, that he has not forgotten his knowledge of philology, and that he has also attained the requirements of his profession in botany, chemistry, pharmacolology, and in the art of preparing and dispensing medicines. He has now reached the age of seventeen or eighteen years. For the next three to five years he must leave the city of his apprenticeship, [wanderschaft,] and exhibit his knowledge of his art in other cities and countries. In many states he cannot receive permission to become overseer of a pharmacy until his twenty-fifth year; indeed, in these states he cannot demand his third examination before this age; and in most of them, as an invariable condition of this so-called state examination, [staats-prufung,] he must previously pass one or two years to a university. In the state examination he must show his theoretical and practical knowledge of chemistry, botany, toxicology, as well as of zoology, and of the laws regulating the practice of medicine and of pharmacy.

After these various examinations (for all which proper fees have to be paid) are at an end; the apothecary must take an oath that he will strictly fulfil his duties as a subject in general, and those belonging to his employment in particular; and he is at length in a condition to look around to see where he can obtain a pharmacy within the reach of his means, or, in some other way, earn his bread.

If an apothecary thus educated has properly used his time, he finds himself in possession of a large body of theoretical knowledge. In botany, he is familiar with the artificial, and with the so-called natural system, and with the names of several hundred officinal and other plants, together with their botanical characters. In chemistry, with the connection, the composition and the equivalent proportions of nearly all the officinal and of many other articles. In the mercantile knowledge of drugs, [waarenkunde,] the distinctive differences, the tests of goodness, and the derivation of officinal drugs. In toxicology, the chief symptoms of the various kinds of poisoning, the most useful antidotes, and the methods of chemico-legal investigation. His practical knowledge is shown in the selection and preparation of his medicines according to the prescription of the physician: but in none of the above-mentioned examinations is he asked regarding the operation of senna, rhubarb, the alkalies, salts, &c., upon the human body, nor in what doses they are to be administered.

He must be well and intimately acquainted with the distinctions between the varieties of rhubarb, bark, sarsaparilla etc., and with their adulterations and falsifications. He must know the botanical names of the plants, whence they are obtained, their nature, country, their chemical analysis, and the pharmaceutical preparations into which they enter; yet how, or in what manner, the remedy in skillful hands is useful or injurious, is none of his business; nay, they do not like that he should make himself acquainted with it. They wish him to be a man who blindly follows his orders, that he may say with Butler, in Schiller's Wallenstein,

I trouble not my brains,—I do my duty.

I must leave to the reader's imagination the situation in which a man formed after this ideal, finds himself when he is suddenly plunged into the American pharmaceutical world.

With the exception of thirty or forty articles, which he is forbidden by law to dispense, a man so formed gives every article to the public which it desires, but he knows nothing of giving advice. He looks down with sovereign contempt upon the sale of all and every patent medicine, and he takes good care not to dispense them himself, since he would otherwise be amenable to the law.

---

## NOTES ON PHARMACY, NO. VI.

BY BENJAMIN CANAVAN.

*Syrup Assafœtida.*—It is sometimes desirable to administer Assafœtida otherwise than in pill or *per anum*, especially to juvenile patients, and consequently in the least disagreeable form possible; for which reasons the following formula, which I have composed, to produce a syrup of the article, may be of some practical use,—

℞ Assafœtida ʒ i.
Aqua. ℥ viss.
fiat emulsio
ad quem adde Sacch: Alb: ℥ viij
et cum calore balnei aquoisa fiant
Syrupi ℥ x quo misa bene
Ol Carui gtt x.

The whole of the Assafœtida, when clean or carefully selected, can be triturated into emulsion, which should not be strained, nor should the syrup, nor the scum be removed; as this and the sediment which is deposited, after standing some time, may be readily re-incorporated by agitation, which should be done before the use or administration of the medicine. I consider this preparation much more artistical, efficient and accurate than that of mixing the tincture with simple syrup, as it is sometimes made.

*Tinctura Kino.*—Having called attention to the discrepancy in the formulas given for the preparation of this tincture, in a letter addressed to the editor of the American Journal of Pharmacy, some two years ago, since when the necessary correction has been silently made in the late editions of the U. S. Dispensatory and Pharmacopœia; and having seen it stated afterwards in a note by the editor, to a communication in the same journal, that he had in his possession a phial of the tincture prepared with the proper menstruum, viz., "spiritus tenuior," or proof spirit, which had become gelatinous in the space of a few months, I forget exactly how many. I desire to state I have now a phial of the article so prepared, which was made sometime previous to January, 1852, *fourteen months* ago, which is as fluid, and in good keeping as when first prepared, and to all appearance is likely to continue so; this is as long, I presume, as it is desirable to keep any tincture which is not *improved* by age.

*Hydroferrocyanas Zinci.*—In making this preparation, according to the method of Schindler, as detailed by Dunglison, I found considerable difficulty in avoiding the blueish cast of the precipitate which is said to arise from the presence of iron in the sulphate of zinc used in the process. After repeated trials, and having ensured the absence of iron from the sulphate of zinc by submitting it to purification, finding the blueish appearance still, I concluded to complete the process, regardless of it, and found that it completely disappeared during the washing; from which circumstance I conceived the color to be owing to perhaps a little sulphate of iron, formed by the elements during their mutual decomposition, and which is dissolved out by the water. The knowledge of this may save other manipulators the loss of much time and material in the operation. Some care is necessary in drying the precipitate to avoid decomposition. By wrapping it in several folds of bibulous paper, and placing it in a temperature of 80° or 90°, it will proceed safely.

*Remarks on Compounding.*—The question of a "compounding department" remotely situated in stores, is treated of in Mohr and Redwood's Practical Pharmacy, and the decision is left to individual discretion. In my experience the reflection has occurred to me that the majority of "mistakes" which are made apart from want of knowledge, experience, or from negligence, are owing chiefly to the circumstance of the compounder's being exposed to the many distractions of attention, which occur in the open store, from the absurd and annoying questionings and discourse of customers. In banks, where the result of error would be comparatively trifling to that in the store of the apothecary, profound silence is observed in all operations and a complete separation of the employée from the visitor maintained. Why, then, where the result to be obtained is so much more important, are not the same precautions adopted by the apothecaries? It is my practice to avoid, as far as possible, short of rudeness, all conversation or other distractions of the attention while engaged in compounding, but as it is impossible to control the loquacity of many, the object would be much more effectually and less offensively accomplished by having a portion of the store set apart specially for the purpose; where the operative, though in view if necessary, would be, at least, beyond the conversation range of the over inquisitive. The very great nervousness and awkward, because unnecessary, perhaps, impracticable explanation which any little oversight or inadvertence give rise to, would be obviated and the main objection which might be urged against the regulation, that the compounder would be deprived of accuracy compelling superintendence of the looker on, is absurd, as this very assumption of superintendence on the part of a customer, is, in itself, mischievous and very desirable to be avoided.

# QUININE AND QUINIDINE.

## REMARKS MADE BY M. O. HENRY, IN THE ACADEMIE DE MEDICINE.

When MM. Pelletier and Caventou obtained quinine from the bark of the cinchona Calisaya, it was easy to foresee the importance of that beautiful discovery. I was sufficiently fortunate, some months afterwards, to aid in its application, by proposing a quick and easy process by which the febrifuge principle of cinchona could be obtained in large quantity. From that time, in fact, its employment became general. Soon every pharmacien prepared quinine and its salts; soon, too, manufactories arose, in which that interesting organic base was extracted on a large scale. We may assert, without fear of contradiction, that for a long time this branch of industry, entirely French in its origin, remained a monopoly of our country, and rendered foreigners tributary to us for this product of the cinchona.

Since, there have arisen in England, Germany, Holland, and the United States, many new manufactories of quinine, and in consequence of this rivalry, as well as of the monopoly of the Calisaya bark, established in Bolivia by an English and Bolivian company, the bark with us has become scarcer, or of a higher price; we may even hear some day of a dearth in the supply of cinchona for our own manufactories. It becomes important, then, not only for the interests of the French manufacturer, but above all, for the necessities of the healing art, to guard against such a danger, and to prevent the bark becoming of a price so high that it would not be within the reach of all classes of society. In consequence, persuaded that quinine, whether extracted from this or that species of cinchona, is identical in a state of purity, we have sought to replace for its extraction, the true Calisaya, by the bark of other species of cinchona esteemed inferior, and therefore of less commercial value. Thus, after having submitted the barks of Peru, o

New Grenada and of Columbia, to diversified and carefully repeated trials, we have obtained, setting aside the cinchonine, which has been perhaps unjustly proscribed, beautiful and perfectly crystallized sulphate of quinine. This has been employed successfully in medicine, and in large proportion, both in the service of the military and in that of the civil hospitals.

We believed then that we had a right to congratulate ourselves on having rendered good service to mankind, in guarding thus against the eventuality of the failure of the Calisaya bark, when fifteen or sixteen months ago, it was announced in England and Germany, that the cinchona barks derived from the sources we have just mentioned, that is to say, from latitudes north of those from which we derive the true Calisaya, do not furnish a pure sulphate of quinine; that they contained a different alkaloid, to which the name of quinidine was given, and that it was consequently necessary to proscribe both such sulphate and the barks from which it was obtained.

It is this proscription that we contend against, in openly defending the cause of the French manufacture of quinine. It is not to give currency to our own products, which might be thought to be mixed with quinidine; for in order to meet the actual exigency, we have been careful to free our quinine, not only from cinchonine, but also from that so-called new substance, when by accident it has been present.

It is a matter of indifference, then, that foreign manufacturers denounce this pretended new organic base, since their attacks do not affect us. But we believe that for the general good, and for the cause of truth, we should not maintain silence; and we protest loudly, repeating that quinidine is nothing but hydrated quinine, or a particular state of crystallization of that alkaloid. What, in fact, is quinidine? The same substance that we discovered twenty years ago, as a product of pure Calisaya bark. In comparing what we published in 1833 and 1834 on that subject with what the English and German chemists have lately written, it will be seen that there is scarcely any difference. All reduces itself to this: quinidine is a hydrate of quinine, containing 2 equivalents of water instead of 3·3, and it differs only in being a little less soluble in sulphuric ether.

In other respects, the same atomic weight, the same elementary composition, the same state of saturation with acids; salts similar in their proportions, etc. Now this quinidine, given up as a new substance twenty years ago, has ever since continued to form part of the quinine of commerce, since it is furnished by the cinchona Calisaya itself. Have any disadvantages been known to follow its employment? Let us add, if the cinchonas termed of inferior value, appear according to the German manufacturers richer in this modified crystallization, in reality it is only the red bark of New Grenada which furnishes it to a marked extent, together with primitive cinchonine and quinidine. The other varieties produce scarcely any of it. We will not, however, stop to discuss this point, but confine ourselves to present the following propositions as conclusions:

1st. It is doubtful whether cinchonine really merits the disfavor in which it is held in comparison with quinine.

2d. Perfectly pure sulphate of quinine can be obtained from a great number of cinchona barks besides that of Calisaya.

3d. The employment of these barks puts the manufacture of that precious medicine on a sure foundation, and obviates the disadvantages arising from its scarcity, and consequently its advanced price.

4th. the substance termed quinidine, which is only a different form of crystallization from quinine, appears to exist in all the cinchona barks, more particularly in that of the red cinchona of New Grenada. It is quinine in a state of hydrate, and the same substance which was discovered twenty years previously, and described under that name.

5th. There are no serious grounds for proscribing the barks of a kind esteemed inferior; doing so, we serve less the interests of truth than the commercial speculations of foreign manufacturers, and we lead France, the creator of the manufacture of quinine, to see herself some day a tributary for that product, one of the greatest benefits of organic chemistry.

After the discussion in which MM. Soubeiran, Guibourt, Bouchardat, H., Gautier de Claubry and Henry took part, and from which there resulted on one hand that the question of the identity, or the difference between quinine and quinidine, is not yet settled by chemists; and on the other that clinical experience has not yet determined the therapeutic value of the barks containing quinidine, the question at the desire of M. O. Henry himself, was referred to the committee on the substitutes for quinine.—*L' Union Medicale, Nov.* '52

---

## POPULINE.

Piria has made some magnificent researches upon populine, the crystalline principle discovered by Braconnot, together with salicine, in the bark and leaves of several species of poplar (Populus tremula, P. alba and P. græca.) By studying the products of its decomposition, he has been led to the conclusion that populine is a combination of *benzoic acid*, *grape sugar* and *saligenine*; thus, $C^{40} H^{22} O^{16}$, 4HO (populine)=$C^{14} H O^{4}$+$C^{12} H^{12} O^{12}$+$C^{14} H^{8} O^{4}$ (saligenine). When populine is acted upon by sulphuric acid and bichromate of potash, hydruret of salicyle is formed in large quantity, just as when saligenine is acted upon by the same agents. When it is boiled with nitric acid, trinitro-phenie (nitro-picria) acid is formed, (just as by the action of nitric acid upon saligenine,) together with oxalic acid (from the sugar.) Finally, when acted upon by dilute acids, populine is actually broken up into benzoic acid, grape sugar, and *saliretine*, which latter substance, according to previous researches of Piria, is a product of the action of dilute acids upon *saligenine*. Anhydrous populine may also be more naturally considered as a combination of benzoic acid with salicine, *minus* two equivalents of water, $C^{4}$ $H^{22}$ $O^{16}$=$C^{14}$ $H^{6}$ O +$C^{26}$ $H^{18}$ $O^{14}$—2HO. For when boiled with baryta-water, there are actually formed benzoate of baryta and salicine. Salicine so prepared perfectly resembled natural salicine in its mode of decomposition under the influence of acids and of synaptase, and gave the same composition on analysis. Piria proposes for populine the name *benzo-salicine.* He has formed, by dissolving populine in nitric acid, a substance which bears the same relation to *helicine* that populine does to salicine, and which he calls *benzo-helicine.* Benzo-helicine may be converted into helicine by boiling with magnesia, which takes up the benzoic acid, and leaves the helicine.—(*Comptes Rendus*, xxxiv. 138.)

The above notice, although at first sight the subject may appear too purely chemical, seems to be worthy of the attention of pharmaceutists in several points of view. The study of the therapeutical relations of populine, of which little or nothing is now known, is invested by these beautiful and surprising discoveries, with great interest. If the salicine obtained by Piria from populine, should prove, as there is little reason to doubt, to be therapeutically, as well as chemically, identical with natural salicine, this indication of a new source of a remedy already so important, and continually becoming more so, is certainly worthy of consideration, and the new source of benzoic acid, at the same time developed, must not be undervalued. In the meantime, these results add new links to the gradually strengthening chain of evidence, which forbids us to despair of the ultimate production of the costly medicinal alkaloids by artificial transformations of cheap organic substances.

H. W.

## FALSE RATHANIA ROOT.

The only important falsification of rathania root hitherto recorded in Germany, has been so satisfactorily described by Martiny, (*Archiv. de. Pharm.* 50, 57,) that there is no difficulty in distinguishing it from the true article; but Prof. Mettenheimer has now described a false rathania root which is not so easily distinguished. Its derivation is wholly unknown to him. He describes it as follows: main stem ½ inch thick, 4 inches long, knotty, with branches 4½ inches long. It consists, however, chiefly of branches separated from the candex, which are nearly half an inch thick. The candex has, indeed, some similarity with that of the true rathania, but it may be distinguished by the branches, which are smoother, show some degree of lustre, and have more abundant and deeper diagonal cracks, which sometimes cut entirely through the bark all around. Wart-formed excrescences are found upon the stem and branches more plentifully, and the branches are still more curved and undulated in their form than in the true root. It is not so tough, breaks easier, and with very short splinters, and, seen in mass, appears of a dirty violet reddish brown color. The bark is thicker, being upon many branches of a thickness of 1½ line, and adheres partly to the wood. Upon the outside the bark is of a dirty dark brownish red color, and granular fracture; upon the inside, lighter in color, fibrous, and a section made with a sharp knife exhibits some lustre. The woody centre is of a dark reddish color, hard, breaking with short splinters, and a section made with a sharp knife is dull, and without the dark central point which occurs so frequently in the true root. The false root is inodorous, and has a stronger astringent taste than the true. Its decoction in eight parts of water is, like that of Martiny's false root, dark reddish brown, and opaque, while that of the true root is light brownish red, and transparent. Mettenheimer has investigated the effects produced upon the diluted decoction by numerous reagents, and the most important reactions are here selected, and compared with the reactions of Martiny's root, and of the true root, the latter being indicated by (1,) Mettenheimer's false root by (2,) and Martiny's spurious article by (3.) Sulphate of copper solution gives with (1) a slight cloudiness, with (2) a dirty dark reddish precipitate, and with (3) a strong cloudiness. Acetate of lead solution with (1) and (2) a flesh colored precipitate, but with (3) a strong dirty dark reddish brown precipitate. Iodide of potassium, with (1) and (3) no change, but with (2) a feeble cloudiness. Chloride of barium, with (1) a feeble cloudiness, but with (2) and (3) a precipitate. Sulphuric acid, with (1) a slight cloudiness, but with (2) and (3) a flocky dirty red precipitate. Oxalate of ammonia, with (1) no change, but with (2) and (3) a strong precipitate.—*Jarhbuch fur prakt Pharm.* xxiii. 193.

---

## CARBONATE OF MANGANESE.

Laming gives results of observations upon the preparation of carbonate of manganese, which are important to pharmceutists. He asserts that by precipitation of a solution of a salt of protoxyd of manganese by carbonate of potash or soda, taking care not to add any excess of the latter, a perfectly neutral carbonate of protoxyd of manganese is obtained, which undergoes no alteration on exposure to the air. If an excess of alkaline carbonate is added, he states that sesquicarbonate or bicarbonate of alkali is formed, and, as a necessary consequence, the precipitate contains in admixture, hydrate of protoxyd of manganese, which becomes brown in the air by oxydation. Carbonate of ammonia, on the contrary, and even caustic ammonia, do not decompose carbonate of manganese. So that a pure product may also be obtained by precipitation with carbonate of ammonia. Also, the precipitates formed by bicarbonates of the alkalies remain unchanged in the air. On decomposition of the pure carbonate by heat, black oxyde is formed, according to Laming, without previous formation of any of the intermediate oxydes.—*Jour. de Chim. Medicale*, 3 *ser*. vii. 706.

---

## MANUFACTURE OF ILLUMINATING GAS FROM WOOD.

Pettenkofer showed, two years ago, by experiments at the convention of the Polytechnic Association of Bavaria, that a considerable quantity of illuminating gas could be obtained from 4 loth (about 2 oz.) of wood. The practicability of manufacturing gas in this way, on a large scale, has since received much attention. Pettenkofer has already introduced his process in Basel, (Basle) and is now negotiating at Zurich, Stockholm and Drontheim. The wood gas will probably be cheaper than coal gas, because it requires little or no purification, and the collateral products are charcoal, wood-tar, acetic acid, and other valuable substances. A commission appointed at Munich to examine Pettenkofer's gas, found it to possess a little greater illuminating power than the coal gas employed to light that city, the proportion being as 11 to 10. An estimate made upon this basis shows the cost of production of the wood gas at Munich to be much less than that of coal gas.—*Knop's Central-Blatt.* 1852, *Bd. I. pp.* 191 *and* 224.

## RESINIFICATION OF OIL OF JUNIPER.

Resinification of oil of juniper commences in the berry itself. Rebling, of Langensalza, has observed, that when fresh juniper berries are cut open, the oil, which is contained in from 6 to 9 colorless, egg-formed receptacles, flows out wholly fluid, but in older berries, is found partially, and in very old berries, wholly resinified. This accounts for the different proportions of oil given by the distillation of berries of different ages.—*Archiv. der Pharmacie*, 2 R. lxvii, 288.

---

## PROCESS FOR THE PREPARATION OF FERROTARTRATE OF POTASSA IN BRACTEÆ.

BY MM. CORNELIS AND GILLE.

Ferrotartrate of potassa is a salt which has occupied the attention of many pharmaceutists; but most have been stopped in their researches by the variation of the product obtained and by the difficulty of constantly obtaining fine bracteæ of perfect solubility. After various and numerous experiments, we have at length arrived at producing regularly bracteæ of a fine deep red, completely soluble in water. We, therefore, publish the process which we have followed, and which has given us such beautiful results:

| | Grammes. |
|---|---|
| Pure crystallized sulphate of iron | 1,000 |
| Sulphuric acid at 66 degrees | 200 |
| Water | 4,000 |

The sulphate is dissolved in the water, the sulphuric acid is mixed with it, and the whole is carried to ebullition in a porcelain or stone-ware capsule. Nitric acid is afterwards added until no more nitrous vapor is produced. When the disengagement has ceased, the liquid is diluted with 10 or 15 times its weight of water, and a sufficient quantity of ammonia, diluted with about 25 times its bulk of water, is poured in. The precipitated hydrate is washed until the washing water becomes perfectly colorless and insipid; it is collected on a cloth, and it is allowed to drain until it is under the form of a jelly. The latter is put into a stone-ware or porcelain vessel, with 680 grammes of bitartrate of potassa. After being carefully mixed, it is heated on a sand bath, at a temperature of 140 to 158° F., until completely dissolved; the liquor is afterwards left to repose, and is then decanted into a vessel in which it is allowed to cool. It sometimes happens that, by cooling, the liquor assumes the form of a reddish yellow mass, and constitutes a precipitate insoluble in water. This phenomenon is due to an excess of cream of tartar; when it occurs, hydrate of potassa is gradually added to the precipitate until it has become entirely soluble. The liquor is filtered, evaporated at a temperature of 122° to 140° F. on plates to the consistence of honey, and it is spread with a brush, in thin layers, on glass plates placed horizontally, in order that the liquor may be spread very uniformly.

In this preparation the hydrate of potassa might be replaced by ammonia; but this alkali presents an inconvenience which is not met with when the hydrate of potassa is employed. Thus, when ammonia is added to the precipitate produced by the cream of tartar in excess, and when it is afterwards heated to a rather high temperature, the ammonia volatilises and the ferrotartrate of potassa again becomes insoluble.—*Journal de Pharmacie*, October, 1852.

# ON THE OCCURRENCE OF BERBERINE IN THE COLUMBA WOOD OF CEYLON, THE MENISPERMUM [COSCINIUM] FENESTRATUM OF BOTANISTS.

BY JAMES D. PERRINS, ESQ.

The following investigation was made in the chemical laboratory of St. Bartholomew's Hospital, under the immediate supervision of Dr. John Stenhouse. Dr. Stenhouse having had for some time past a quantity of wood of the *Menispermum fenestratum* in his possession, suggested to me this investigation. I am anxious, therefore, to acknowledge my obligation to him, not only for the material, but also for several valuable suggestions in the course of the inquiry.

Hitherto the chief source of the alkaloid berberine has been the root of the barbery, *Berberis vulgaris*. Bodeker, however, about four years ago, ascertained its existence in the columba root of pharmacy, the *Cocculus palmatus*, where it occurs in small quantity associated with columbine.

The following remark is made in the *Chemical Gazette* for 1849, vol. vii., p. 150:—

"The occurrence of berberine in *Berberis* and *Cocculus* is remarkable in a physiological point of view. Bartling places both of these families, the Menispermeæ and Berberideæ, in the class of the Cocculinæ, which is in accordance with the fact of both containing the same principle.

As berberine has now also been found in another of the Menispermeæ, the accuracy of Bartling's view seems to be greatly confirmed.

The following was the process adopted for the extraction of berberine from the *Menispermum fenestratum*. A quantity of the wood, which had a bright yellow color resembling that of quercitron, was rasped, and then treated with successive portions of boiling water till it had become nearly tasteless. The aqueous decoction acquired a deep yellow color and an intensely bitter taste. It was next evaporated carefully to the consistence of an extract, then introduced into a flask and boiled with ten or twelve times its bulk of rectified spirit of wine, filtered while hot, and the residue boiled with a further quantity of spirits, which dissolved the berberine, and also a quantity of resinous matter by which it was accompanied. The alcoholic solution was then introduced into a retort, and the spirit carefully distilled off, until the residue on agitation appeared to have nearly the consistence of oil of vitriol. It was then set aside in an open vessel, and in the course of twenty-four hours the liquid became filled with a mass of impure crystals.

After draining off the mother-liquor, these crystals were washed with a small quantity of cold spirit redissolved in boiling alcohol, and set aside to crystallize. Their complete purification was attempted by repeated crystallizations. It was found, however, that a small quantity of resinous matter adhered obstinately to the cryatals, causing them to remain of a brownish-yellow color. This brownish tint was ultimately entirely removed by solution in spirit of wine and digestion with a little purified animal charcoal, the pure berberine crystallizing from the solution in beautiful bright yellow needles. The crystals were found to contain nitrogen, and their behaviour with various reagents corresponded exactly with those of berberine.

As these crystals were very soluble in boiling water, a quantity of them was dissolved in that menstruum; and on the addition of the requisite amount of hydrochloric acid, a crystalline precipitate was immediately obtained in the form of long, slender, golden-colored needles, of a fine silky lustre.

This salt was dried in a water-bath at 212° F., and subjected to analysis with the following results:—

6·25 grs. ignited with chromate of lead, gave 14·398 grs. of carbonic acid and 3·2 grs. of water.

The nitrogen was determined by Wills's method. 8·18 grs. of salt gave 4·94 grs. of the double chloride of platinum and ammonium.

The chlorine was determined as chloride of silver. 3·59 grs. gave 13·5 of chloride of silver.

HYDROCHLORATE OF BERBERINE.

| | Calculated numbers. | | Found numbers. |
|---|---|---|---|
| 42 equivs. Carbon........ | 3150.. | 62·75 ........ | 62·79 |
| 20 equivs. Hydrogen...... | 250.. | 4·98 ........ | 5·67 |
| 1 equiv. Nitrogen....... | 177.. | 3·53 ........ | 3·78 |
| 1 equiv. Chlorine........ | 442.. | 8·85 ........ | 9·02 |
| 10 equivs. Oxygen........ | 1000.. | 19·90 ........ | |
| | 5019 | 100·00 | |

These results correspond pretty closely with the formula of hydrochlorate of berberine, which, when dried at 212° F., contains one equiv. of water, and is consequently $C^{42}H^{18}NO^{9}$, $HCl+HO$.

The hydrogen in this determination is considerably too high, which, however, is easily accounted for, as the hydrochlorate of berberine, after being dried in the water bath, is eminently hygroscopic, and consequently absorbs moisture rapidly, while being mixed with the chromate of lead. This observation has already been made by Fleitmann, who, while analysing this salt, obtained an equally great excess of hydrogen.

A quantity of the double platinum salt was also prepared by mixing a solution of the hydrochlorate of berberine with one of chloride of platinum. The compound obtained corresponded precisely in its appearance and properties with the salt prepared in the same way by Fleitmann.

2·80 grs. of salt gave 0·49 gr. of platinum=17·5 per cent. the calculated quantity being 17·55 per cent.

A small quantity of the acid chromate of berberine was also prepared by adding a solution of bichromate of potash to one of hydrochlorate of berberine. The salt which precipitated likewise perfectly agreed in its properties with the acid chromate examined by Fleitmann.

The results of these analyses and reactions leave no doubt as to the identity of the alkaloid, and also serve to corroborate the correctness of Fleitmann's formula for berberine, which I briefly subjoin:

Berberine crystallized at the ordinary temperature, $C^{42}H^{18}NO^{9}+12HO$.

Berberine dried at 212° F., $C^{42}H^{18}NO^{9}+2HO$.

The hydrochlorate dried at 212° F., $C^{42}H^{18}NO^{9}+HCl+HO$.

Double chloride of berberine and platinum, $C^{42}H^{18}NO^{9}+HCl+PtCl^{2}$.

The *Menispermum fenestratum* is, according to Ainslie, a large tree, which is very common in Ceylon, and an infusion of which has long been employed by the Cingalese as a valuable tonic bitter.

Gray, in his *Supplement* to the Pharmacopœia, informs us that this tree is known to the Cingalese by the names of Woniwol and Bangwellzetta.

Berberine may easily be obtained in very considerable quantity from columba wood, the whole of which it pervades, and of which it is the coloring principle; and if, as I suspect, the resinous matter accompanying it consists chiefly of altered berberine, improved methods of extraction, such, for instance, as the employment of a vacuum pan apparatus, would in all probability still further augment the amount of product.

I am informed that berberine is employed as a remedial agent on the continent, but its scarcity seems hitherto to have prevented its introduction into the medical practice of this country. As a good source for it has now been pointed out, it may be expected that berberine will take its place with the other alkaloids in our materia medica.

To prevent misconception from the similarity of names, it may, perhaps, be well to remark, that berberine and berbeerine are very different substances; the latter being the active principle of the bark of the bebeeree tree of Guaiana, and as yet has not been obtained in a crystalline form.—*Phil. Mag.*, Aug.

*St. Bartholomew's Hospital,*

*July* 20, 1852.

# ON THE MICROSCOPE AS A MEANS OF DETECTING THE ADMIXTURE OR ADULTERATION OF DRUGS.

"You are doubtless conversant with the recent very extensive employment of the microscope for disclosing the adulteration of food. No less useful—no less powerful is it in disclosing the contamination of drugs; and I cannot too strenuously recommend you to employ it." Such was the language used by Dr. Pereira, in his introductory lecture on Materia Medica, delivered this year at the Pharmaceutical Society.

Many persons of no mean skill in chemistry, smiled incredulously at the results obtained, when they ascertained that the principal instrument employed by Dr. Hassal, the *Lancet* commissioner, in detecting the adulteration of substances used as food, was the microscope. We confess that we entertained considerable doubt as to the accuracy of the extraordinary revelations that he gave, confidently, to the public in the pages of the *Lancet.* Every person conversant with chemistry was well aware what a useful adjunct the microscope has been to the chemical analyst, in distinguishing the form of minute crystals, and thereby determining their true character, when mixed with organic or inorganic bodies; but few foresaw that it might be employed as a means of analysis itself, in mixtures of organized substances.

In fact, in physiological chemistry, the microscope is preferred to every other resource as a means to detect the presence of minute quantities of organic crystalline compounds in the complex fluids secreted by animals.

Dr. C. G. Lehmann, a very high authority, observes, when speaking of the tests for the detection of urea, that the best method to ascertain its presence, is by the formation of its salts with nitric and oxalic acids, and to submit the salts so formed, when crystallised by the evaporation of their menstruum, to microscopic examination, and thus to a scertain the correct shape of the crystals, "of which, if the investigation is to be unquestionable, the acute angles must be always measured;" for, as he farther remarks, that "a good crystallometric determination yields the same certainty as an elementary analysis, which, in these cases, would never or extremely seldom be possible."* These evidences of the value of the microscope as a means of testing by the physical characteristics of a crystalline substance, might be multiplied almost innumerably from the same and other authorities.

However extraordinary the statement may appear, that Dr. Lehmann and others prefer the microscope as the agent by which the composition, or some of the ingredients, of a complex body are to be determined, when those ingredients are crystalline, the results of the investigations of Drs. Hassal and Pereira, and Mr. Quekett, are yet more remarkable and worthy of attention; for they prove that the microscope is the only, or at least the only good means which science has at present discovered to detect the admixture or adulteration of non-crystalline organic substances.

Dr. Pereira first impressed on the attention of pharmaceutists the value of this instrument for discriminating between the numerous varieties of starch which are offered to the public for domestic purposes, under an equal variety of names; but it remained for Dr. Hassal to show its unlimited valuable applications.

The conclusions that may be drawn from the *Lancet* commis-missioner's laborious researches are, that the solid portions of all organized structures present to the eye, when aided by the microscope, such distinguishing characteristics, that, by an experienced observer, they can be referred to their respective origins; and that when even these portions are in a state of minute subdivision, the form of the cells, the shape of the starch granules, and the condition of the spiral vessels, and other indications, afford an equally accurate result.

To assert that Dr. Hassal has never arrived at an erroneous conclusion in his investigations, would be to ascribe to him something more than human; but to state that his results are sur-

* Lehmann's Physiological Chemistry, vol. i. pp. 150 and 160.

prisingly accurate, would be within the limits of truth; to which statement even the victims, as no doubt they consider themselves, of his indefatigable and ruthless microscopic skill, have repeatedly borne testimony.

As this paper is written for the student, and not for the initiated in these matters, we shall here briefly indicate the method by which skill, when aided by perseverance, may be acquired in detecting the adulteration of drugs, by microscopical observation. It is unnecessary to describe the construction of the microscope, as it is an instrument that most persons are familiar with, and a description of it may be found in many standard works; but it may be observed that the instrument necessary for this purpose should possess a magnifying power from 200 to 400 diameters.

We shall assume, to illustrate the method, that a sample of suspected powdered rhubarb has been taken for examination; but before the investigator can pronounce an opinion, or form a judgment of the suspected sample, it is necessary that he should be well acquainted with the characteristics of powdered rhubarb of authenticated genuineness, which he can readily prepare for himself.

It is by a comparative examination of the genuine and the adulterated article under the microscope, that the presence of foreign substances in the adulterated powder, can be distinguished; because, as previously stated, the form of the starch granules, the shape of the cells of each organic substance, have a character peculiar to themselves, by which their source may be determined.

By a similar process the question can be answered, when it is thus ascertained that a drug has been adulterated—by what substance or substances has this drug been contaminated?

The investigator will know, from previous experience, those materials which are most suitable for the sophistication of the genuine article, and by rendering himself familiar with their appearances in a pulverized state, when viewed by the microscope, he will readily detect their presence in the adulterated powder, and be able to refer them to their origin. But in this instance, and all others, he must learn the microscopical characteristics of any substance whose detection is desirable, from specimens, the genuineness of which he can vouch for.

To avoid a constant repetition of the examination of every substance whose microscopical characteristics it may be desirable to be acquainted with, and which are difficult to commit to memory, it will be advisable, for the purpose of reference, to obtain drawings of them, which is most readily and perfectly accomplished by the aid of the camera lucida.

Moreover it should be borne in mind, that the microscope can never supplant chemical analysis in detecting the admixture or adulteration of such drugs as opium, scammony, and others, which are the concrete juices or exudations of plants; but for powders of barks, roots, leaves, and such organized substances as consist of cellular tissue, ligneous fibre, &c., it is in the highest degree superior to every other known or available means for the discovery of their sophistication.

In conclusion, it may be remarked that, although investigations by the aid of the microscope require less time for their performance, and certainly not greater ability for the acquirement of the necessary skill, than chemical analyses, yet no one can expect to be *au fait* in the application of this instrument for the purposes described, except by the devotion of much time and attention to its study.—*Annals of Pharmacy, Jan.* 1852.

---

## FACTS AND DISCOVERIES IN SCIENCE.

*Iodine in Plants.*—M. A. Chatin has arrived at the following conclusions, from an extensive series of experiments on this subject:

1. That the proportion of iodine present in plants is gener-

ally independent of their nature, but closely connected with the localities in which they are to be found growing. Thus, the *Confervæ*, the *Nymphæa*, the *Ranunculi*, the *Patamogetans*, and the varieties of cresses, contain much more iodine in running streams, than when they are growing in marshy places.

2. That the iodine is present in the juice or sap of the plants as an alkaline iodide, and altogether uncombined with the tissue of which the plant is composed.

3. That iodine is not universally present in terrestrial plants, but that it exists, in more or less abundance, in all aquatic plants.

4. That in aquatic plants, those that are growing in stagnant waters are found to contain far less iodine than those that are growing in running streams.

5. That in such collections of water as are large enough to be strongly moved by the action of the winds, the plants growing therein contain much more iodine than those growing in waters at all times stagnant, and not agitated on their surface.

*Chlorinated Merino; a Test for ascertaining the Presence of Sugar in Liquids.*—Strips of white merino, after being soaked three or four minutes in an aqueous solution of bichloride of tin, made with 100 parts of the bichloride of tin and 200 parts of water, and subsequently carefully dried, are convenient as a test for this purpose. By employing this chlorinated merino, the physician is able, without the least trouble, to ascertain whether the urine, or other fluid contains any trace whatever of sugar in it. All that is required is to drop a very little of the urine, or fluid to be tested, on a strip of the chlorinated merino, and to hold it over the flame of a spirit-lamp, when, if any sugar be present, a very distinct black spot will be produced.

M. Maumene, to whom we are indebted for this reagent, says that it is a most delicate test. Ten or a dozen drops of diabetic urine, containing sugar, mixed with a large quantity of water, will produce a dark brown stain, on the introduction of a strip of this prepared test; whereas healthy urine, urea, and lithic acid, are not thus discolored by the addition of chloride of tin.

*Preparation of Atropia by means of Chloroform.*—M. Rabourdin recommends the following process for the preparation of atropia, the active principle of the *Atropa belladonna*:—

Take fresh belladonna, as soon as it begins to flower, bruise it in a marble mortar, and press out the juice, which is to be heated so as to coagulate the albumen. When the juice thus clarified is cold, add to every litre four grammes of caustic potash, and thirty grammes of chloroform; the mixture is then to be shaken for a minute or two, and suffered to stand. In half an hour, the chloroform, holding the atropia, is deposited, having the appearance of a greenish oil. The supernatant liquor is then to be poured off, and replaced by a little water. This is afterwards poured off, and the washing is to be continued till the water comes away quite clear. The chloroform solution is then to be put into a small tubulated retort, and distilled in a water-bath, until all the chloroform has passed into the receiver. The residue in the retort is to be heated with a little water, acidified with sulphuric acid, which dissolves the atropia, and leaves a green resinoid matter; the filtered solution is colorless. To obtain the atropia in a pure state, it is only requisite to pour into the acid solution a slight excess of solution of carbonate of potash, and to dissolve the precipitate in rectified alcohol. This solution yields, by spontaneous evaporation, fine groups of acicular crystals of atropia. M. Rabourdin supposes, that this mode of operating with the *Atropa belladonna* may be applied to many other substances containing vegetable alkalies, as the cinchonas and other plants.

*Nitro-mercurial Test for Albumen and other Protein Compounds.*—The nitro-mercurial solution of M. Millon is prepared by adding to the metal mercury, an equal weight of nitric acid, containing four and a half equivalents of water. This mixture is to be gently heated until the metal is completely dissolved, when two volumes of water are to be added to one volume of the nitro-mercurial solution. After standing some time, the clear liquid is to be poured off. This acid solution of mercury, M. Millon says, is a very delicate test for all albuminoid substances, as well as for many secondary products connected with it. It imparts a deep red color to such substances, and by its application as a reagent, the ten-thousandth part, or even less, of albumen may be detected. He affirms that cotton, various kinds of starch, and gum-arabic, assume a very distinct rose tint when brought into contact with it. The urine is almost immediately rendered of a rose-red color. The albumen of the blood, and of vegetables, fibrine, casein, gluten, legumin, silk, wool, feathers, horn, the epidermis, gelatine, chondrine, protein, the cornea of the eye, &c., are all rendered more or less red by the application of this test.

*Ballota Lanata.*— This plant has been highly extolled by Professor Brera as a diuretic. It is indigenous in that part of Siberia adjoining China. It is collected at the time of flowering, and brought by the Russians to market in bales covered with fur. The whole of the plant is useful in medicine. It has a smell very much resembling that of tea, whilst its taste is slightly pungent and bitter. The infusion of the plant is of a pale greenish-yellow. The tincture made with weak spirit contains all the active properties of the plant. Decoction is said to be the most efficient form in which this medicine can be administered. This preparation is directed to be made by boiling in an unglazed vessel, for a quarter of an hour, half an ounce of the plant, in as much water as, when strained, shall amount to eight fluid ounces; and this quantity is considered as four doses, which may be taken during twenty-four hours.

To show the very high opinion Professor Brera entertains of this drug, he remarks, that "the *Ballota lanata* is the most efficacious plant to supply the blood with what is required to relieve it from all morbid supersaturation, and to prevent its reproduction."

*Cainca.*—The diuretic properties of this plant have been long known in the Brazils, and some other parts of South America; but it was first made known to European practitioners by one of the Russian consuls, stationed at Rio Janeiro. It is the *Chiococca racemosa*, in the Linnæan and of the family *Rubiacœa*, in the Jussieuan systems of botany. The root of the plant consists in a great part of a delicate cortical portion, enclosing a woody centre; but it is in the cortical portion only that the medicinal properties of the plant reside. This has a slightly bitter, pungent, and astringent taste, and breaks with a resinous fracture. The root, or rather the cortical part of it, possesses remarkable tonic properties, whilst it is, at the same time, slightly purgative, and powerfully diuretic. It is usually administered in the form of decoction, prepared by boiling a drachm of the root in a pint of water, which may be taken in the course of twenty-four hours.

*Seeds of Phellandrium Aquaticum.*—Dr. Recamier, of Paris, recently deceased, physician to his late Majesty, Louis Philippe, and other medical authorities, have recommended and employed these seeds extensively in various kinds of pulmonary affections, particularly in that form of chronic bronchitis which so frequently attacks the aged in cold, damp weather, and which causes them so much annoyance, and sometimes so much suffering, until the weather undergoes a change. These seeds may be administered twice a day, either in the state of powder, or in the form of syrup, of which latter from two to four spoonfuls may be taken during the day, and continued for some few weeks, until relief is obtained. The powder is usually given to the patient mixed with a little sugar.—*Annals of Pharmacy, December*, 1852. C.

---

## ARTIFICIAL FRUIT ESSENCES.

BY FEHLING.

*Pine-apple Oil* is a solution of one part of butyric ether, in eight or ten parts of alcohol. For the preparation of this ether, pure butyric acid must be first obtained by the fermentation of sugar, according to the method of Bensch*. One pound of this acid is dissolved in one pound of strong alcohol, and mixed with from a quarter to half an ounce of sulphuric acid; the mixture is heated for some minutes, whereby the butyric ether separates as a light stratum. The whole is mixed with half its volume of water, and the upper stratum then removed; the heavy fluid is distilled, by which more butyric ether is obtained. The distillate and the removed oily liquid are shaken with a little water, the lighter portion of the liquid removed, which at last, by being shaken with water and a little soda, is freed from adhering acid.

For the preparation of the essence of pine-apple, one pound of this ether is dissolved in 8 or 10 pounds of alcohol. 20 or 25 drops of this solution is sufficient to give, to one pound of sugar, a strong taste of pine-apple, if a little citric or tartaric acid has been added.

*Pear Oil.*—This is an alcoholic solution of acetate of amyloxide and acetate of ethyloxide. For its preparation, one pound of glacial acetic acid is added to an equal weight of fusel oil (which has been prepared by being washed with soda and water, and then distilled at a temperature between 254° and 284° Fahr.), and mixed with half a pound of sulphuric acid. The mixture is digested for some hours at a temperature of 254°, by which means acetate of amyloxide separates, particularly on the addition of some water. The crude acetate of amyloxide obtained by separation, and by the distillation of the liquid to which the water has been added, is finally purified by being washed with soda and water. 15 parts of acetate of amyloxide are dissolved with half a part of acetic ether in 100 or 120 parts of alcohol. This is the essence of pear, which, when employed to flavor sugar, to which a little citric or tartaric acid has been added, affords the odour of bergamot pears, and a fruity, refreshing taste.

*Apple Oil* is an alcoholic solution of valerianate of amolyxide.

*See this journal, No. 2, p. 13.—*Editors of " The Annals."*

It is obtained impure, as a by-product, when, for the preparation of valerianic acid, fusel oil is distilled with bichromate of potash and sulphuric acid. It is better prepared in the following manner:—For the preparation of valerianic acid, 1 part of fusel oil is mixed gradually with three parts of sulphuric acid, and 2 parts of water added. A solution of 2¼ parts of bichromate of potash, with 4½ parts of water, is heated in a tubulated retort, and into this fluid the former mixture is gradually poured, so that the ebullition is not too rapid. The distillate is saturated with carbonate of soda, and warmed, when a solution of 3 parts of crystallized carbonate of soda, 2 parts of strong sulphuric acid, diluted with an equal quantity of water, are added. The valerianic acid separates as an oily stratum.

One part, by weight, of pure fusel oil, is carefully mixed with an equal weight of sulphuric acid. The cold solution is added to 1¼ parts of the above valerianic acid; the mixture is warmed for some minutes (not too long or too much) in a water-bath, and then mixed with a little water, by which means the impure valerianate of amyloxide separates, which is washed with water and carbonate of soda. For use as a essenc e of apples, one part of this valerianate of amyloxide is dissolved in 6 or 8 parts of alcohol.—*Annals of Pharmacy, Dec.*, 1852.

# EDITORIAL—VARIA.

QUINIDINE.—The new alkaloid of Winckler bids fair to become a fruitful source of controversy. In our last number, (p. 43) we extracted an article by Leers, a German chemist, on its chemical composition; in our present will be found a translation from *L'Union Medicale*, of some remarks made by M. Henry at the Academie de Medicine, of Paris. The statements of M. Henry derive great weight from his character and position, as well as from the extensive experience he has had upon the subject. They possess an especial interest here, from the bearing which they have upon the value, and consequently upon the admission into our ports of the Carthagena barks. They are, however, merely assertions, and must be received as such, while the counter-testimony of Leers, Winckler, Zimmer, &c., is of great weight. Whichever way it may be decided, we must not forget that there are two distinct questions to be solved: 1st. As to the existence of quinidine as a distinct principle, and its chemical composition and relations; and 2d. As to its therapeutic properties. The first is of much less importance to the physician and to the community than the second. No matter whether quinidine be or be not a distinct principle, if it produces the same effect on the human body as quinine, the bark in which it exists in so large a proportion must speedily rise in commercial value, and a new source will be opened for obtaining a remedy, the demand or which bids fair far to exceed the supply. Every advance made in bringing the new lands of the west and south-west under cultivation, every movement by which the travel through Central America is increased, causes an additional consumption of quinine, and the progress of civilization in India, in Algeria, in Central Africa, and South America, all have the same effect. The importance of the point at issue cannot then well be overrated, and we hope that the committee of the National Association, as we suggested on a previous occasion, will cause therapeutical experiments to be instituted, which will help to set it at rest.

AN ACT RELATING TO THE SALE OF DRUGS AND MEDICINES.— We would call the attention of our readers to the following act which has been introduced early in the present month, into the Assembly of our State, been reported on favorably by the Committee on Trade and Manufactures, and committed to the committee of the whole:—

"*The People of the State of New York, represented in Senate and Assembly, do enact as follows:*

SECTION 1. It shall not be lawful for any physician, druggist, apothecary or any person or persons engaged in preparing or manufacturing any medicine or compound, to be given or administered as a medicine, (except such medicines and compounds as are published in standard works of chemistry, materia medica or pharmacopœia,) to offer the same for sale, either himself or by his agent, without first filling in the office of the county clerk in the county where he resides, a receipt of the medicine, compound or nostrum, written or printed in the English language, stating the name of the drug or drugs, medicine or medicines or ingredients of which it is compounded, together with the proportions of each, with an affidavit attached, taken and subscribed before some officer who is by law authorised to take the acknowledgment of deeds, stating that the receipt to which said affidavit is attached is a true receipt of all the medicines and their proportions of which the said medicine or compound is composed.

§ 2. It shall not be lawful for any druggist, apothecary, or other person or persons, to sell or offer for sale any preparation, medicine or compound intended to be administered as a medicine, except such as are published in standard chemical or medical works as provided in the first section of this act, unless there shall be affixed or attached thereto in a conspicuous manner a receipt written or printed in the English language, stating the names of all the ingredients with their proportions of which said preparation or compound is composed, and signed by the maker or manufacturer in his own handwriting, or by a fac simile of his handwriting, and referring to the office where a true copy of said receipt, with an affidavit attached, is filed according to the first section of this act.

§ 3. The provisions of the first and second sections of this act shall not apply to the prescriptions of practicing physicians, nor to druggists or apothecaries in preparing the prescriptions of practicing physicians in the ordinary course of their business.

§ 4. Any person who shall counterfeit the handwriting or fac simile, as referred to in the second section of this act, shall be deemed guilty of felony, and on conviction thereof shall be punished according to law.

§ 5. Any person who shall make a false affidavit in relation to any such medicine or compound, shall be deemed guilty of perjury, and on conviction thereof shall be punished according to law.

§ 6. Any person or persons who shall violate the provisions of this act, shall be considered guilty of a misdemeanor, and on conviction thereof shall be fined for each offence a sum not less than ten dollars, nor more than one hundred dollars, or be imprisoned for a term not exceeding three months in a county jail.

§ 7. This act shall not take effect until the first day of January, eighteen hundred and fifty-four."

As will immediately be seen, the act is levelled at quack, or as they are termed, patent or proprietary medicines; its strict execution would, however, be calculated to give apothecaries some annoyance in the legitimate prosecution of their business. We doubt greatly, too, whether it would ever be effectually enforced, and our statute books are already sufficiently lumbered with laws which are a dead letter. Every man, learned or unlearned, with a diploma or without one, is permitted to practice medicine, and all, by the law, are placed upon a footing of equality. The same thing practically prevails with regard to apothecaries, for though a law, we believe, exists, regulating the sale of drugs and medicines, it is never enforced. The public, so far as its health is concerned, seems bent upon seeing where the doctrines of free trade will carry them, and we doubt therefore the wisdom, and question the success of any partial crusade against quack medicines.

Death of Dr. Pereira.— Late English papers announce the death of Dr. Jonathan Pereira, well known as the author of the Elements of Materia and Therapeutics, and of numerous contributions to Pharmacology. He died at his residence, in Finsbury-square, London, on the 21st of January last.

NEW YORK

# JOURNAL OF PHARMACY.

APRIL, 1853.

## GERMAN AND AMERICAN PHARMACY.

BY FERDINAND F. MAYER.

(*Continued.*)

WHEN we bear in mind the course of study just described, of the German Pharmaceutist, we might readily conclude that the State might entrust the direction of an apothecary's shop to a man thus educated with perfect confidence and security, without further supervision or precautionary regulations. Far from it; for now first commences a still stricter control, which consists in periodic inspections. These inspections, for the most part annual, are made by the district physicians, and at longer intervals by the so called Government physician (Regierungsarzt). These gentlemen are seldom familiar with the specialities of pharmacy, so that it is not easy for them to execute these inspections in a practical manner; this is easily conceived when it is understood that they should examine thoroughly some twelve chemical preparations. The inspection, for the most part, then, is a form; for example, they enquire whether the apothecary makes or purchases his preparations? The mercurial preparations, with the exception of the corrosive chloride and the red oxyde, he must prepare all himself, and so with the preparations of zinc, iron, silver, antimony, potash, soda, ammonia, &c. With regard to the organic alkaloids, the law is not so strict, yet it is preferred that even these should, at least in part, be prepared by the apothecary personally. For example, that he should purchase pure morphia, and prepare its various salts from it, &c. In short, it is the desire of the Government that the apothecary shall not be a mere dealer in drugs, but that he shall constantly employ himself in the manufacture and purification of compound medicines. In order to attain this end and render the supervision practicable, the apothecary is required to keep a record of his labors, in which he must state the number, mode of preparation, results and remarks upon his pharmaceutico-chemical labors. The official visitor looks *closely* to this "elaborations" book, in order to form an opinion of the diligence of the apothecary.

In a similar book he must enter all his purchases, and this book helps the visitor to draw conclusions as to the goodness of the drugs, as well from the prices which are paid for them as from the sources from which they are obtained, since a high price or a house of established reputation may be a better warrant for the goodness of an article than his own judgment.

I may here compare an occurrence which took place in Germany with the case which is related in this journal (Vol. 1, No. 11) under the head of "Accidental Substitution of Extract of Belladonna for Extract of Dandelion." In most States in Germany an apothecary would be severely censured who did not prepare all his extracts himself, not excepting the Extract of Rhatany. In case of a substitution, such as is alleged of the Extract of Belladonna for that of Dandelion, the pretext that the extract had been purchased would have had no other effect than to render the punishment of the apothecary, on account of such negligence, more certain. If an apothecary, in case of urgency, should be unable personally to make the preparation, he must purchase it for the occasion from one of his colleagues only.

More than forty years ago an accidental substitution of the

herb of Belladonna for that of viola tricolor occurred, which was followed by fatal results. The following, according to my recollection, are the material points in the case: A prescription for an infusion of herba violæ tricoloris, which enjoys some reputation in diseases of the skin, was directed for a child, and sent to a pharmacy, which, being under the immediate patronage of the king, was termed the court-pharmacy, (Hof-apotheke). Its employment was followed by the symptoms of narcotic poisoning, and the death of the child ensued. On investigation it was discovered that in the compartment of the pharmacy which was labelled Herba Violæ Tricoloris, or Jaceæ, Herba Belladonnæ was placed—a change which had its origin in the fact that the supply of the first herb was placed together with the last in one and the same chamber, in which the more active medicinal agents were stored; Herba Jaceæ was already, on account of its nauseating properties, somewhat related to these agents. The blame of the substitution could not be ascribed personally to any one, since it was not known which of the assistants had made it, and yet some one must be punished for it, such was the will of the ruler. Thus it happened that the assistant, who, from the nature of his duties, is termed Defectarius, was singled out for punishment, not because he had himself made the substitution, but because the task of filling the empty vessels fell to his duty, and he, at least, was so far answerable, even if another, in his place, had committed the oversight. The sentence was imprisonment for a period, and a prohibition to exercise again the business of an apothecary.

The convict became afterwards an excellent chemist, and the head of a manufacturing establishment, in which his position was better than if he had remained an apothecary.

For the thorough understanding of this case I must add that in Germany, whenever an error arises of any kind, it is the dispensing apothecary who is always the first to be punished. In the substitution which occurred through the purchase of

Dandelion Extract, the blame would scarcely have fallen upon any other than upon the overseer of the apothecary's shop. The merchant and the manufacturer would have come off with a slight reproof for the unintentional change of the label.

In Germany they are accustomed to load the shoulders of the pharmaceutist with the responsibility for all manner of errors, and, in all probability, chiefly from this cause, that while medicine is fully represented in the governing colleges and in those of justice, (Regierung und Justiz Collegien,) pharmacy is not. A society of physicians prescribes to the apothecary the manner in which he shall prepare his medicines, makes the laws by which he is governed, puts a price upon his articles, and sets a value upon his labor. A physician examines the young man when he desires to become an apprentice ; (Lehrling, a learner)—again a physician examines him when he has completed his studies, and a medical college takes part in the last examination before he is capable of becoming the overseer of a shop. In fine, we can thus understand the open declaration of a professor of medicine and surgery in a German University, when he said, " The apothecary is of no farther signification to the physician than as a fulfiller of his orders—he stands in the same rank with the mechanic that prepares and sharpens my surgical instruments."

This condition of things appears to me to have had its origin in the times in which princes first began to entertain physicians, who had their servants for the preparation of their medicines. From these servants, perhaps, the apothecary has gradually been unfolded, and he still preserves the same subordinate place to the physician and to the State to this day, whilst the physician, standing from the commencement in immediate connection with the leaders of the State, in this manner secured the preponderance of his own position. In later times the more the apothecary has added theoretical knowledge to his practical skill, the further he has won above his subordinate position, so that already, in many States, the pharmaceutist is at least heard in the preparation of a new pharmacopœia or of an ordinance relative to apothecaries. To this time, however, his opinion is only advisory, and otherwise of no influence in the result. What effect would it have on the developement of medicine if it were placed under a similar supervision of pharmacy, which, at least, comprehends within itself more positive knowledge than her elder sister? How moderate a price, for instance, would be set upon the labors of physicians if they were to be valued by pharmaceutists?

Now that I have previously, in the most cursory and condensed manner, unfolded the course of education and the relative position (aussere stellung) of an apothecary in Germany, I come to the arrangement of a pharmacy as it is there required.

In a perfect arrangement there is required—1st, the shop; (officin); 2d, the laboratory; 3d, the room for pulverizing; (stoss-kammer); 4th, the water cellar; 5th, the store room; (material-kammer); 6th, the herb room; (kräuter-kammer); 7th, the room for poisons (gift-kammer); 8th, the room for implements; (geschirr-kammer).

1st. To the shop proper (officin) belong—1st, scales, weights, measures, which must not only be in sufficient number but also of a proper degree of justness. The limits of their exactness are from one to two parts in a thousand; that is scales, loaded with from one to two ounces must show a weight of from one to two grains. An ounce may at the most be half a grain too light or too heavy, and a similar proportion holds in regard to measures. Farther, nothing must be measured except, at the most, watery fluids, and in Prussia not even these, since it is expressly forbidden in the pharmacopœia to define the quantity of a fluid by measure, much less to dispense by it. [The words are—Mensuris nunquam, sed semper ponderibus, liquorum quantitas indicanda est.]

2nd. Dishes for trituration, (Reibschalen) of porcelain; iron mortars (brass is not favorably looked on); Spatulas, spoons, of horn and iron, but not of compound metal.

A special trituration dish is required for musk and poisons, as well as separate scales for both these substances. Besides the metallic pill machine, there must be similar ones of wood and horn.

3rd. Further, a proper quantity of earthen vessels, boxes, pots, and glass-ware, are required.

4th. The vessels for containing the drugs must not be disproportionately large, the glass-ware must shut tight, the drawers be properly covered, the *covers* of the pots fitting well. It is required that the more active medicines shall be placed in a separate compartment. For instance, the mercurials, the antimonials, and other metallic preparations, narcotic drugs, even aloes and jalap. The extent to which this is carried is seen in the case we have cited of the substitution of HBa Belladonna for HB Jaceæ, since the last, as causing nausea, had been associated with the more active drugs. For some time it has been particularly provided that many articles must be properly protected by the vessels which contain them, from the light. For example, the most of the preparations of iodine, together with the subnitrate of bismuth, aqua amygdalarum amar, ammonium, carbonic pyrooleosum, ferrum sesquichloratum, &c. Besides this and the general order in the placing of the medicines, there is still a special "noli me tangere" in the shop, that no pharmaceutist yet rightly understands how to manage—I mean the poison chest, (gift-schrank). In this are secured the Arsenicalia and the Corrosiva; to wit, arsenious acid and the sulphurets of arsenic, the corrosive chloride and red iodide of mercury, phosphorus, veratria, strychnia, etc. As I myself had something to do with the inspection of shops, I know from my own experience as well as from communications from my friends, that the apothecary can scarcely ever succeed in meeting the demands of the inspectors in regard to this poison chest. Now he has too much, now too little, secured in it. The special scales and weights enclosed in it are rusted or injured, or the chest itself is not in the right place!

The character of the labels is a strong point for the visiting physician. They must, throughout, be regulated by the pharmacopœia which is authorized by the particular State. As the nomenclature of the preparations is, to a great extent, changed on every revision of the pharmacopœia, the inspector may thus drive the apothecary to despair. I know this from experience. Scarcely two years before the appearance of a new pharmacopœia I arranged my shop anew, procuring all my glass ware from Prague, in Bohemia, with the labels burned in. A rather ignorant inspector, *who* was in no condition to discover an error of real consequence, and who yet desired to show his authority, discovered that my vessels were not labelled exactly according to the last edition of the pharmacopœia. This gave him a good source for a series of annoyances, which I esteem myself happy to have escaped.

2nd. The laboratory is one of the most essential of the appurtenances. It must be arched, fire-proof, light, dry and roomy. It must be provided with several furnaces, sand, water and steam baths, a *drying place*, and a good press. Besides the ordinary pans, boilers and dishes, the apparatus for distilling is placed here, with a blast furnace for crucibles.

If there is no special place for preserving the utensils, then evaporating dishes of porcelain and metal, the before-mentioned dishes, pans, crucibles for melting, filtering apparatus, and, finally, thermometers and specific gravity bottles must be placed in the laboratory.

3d. The room for pulverising must be separated from the laboratory on account of the dust which that kind of work occasions. In it should be found, mortars of iron and stone, the last for comminuting fresh herbs, almonds, &c., a proper number of sieves, of which many must be employed only for single articles, as for sugar, assafœtida, narcotica, virosa, metallica, a variety of knives for cutting roots, rasps, files, a machine for pulverizing, &c. The German pharmaceutist is strictly forbidden to purchase a substance in the form of powder when it is possible to avoid it.

# ON PHELLANDRINE, OR THE ACTIVE PRINCIPLE OF PHELLANDRIUM AQUATICUM.*

The researches of MM. Devay and Guillermont on the active principle of Hemlock, those of Buchner on that of Digitalis tend to confirm the opinion, that in those two substances the active principle is found chiefly in the fruit. It is natural to suppose that for Phellandrium, whose seeds we know have for some years been largely employed in medicine, the active principle should likewise be found in them, and might, in consequence, be extracted without difficulty. An apothecary of Lyons, M. Hutet fils has proved that this supposition is correct.

The active principle of phellandrium, which he terms phellandrine, is easily obtained. The seeds from which it is procured contain, judging by the result of several operations, on the average two or three per cent. To procure it, the fruit, previously bruised, is exhausted by sulphuric ether; the ethereal solution is treated with an excess of caustic potash, is distilled until the greater part of the ether employed is again obtained; the residuum is treated with water acidulated with sulphuric acid, and submitted to distillation at a temperature of from 176° to 212°F. A neutral liquid is thus obtained, almost colorless at the commencement of the distillation, afterwards of a light amber tint, of an oily appearance, lighter than water, in which it is slightly soluble, of a strong nauseous and slightly ethereal odour, soluble in ether, in alcohol and fats, less soluble in fixed than in volatile oils—this is phellandrine.

---

* The phellandrium aquaticum, an umbelliferous plant, indigenous over the greater part of Europe, is much used in France, and particularly in Germany. The seeds are chiefly employed; they are esteemed narcotic, diuretic, and febrifuge, and have been much used in phthisis.—Ed. *New York Journal of Pharmacy.*

Its effect on animals proves it is the active principle of phellandrium. Fifty centigrammes (7½ gr.) of phellandrine, injected into the veins of a dog, produced, in a few instants, difficulty of respiration, nervous tremblings and anxiety, lasting some hours. The animal recovered, but two birds, into whose beaks the same dose was introduced, died in fifteen or twenty minutes. It has also the theraupeutic effect of phellandrium, for M. Devay, who employed an ointment composed of one part of phellandrine united with fifty parts of lard, thinks that by its anodyne and sedative effects it resembles the balm of conicine, and that the preparation merits a careful trial, that we may arrive at certain conclusions regarding its resolvent action.

It may be employed internally in granules, containing each a milligramme of the active principle, or in syrup, containing a centigramme in each spoonful.—*Bulletin de Theraupeutique, Aug.*, 1852.

---

## PASTILLES CONTAINING IODINE, OR VOLATILE IODIDES.

Dr. Langlebert has recently communicated to the Academy of Sciences a note upon a new method of administering iodine and the volatile iodides, by means of lozenges, similar to those known under the name of "pastilles du sérail." The following is his formula:

℞—Freshly burned charcoal, pulverized.......20 grammes.
Nitrate of potash......................3 grammes.

Mix intimately and pass through a fine sieve, then add—
Iodine..............................10 grammes.

Mix by trituration.

The ingredients being thoroughly mingled, add a sufficient quantity of very thin mucilage of gum tragacanth to make a paste, which is to be divided into twenty pastilles.

Dry them rapidly in the sun or in a stove, and keep in a well stopped bottle. Each pastille contains fifty centigrammes of iodine.

To employ the pastilles it is only necessary to kindle them at the top, and place them upon the mantel-piece or table. The combustion goes on of itself, slowly volatilizing the iodine in the atmosphere of the room.–*Bulletin de Therapeutique*, *Aug.* 1852.

---

## ON THE REDUCTION OF CHLORIDE OF SILVER BY AN ELECTRO-CHEMICAL PROCESS.

BY F. WANDERSLEBEN, APOTHECARY.

The reduction of Chloride of Silver by iron or zinc, as is the general custom, is a very tedious operation, and attended with great waste of time. The following method of preparing chemically pure silver for medicinal use, is a very simple, short, and delicate one, and may therefore be recommended:

A square piece of zinc is laid on the bottom of a tumbler, and upon the zinc a platinum or copper dish, containing the precipitated Chloride of Silver, taken from the filter; afterwards some very dilute sulphuric acid is poured from the edge of the tumbler, until it has exceeded the level of the platinum or copper dish: the metallic reduction commences immediately from the under surface of the Chloride of Silver, and spreads slowly over the whole surface. The end of the operation, that is, the reduction of the Chloride of Silver to the metallic state, is determined very nicely by the commencement of the decomposition of the water, a very rapid evolution of hydrogen gas appearing at the negative pole, (platinum or copper). The whole operation may be done in a shorter time, the electric current being increased, if the dish of platinum or copper is covered with wax on the outside to the level of the Chloride of Silver. It is evident that this process is equally useful for the quantitative definition of Chloride of Silver.—*Journal der Pharmacie und Chimie*, *August*, 1852.

## SUCQUET'S METHOD OF PRESERVING BODIES IN ANATOMICAL INSTITUTES.

Sucquet, of France, received a medal at the exhibition in London, and lately a premium of 2000 francs from the Academy in Paris, for his invention to preserve corpses, and to prevent infection in anatomical institutes. The method, proving to be a good one, is introduced now in almost all academies or anatomical theatres abroad. The liquid injected into the body is prepared as follows: Sulphurous acid, obtained by heating sulphuric acid and wood-raspings, is passed into a solution of carbonate of soda (of 22° Baumé) until all carbonic acid is expelled, and the sulphurous acid is in excess, the solution has 24° Baumé,) then it is poured upon zinc filings, until it becomes neutral. (A polished iron dipped into it and then exposed to the air for some time, should not become brown.) Of this liquid, about one gallon is injected through one of the arteries of the neck. The section may then be commenced either after 24 hours, or postponed for 20, 30, and even 40 days, without any disadvantage. Those parts which are already separated from the body and more exposed to the air, are impregnated with a solution of chloride of zinc, a precaution which is likewise to be applied to those bodies which have been opened before being injected with Sucquet's liquid. In these cases, the vessels are tied up, to prevent the escape of the injection. Sucquet's liquid must be applied to recently dead bodies, because it does not prevent putrefaction, if they have commenced to decompose. The instruments, knives, etc., are not much acted on by Sucquet's liquid, and are therefore easily cleaned again. It is stated, too, that dissection-wounds have never proved fatal when Sucquet's liquid has been used —*Polytechnisches Journal, Jan.*, 1852.

# ON CATHARTIN OBTAINED FROM THE BERRIES OF RHAMNUS CATHARTICA.

BY F. L. WINKLER.

To obtain the purgative principle of these berries, fifteen pounds of them, when quite green, (collected in September,) were bruised and expressed. The juice had a dark violet color, an extremely bitter taste, and evaporated by means of a water-bath, remained as a dark brown syrup. This was then exhausted several times by boiling hot alcohol (absolute) until the latter had but a slightly bitter taste. The united tinctures became turbid after cooling; they were then filtered and mixed with four times as much sulphuric ether. A large quantity of a slightly bitter, dark-colored, extractive matter separated, containing no sugar. The filtered solution of cathartin in ether and alcohol was distilled in a water-bath, the cathartin remaining with the coloring matter, then treated again in the same way, and 2½ ounces of pure cathartin were obtained.

The residuum of the expressed berries was boiled with six or eight times its weight of water, set aside for several days, and a good quantity of impure RHAMNIN obtained. This was then collected on a filter of dense linen, washed with water, dried, and appeared as a greenish gray mass, of a slightly bitter taste, loosely coherent. This, again dissolved in alcohol, was decolorized by animal charcoal, separated by the addition of water, and thus obtained in a pure state. The dry mass was dissolved again in absolute alcohol, and by slow evaporation ten drachms of pure Rhamnin, crystallized in pale yellow crystals, similar to cauliflowers, of a peculiar taste, little distinct, almost like dough; it is not soluble in cold alcohol nor ether, but readily soluble in boiling alcohol, and forms a mucilage, if boiled in water.

It is dissolved by caustic alkalies and their carbonates, with saffron yellow color, tasting almost like grape sugar, and decolorized by acids, by which operation the Rhamnin is precipitated. It is likewise dissolved by strong chlorohydric and sulphuric acid, with the same color, and precipitated by a large quantity of water. Hot nitric acid converts the Rhamnin into oxalic acid, a yellow, bitter substance, (perhaps picrinic acid), and a new crystalline substance.

Ripe buckthorn berries yielded Cathartin, but no Rhamnin; and it is probable that the Rhamnin, by the ripening process, is converted into Cathartin and grape sugar.

Cathartin is a pale yellow powder, soluble nearly in any proportion of water and spirits, (not in pure ether), has a disagreeable, bitter taste, like aloes, is neutral, turns of a dark, brownish green by deutochloride of iron, gold yellow by liquor subacetatis plumbi and the alkaloids, fuses by heat, and is decomposed at a high temperature; acted on by nitric acid, it yields a good quantity of picrinic acid.

The resemblance of Cathartin to pure Aloin is extended, likewise, to its physiological properties. Dr. Graff, president of the medical board, (medical director), wrote to me as follows:

"Since I had the honor to receive your compound pills of cathartin and liquorice, I have experimented with them frequently and with good effect. Pills containing one grain of cathartin, cause, in strong persons, one or two stools; in weaker ones, three or four, without any griping. In many cases the dose had to be repeated after three or four hours, to operate well. A young, stout mechanic, 20 years of age, suffering under an affection of the liver, had to take three pills pro dose, two or three times a day, to produce one or two large discharges; after taking them continually, he wanted but one dose of three pills for the same effect. In general, it is advisable to commence with one grain of cathartin, and then to increase the dose, if necessary. On a sick man, one grain of cathartin had no effect at all, but taking two, he had four or five moderate stools, etc., etc. This remedy is certainly very valuable in constipation of the bowels, obstructions of the liver and spleen, in hæmorrhoids, hydropsy, and gout."

If the juice of unripe buckthorn berries be evaporated to the consistence of a syrup, and then treated with liquor Hoffmanni, (one part of ether and two parts of alcohol of 80°), cathartin is obtained in an impure state; but being very powerful, it will answer any purpose better than aloes, and should be administered, because it can be obtained at a moderate price, twelve pounds of fresh expressed juice yielding about eight ounces of cathartin.—*Jul. Ruthardt, Pharmaceut.*

---

## NOTE ON THE TANNATES OF QUININE AND CINCHONINE.

The increasing scarceness of the better varieties of cinchona and the increasing price of the sulphate of quinine, have latterly given rise to much research after substitutes for this latter product. Thus in turn experiments have been made with sal ammoniac, already used by the ancients, marine salt, hydroferrocyanate of potassium and urea, arsenious acid, tannate of quinine, &c. If experience has already decided with regard to some of these products, there are others on which it has been silent, and amongst these is tannate of quinine. Although long known to chemists, it is only recently that this salt has been introduced into therapeutics, and this was owing to the opinion first expressed by Berzelius, that it approaches at once sulphate of quinine by the fixity of its composition and cinchona by the nature of its constituent principles. And, in fact, this compound is a perfectly definite salt, closely allied to what chemists call red cinchonic, a product which arises in all cases where cinchona is found in presence of an aqueous or alcoholic vehicle, and which is formed of tannin and the alkaloids peculiar to this bark.

Tannate of quinine is obtained by the decomposition of a cinchonic salt by means of tannic acid. Thus, on pouring a solution of tannin into a solution of a salt with a base of quinine, a precipitate of tannate of quinine is formed; but the best mode of preparing this compound consists in treating the acetate of quinine obtained from the pure sulphate with the tannin of Pelouz, collecting the precipitate, washing and drying it. Thus obtained, the tannate of quinine is an amorphous powder, of a yellowish white, slightly soluble in water, and, like sulphate of quinine, undergoing no change by keeping. It is composed of two equivalents of tannic acid and one of quinine, or, in decimals, of—

| | |
|---|---|
| Tannic acid | 69.55 |
| Quinine | 30.45 |

On account of its pulverulent and amorphous form, tannate of quinine admits of adulteration more easily than sulphate of quinine, which is always in crystals; it is, therefore, indispensable, before using it, to be assured of its purity. This is done in the following manner: Take 5 grammes of the tannate to be tested, reduce it to a fine powder, and incorporate it well with 8 grammes of slaked lime, and a sufficient quantity of water to make a soft paste, after which, submit the whole to ebullition, with 40 or 50 grammes of rectified alcohol. After some moments of ebullition, filter the liquor, and then evaporate it by a gentle heat. Towards the close of the operation it is saturated with a slight excess of sulphuric acid, then precipitated by ammonia. The alkaloid, being well washed, is again combined with sulphuric acid, to obtain the sulphate, which is then submitted to the various means employed to ascertain the purity of this substance. We may, besides, after the precipitation by ammonia, treat the precipitate with ether, which dissolves the quinine, decant the etherized product, evaporate it to dryness, and, from the weight of the alkaloid obtained, deduce the pureness of the tannate subject to trial. Five grammes of tannate ought to give 1.52 of pure quinine.

The tannate of quinine is generally administered under the form of pills or enclosed in wafers; but it may also, on account of its slight bitterness, be taken in lozenges, or in powder mixed in syrup. We may, however, say that, for certain very impressionable people, its bitterness, which cannot be compared to the very intense taste of sulphate of quinine, is still sufficiently marked to prevent their using it under these latter forms.

The tannate of cinchonine has been also indicated as a substitute for sulphate of quinine, and in the same degree as the tannate of that base. Some experiments tried in Italy have induced us to place before our readers the mode of preparing these new salts of quinine.

Tannate of cinchonine, whose properties are formed, if we may so speak, on those of tannate of quinine, is obtained in the same way, and administered in the same doses.—*Bulletin Therapeutique*, *Nov.*, 1852.

---

## ITALIAN "CACHOU AROMATIQUE."

Extract of liquorice by infusion..100 grammes.
Water........................100 grammes.

Dissolve in water bath, and add:

Powdered catechu...............30 grammes.
Powdered gum..................30 grammes.

Evaporate to the consistence of an extract, and then incorporate the following substances, reduced to powder:

Mastic.........................2 grammes.
Cascarilla.....................2 grammes.
Charcoal.......................2 grammes.
Orris root.....................2 grammes.

Concentrate the mass, remove it from the fire, and then add:

Oil of peppermint................2 grammes.
Tincture of musk................5 drops.
Tincture of amber................5 drops.

Pour it on a marble, previously oiled, and roll it by means of a roller to the thickness of a piece of fifty centimes.* When the mass is cold remove the oil from both surfaces by means of unsized paper, moisten it slightly, cover it with silver paper, let it dry, and then cut it into narrow strips, and divide these into minute squares or lozenges.

This preparation, much used by smokers, to destroy the smell of tobacco, is also a stomachic and carminative of a very pleasant flavor.—*Bulletin de Therapeutique*, *Aug.*, 1852.

---

## REMARKS ON THE PREPARATION OF HYDRATED SESQUI-OXIDE OF IRON AS AN ANTIDOTE, AND ON THE DUTY OF THE PHARMACEUTIST IN REGARD TO IT.

By William Proctor, Jr.

There are few antidotes to active poisons that have proved more uniformly successful than the hydrated sesqui-oxide of iron, for poisoning by arsenious acid. Where it has failed, the ill success can, in most instances, be traced to the delay in obtaining it; to its age, and consequent dehydration, when kept ready prepared; to the excessive quantity of the poison, or to the neglect of a proper preliminary use of emetics to

* A coin about the size of a ten cent piece.

throw off undissolved portions of the poison. From the facility with which arsenious acid can be procured in this and other cities, this poison, from its widely known reputation for virulence, is but too frequently resorted to by the suicide. The slowness with which it dissolves in water is a circumstance favorable to the success of treatment; and as, when ingested by design, it is merely suspended in some liquid, the sooner emesis is excited the better.

The object of these remarks has reference mainly to recall attention to a few suggestions made some years ago,* which will enable any apothecary, who will attend to them, to prepare the antidote in its most eligible form in fifteen or twenty minutes' notice; and also to urge, that it is his conscientious duty to be always ready to furnish the antidote, no matter how few may be the calls for it.

The following formula, which is somewhat different from that proposed in 1843, is easily executed, and furnishes a concentrated solution of the ter-sesqui-sulphate of iron of known strength, so that the operator can graduate the precise quantity of oxide by means of his measure glass:

Take of (proto) sulphate of iron, (well crystallized,) sixty-four ounces Troy.

Sulphuric acid, seven fluid ounces.

Nitric acid, sp. gr. 138, twelve fluid ounces.

Water, a sufficient quantity.

Reduce the sulphate of iron to moderately fine powder in an iron mortar, mix together the acids and five fluid ounces of water, put the mixture in a large porcelain capsule on the sand bath or other regular source of heat, and add the powdered sulphate, about two ounces at a time, stirring after each addition, till the effervescence ceases, until all has been added and the elimination of nitrous fumes has ceased. In the absence of a porcelain capsule and sand bath, the operator may use a gallon glass jar supported in a vessel of boiling water;

* American Journal of Pharmacy, vol. xiv., p. 35.

in either case, the vessel should be large enough to allow for active effervescence, and it is hardly necessary to say that the operation should be performed under a chimneyhood, or in the open air, to avoid the noxious fumes of nitrous acid. The dense solution thus obtained should then be diluted with water until it measures four and a half pints, (wine measure,) and then filtered through thick muslin.

Solution of ter-sulphate of iron, thus prepared, has a dark, reddish-brown color in quantity, the specific gravity of 1.587 at 60° F., but little if any odor, a powerful styptic taste, and mixes readily with water, so as to form a solution with more color in proportion to its dilution than the strong liquid. Each fluid ounce of this solution contains a fraction more than 120 grains of sesqui-oxide; each fluid drachm 15 grains, and each minim a quarter of a grain; and as it is equally applicable for preparing the oxide for chemical as for antidotal purposes, this correspondence of weights with measures gives great facility in calculating any precise quantity desired.

It is this solution which I have proposed should be kept by *every* apothecary as the source of hydrated sesqui-oxide of iron. Its strength is such that it requires about an equal measure of commercial solution of ammonia (sp. gr. .940,) to decompose it. The apothecary who is suddenly called upon for the antidote will proceed in the following manner:

Take of Solution of ter-sulphate of iron, half a pint.
" Solution of ammonia, half a pint, (or a sufficient quantity).
" Water, a sufficient quantity.

Pour the solution of iron into a half gallon jar, add two pints of water, and then add the ammonia, stirring constantly until in slight excess. This is known when, after displacing the air in the jar by blowing, it continues to smell slightly of ammonia. The contents of the jar are then thrown on a piece of strong muslin, previously well moistened, and the liquid, holding in solution sulphate of ammonia, expressed from it as quickly as possible, until the oxide remains in the cloth of a pasty consistence. The cloth is then opened on a dish, water added and incorporated with the oxide by means of a spatula, and then again expressed. If the demand is urgent, the oxide may be sent without further washing, if not urgent, the washing may be repeated twice more. It is then quickly removed by a spatula from the cloth to a quart mortar, and water mixed with it by trituration, until it measures a pint, when it should be poured into a wide mouthed bottle, corked, and the following label attached, viz. :

---

**HYDRATED SESQUI-OXIDE OF IRON.**

**(Ferri Oxidum Hydratum U. S. Pharm.)**

*Antidote to Arsenic.*

This preparation consists of Hydrated Sesqui-oxide of Iron and water, in such proportion that each table spoonful contains *thirty* grains of the dry oxide ; and is intended to neutralize the poisonous effect of *Arsenious acid*, or *common white arsenic*, when taken into the stomach. It is well to precede the administration of this antidote by an active emetic of ipecacuanha or mustard, so that any undissolved arsenic may be thus mechanically removed, if possible. If, however, this has not been done before obtaining the *antidote*, no time should be lost in giving it. The patient should take a table spoonful for a dose every five or ten minutes, but, if vomiting should intervene, let a dose be given immediately after each attack, unless otherwise directed by the physician in attendance.

When the poisoning has been caused by *arsenite of potassa*, (Fowler's Mineral Solution,) *soda*, or *ammonia*, or by the salts of *arsenic acid*, after giving the first dose add six table spoonfuls of vinegar to the contents of the bottle, and shake it a few minutes, until the acidity is neutralized, and then give it as above.

---

When the oxide is intended for other ferruginous preparations, as, for instance, citrate of iron, it should be washed by displacement on a cloth filter, till the washings cease to precipitate chloride of barium. The small amount of sulphate of ammonia remaining in the oxide, when prepared hurriedly as above, is of no account in a case of poisoning.

The detail in the above label is not objectionable, as it will be often of use even to the experienced physician, not to speak of the very many who have had little if any experience in poisoning cases, and will likewise enable any person of ordinary ability to administer the antidote without loss of time.

And now a word in reference to the obvious *duty* of apothecaries, and their *actual* practice as regards a state of preparation to meet the emergencies requiring this antidote. In this country no law compels the pharmaceutist to keep *any* preparation; he may be without remedies of the first importance, may decline compounding prescriptions on the score of not having the material, or from any other cause, without any legal risk, and no impelling motive to the contrary exists, except self-interest and a feeling of duty. The *former* of these motives is not always appealed to; it has often happened in my experience that no reward, except moral satisfaction, has followed the trouble and expense attendant on supplying a demand for the antidote; as the sufferers too often belong to the utterly miserable poor, or the messengers come, unprovided with the means of payment, from a great distance, and, in the agitation of the moment, forget the due of the apothecary. In this city it has become a practice with many apothecaries to send applicants for hydrated sesqui-oxide to other stores; I have repeatedly been called on, after the messenger had made a circle of four, five or six stores, and walked a long distance, thus greatly delaying the application of the antidote. When it is so easy to be prepared for these occasions, it is greatly to be desired that every apothecary, who has a proper regard for his reputation and duty, will provide the means as above detailed, and be ever ready.

[While commending the suggestions of Mr. Proctor to the attention of our readers, we can by no means agree in his view of the efficacy of the Hydrated Sesqui-Oxide of Iron as an antidote for poisoning by arsenious acid. When the arsenic is in solution it will be precipitated in a comparatively insoluable, and consequently innocuous, form, by the Hydrated Sesqui-Oxide. But arsenic is rarely taken in the form of solution, either in cases of criminal poisoning or of suicide, and when it is in the form of powder or small lumps, the vaunted antidote can be of no use except mechanically, by enveloping the particles of the poison, and thus shielding the coats of the stomach. In many cases in which the cure of the patient has been attributed to the sesqui-oxide, it has been in reality due to the vomiting which was produced by the poison, and which removed it from the stomach before it had time to exert its noxious influence. In all cases where solid arsenious acid has been taken, the first object is to remove the poison from the stomach by means of an emetic or stomach pump. Time must not be wasted in waiting for the sesqui-oxide; lime-water and oil, flour and milk, &c., will answer equally well to envelope the poison during the operation of the emetic. The true antidotal effect of the hydrated oxide is, as was before observed, confined to the few cases in which the poison is taken in the form of solution.—Ed. *N. Y. Journal of Pharmacy.*]

---

# ON THE PREPARATION OF IODIDE OF AMMONIUM.

By John A. Spencer.

(*Read before the Chemical Discussion Society.*)

The salt, iodide of ammonium, having lately been used, and from its possessing certain advantages over the similar compound of potassium, being likely to come into more extensive use among those practicing photography, I am induced to lay before the Society a method I have adopted for preparing the substance in question, of greater purity and with more facility than those processes which are given in most works on chemistry, viz., by the double decomposition of solutions of iodide of iron or zinc by carbonate of ammonia, filtering, washing the precipitate, and evaporating the solution to dryness. These methods do not usually yield an unexceptionable product, as it is generally of a yellowish color, while the pure salt is perfectly white; they also require a comparatively large quantity of water, to prevent losing much of the salt in the precipitate.

The action of iodine on solution of ammonia, differs, as is

well known, from that upon the fixed and caustic alkalies; in the latter case, an iodide and iodate of the metal is formed, which may be separated either by alcohol, which leaves the iodate untouched, or the iodate may be converted, by exposure to a red heat, into iodide. By acting on *ammonia* with iodine, only a small portion of iodide of ammonium is formed, accompanied by that most formidable substance, iodide of nitrogen, a substance whose explosive properties render it an operation of danger to prepare it in large quantities; but if, instead of using caustic ammonia, a solution of *sulphide of ammonium* be used, the reaction which ensues is perfectly safe, and gives us the salt in question very readily. The operation is very simple. A quantity of pure iodine is placed in a flask with a small quantity of water, and sulphide of ammonium added to it till the liquid loses its red color, and is turbid only from separation of sulphur; the flask is then agitated till the sulphur, for the most part, agglomerates into a mass, the liquid poured off, and, if necessary, ammonia added to it till it manifests a slightly alkaline reaction, and then boiled till all odor of sulphuretted hydrogen and of ammonia is lost, then filtered, which is done with great facility, and evaporated at a boiling heat, constantly stirring from the edges of the vessel, till it becomes a pasty mass, when it is immediately transferred to a water bath, and the stirring continued till the salt is dry. It then forms a beautifully white and crystalline powder, which will keep for some time, if carefully excluded from the air, but which, after the lapse of a few weeks, becomes yellowish, and at last brown; it may, however, be easily restored, by adding a little solution of sulphuretted hydrogen till colorless, filtering and evaporating to dryness. By means of this process, a pound of the substance may be procured, in a perfectly pure condition, in a couple of hours, while, by the old method a much longer time would be necessary and the product be not so good.—*Annals of Pharm.*, Jan., 1853.

# ON SABADILLINE.

By Fr. Hubschmann.

It is known that Couerbe has discovered in sabadilla seed, besides veratrine, a second organic base, which he has named sabadilline. He obtained it by boiling the impure veratrine, precipitated by potash or soda, with water, from which it crystallizes out by cooling. E. Simon afterwards regarded this sabadilline of Couerbe as a double compound of resin and soda with resinous veratrine, from whose solutions in sulphuric acid, pure veratrine could be precipitated by means of ammonia.

The author now shows, by the following research with a body which he had obtained, by treating his veratrine with ether, as a residue, that this residue is sabadilline, and thus proves the existence of this alkaloid.

Sabadilline is a white amorphous powder, which, when rubbed in a mortar, does not cause sneezing; whereas, veratrine, as is well known, irritates the nose.

Sabadilline is only taken up as a trace by ether, whilst veratrine is extremely soluble therein.

Sabadilline dissolves in 143 parts of boiling water. This solution is not rendered turbid by ammonia; but very much so by carbonate of potash, which, however, precipitates only two-thirds of the dissolved alkaloid; this precipitate, by heating the solution, forms into a resinous mass. Veratrine does not dissolve in water in an observable degree.

A solution of 1 part of sabadilline in 4 parts of diluted sulphuric acid, and 100 parts of water, does not become turbid with ammonia. A similarly prepared solution of veratrine gives, with ammonia, a strong turbidity.—*Annals of Pharmacy, Jan.*, 1853.

## LETTER OF M. ORFILA TO THE DIRECTOR OF THE "ECOLE SPECIALE DE PHARMACIE" OF PARIS.

Paris, January 1st, 1853.

MONSIEUR LE DIRECTEUR AND MY DEAR COLLEAGUE,

An Examiner for thirty-two years of the Special School of Pharmacy of Paris, I have been able to appreciate the distinguished merit and the honorable zeal of its professors, as well as the remarkable aptitude of most of the candidates who have attentively followed their courses of instruction. I will retain during my life a grateful recollection of the relations which have always existed between you, your colleagues and myself, and I esteem myself happy at this time to be able to give you a proof of the desire which animates me to contribute somewhat to elevate the renown of an institution which does honor to France, and of which you are a worthy director.

I place at your disposition an inscription of 500 francs per annum in the three per cents, destined to found a prize of 1,000 francs, to be awarded every two years, dating from the first session of the year 1856. This inscription represents a sum of 14,000 francs (at 84, the price at which it was purchased).

The prize is never to be divided. If it is not awarded, the same question is again to be submitted for competition, and the prize will then be 2,000 francs. If a second time the prize is not awarded, the same question is to be proposed a third time, and the prize will be 3,000 francs; if, despite these delays, the question is not properly resolved, and the prize is not adjudged, the sum of 3,000 francs is to be paid into the Treasury of the Association of the Physicians of the Department of the Seine, which I founded in 1833.

Permit me to indicate summarily, a certain number of questions which *appear to me* should be first proposed.

1st. To extract from the most important composite medicinal substances all the immediate principles or other active substances which enter into their composition. We must not believe because we have obtained from a medicine an alkaloid or other body endowed with a certain activity, that science has exhausted it; in fact, the substance extracted from a composite medicine may account for a certain number of the therapeutic effects of the article, but often numerous other effects depend on matters not yet isolated. It is necessary to be very sure in this respect in order to complete every thing which is concerned in the action of composite medicines upon the human body, and the part which the different active elements it contains take in this action. This question will furnish, without doubt, a goodly number of subjects for prizes.

2nd. To determine, by experiment, what substances in the different kingdoms, should never be united in the same formulas, because they mutually decompose each other, and the products which result from them are entirely inert. To determine, on the other hand, the substances, which, by their combination, even when decomposition ensues, produce substances endowed with a certain activity, and useful in the practice of medicine. To indicate the kind of alteration the different substances undergo, and the nature of the new compounds which are formed.

3rd. To expose the methods proper to recognise certain sophistications which have not hitherto been the subject of careful examination.

4th. To ascertain the modifications which certain animal and vegetable drugs undergo on prolonged exposure to heat and light, to dry and moist air, etc., and to state if the products which result from this alteration may give rise to accidents in the cases in which these drugs are employed as remedies.

5th. To analyse the saliva, the urine and the perspiration, in the principal acute diseases termed specific, in order to state the changes which these fluids undergo; to join to this the examination of the air expired.

6th. To seek if, in lying-in women, the milk in part abandons the galaktopherous vessels, or other channels, and, especially, if in what are termed milk diseases, to which sometimes women recently confined are subject, the milk has really been carried into the urine, into certain serous cavities, &c., &c.

7th. To submit to analysis the mineral waters that are still but little known, and again to take up the examination of those which enjoy a great reputation, in order that we may ascertain if they do not contain some new active substance.

Such, M. le Directeur are the questions which it is necessary to elucidate. The demands of science will lead you to propose others either before or after those which have been indicated; I rely in that respect confidently on the sagacity of the professors, whose programmes, whatever they may be, I accept beforehand.

Receive, M. le Directeur, the assurance of my distinguished consideration and affectionate esteem.

ORFILA.

—*Journal de Pharmacie*, *Feb.*, 1853.

---

## NEW REMEDIES FOR FEVERS AS SUBSTITUTES FOR QUININE.

It is well known that the *Société de Pharmacie*, at Paris, in November, 1849, instituted a prize of 4,000 francs to be given to the person who should succeed in preparing an artificial quinine, under the condition that it should be derived from a material which does not contain quinine already formed by nature therein. It was further determined that, in case this problem should not be solved, the prize should be decreed to the person who should furnish the best substitute for quinine, which should be equivalent to quinine in its therapeutical relations. The Commission which was charged with the decision between the competitors for this prize, consisting of Bussy,

Guibourt, Gaultier de Claubry, Bouchardat, Quevenne and Brignet, have now reported upon the matter as follows:

(1). In the first treatise presented to their notice, it is proposed to use roasted vegetable substances as remedies for fevers; that is, by roasting, to impart to vegetable substances febrifuge power, without giving more particular information on the subject.

(2). This treatise proposes sulphates of brucine and strychnine, without announcing anything new.

(3) & (4). These are not more successful than the preceding, one of them proposing the second bark of the oak, the other an extractive matter.

(5). This one proposes, under the denomination of *modified colophony*, the powder which he has obtained by a particular method of treating powdered colophony with nitric acid. The author of this treatise alleges 55 cases in which this remedy has proved effective. The commission requires still more satisfactory evidence.

(6). This one proposes the seeds of parsley and celery (*graines de l'apiol*). This remedy has been found to be important, and accordingly this treatise is particularly distinguished by the Commission.

(7). This proposes the fruit of the olive.

(8) & (9). One of these proposes a not-particularly-well-defined form of starch, and the other a material which is called *true tannin*. All these propositions are of no importance.

The Commissioners have submitted the remedy proposed in No. 6 to various distinguished physicians in France and in the French army, whereby it has been established that the parsley-seed has a decided power against fever, although its operation is not equal to that of quinine. The author obtained a sum of 1,000 francs as a reward for his treatise.

A prize is now, however, offered anew, of 6,000 francs, for a treatise which shall solve the problem to the extent that the original proposition requires, to be awarded at the meeting of 1854.—*Journal de Pharmacie et de Chimie*, 3 *Ser.* xxii., 81.

H. W.

## HYPOSULPHITE OF SODA AND SILVER AS AN OCCASIONAL SUBSTITUTE FOR NITRATE OF SILVER.

Dr. J. Delioux, of Cherbourg, brings the hyposulphite of soda and silver under notice, as a therapeutic agent, in the *Bulletin Général Thérapeutique* for October 15th and November 15th, 1852. He prepares it by pouring a solution of hyposulphite of soda on oxide of silver, recently precipitated by potassa, until it is completely dissolved. On evaporation, minute crystals of hyposulphite of soda and silver are left. The salt appears as a greyish-white crystalline powder, of sweetish taste, leaving a slightly styptic flavor: it is very soluble in water, but insoluble in alcohol. It becomes black on long exposure to light, but preserves its color indefinitely when kept in bottles of colored glass, or covered with paper. The solution becomes black when exposed to diffused light, but much more slowly than that of the nitrate of silver. When pure, it does not discolor the epidermis nor linen. Its power of coagulating albumen, and hence its astringency, is small compared with that of the nitrate; and its local action is less irritating.

From various experiments, Dr. Delioux concludes: First, that for external use, the hyposulphite of soda and silver may be employed in larger doses than the nitrate of silver; and that in these doses it is much less irritant, and incapable of producing a true eschar: Secondly, that for internal use, if it is sufficiently diluted, there is no risk of injuring the mucous membrane of the stomach. Moreover, as the solution does not coagulate albumen, nor form a precipitate of chloride of silver, it will be readily absorbed by the veins of the stomach.

Dr. Delioux has had an opportunity of administering the salt in only one case of epilepsy. Here it was unsuccessful as far as the epilepsy was concerned; but it produced no blackening of the skin, nor any physiological disturbance beyond excessive hunger. But the author very justly points out that no inference can be drawn from a single case. He gradually increased the daily dose from 5 to 60 *centigrammes* ($\frac{3}{4}$ of a grain to 9 grains).

As an external application, Dr. Delioux uses the hyposulphite as a substitute for nitrate of silver, in cases where a local alterative is required which shall produce less irritation, and act chemically on the tissues less than the latter salt. It should be tried in obstinate ulcers, as an injection into purulent collections and into sinuses, in chronic fluxes of the external ear and of the nasal fosse, and as a collyrium in diseases of the eye. Among the latter, Dr. Delioux can only cite from experience cases of acute conjunctivitis, which he has often found benefited, after the inflammatory stage has passed, by a dilute solution of this salt.

Dr. Delioux has employed the hyposulphite of soda and silver most frequently in acute and chronic urethretis ; and here he has found it most efficacious, especially in chronic cases, and at the end of the acute stage. He does not set it forth as a specific, nor as pre-eminent among local remedies; but as one to which recourse may be had among others. He generally uses an injection of from 50 *centigrammes* to a *gramme* ($7\frac{1}{2}$ to 15 grains) of the salt in 100 *grammes* (about three ounces) of distilled water. It produces little or no pain, and does not act as an astringent.—*Association Medical Journal, January* 14, 1853.

---

## NON-ARSENICAL FLY POISON.

Quassia..............................8 parts
Water............................500 parts
Molasses..........................125 parts

Boil the quassia with the water for ten minutes, strain and add the molasses.

Flies attack this preparation with avidity, and are quickly destroyed.—*Bulletin de Thérapeutique.*

# EDITORIAL—VARIA.

Letter of M. Orfila.—The Letter of M. Orfila to the Director of the Special School of Pharmacy of Paris not only exhibits an example of noble munificence on the part of the veteran professor, but shows his views as to some of the points which remain to be settled by pharmaceutical chemists. It shows, too, the kind of questions which are proposed for resolution to the pharmaciens of France. Besides the sum of 53,200 francs to the School of Pharmacy, M. Orfila leaves for other scientific purposes the sum of 67,500 francs, the greater part of which is devoted to the completion of the Orfila Museum.

Ancient Greek Vases.—Dr. J. Y. Simpson gives, in the January number of the *Monthly Journal of Medical Science*, a description, accompanied by drawings, of four ancient Greek vases, which, as shown by the inscriptions on them, were employed to contain Lykion, a celebrated ophthalmic remedy, treated of by Dioscorides, under the name of Indian Lykion, and much used by the Greek physicians. The same substance, "an inspissated extract, prepared from the wood or roots of several species of Berberis, as the Berberis Lycium, Aristata, &c., growing on the mountains and plains of Upper India," is still used for similar purposes by the native medical practitioners of India under the name of Rusat or Ruswut, and, from trials made by European physicians, appears, in cases suited to its employment, to be possessed of decided remedial properties. Independent of the interest felt in the vases themselves, as monuments of our art of so remote an antiquity, the subject is curious as another proof of the early commerce which subsisted between the remote east and the southern parts of Europe.

Iodide of Sodium.—Ruspini, an Italian physician, recommends the employment of the Iodide of Sodium in preference to the Iodide of Potassium, as more directly assimilable by the system, and less repugnant to the palate, it being entirely free from the acrid and ley like taste of the latter salt. For its preparation, he directs three ounces of iron filings to be added to two pounds and a half of distilled water; to this a pound of iodine is gradually added, the whole being constantly stirred. As soon as the mixture has acquired a uniform greenish color, it is to be filtered, and quickly treated with a solution of carbonate of soda, until all the iron is thrown down. The carbonate of iron is then separated by filtration, and the filtrate evaporated to dryness. The salt is re-dissolved, evaporated until a pellicle is formed, and set aside to crystallize. The crystals are white rhomboidal prisms, deliquescent, and of a saltish taste. The dose is about the same as that of the iodide of potassium, and the preparation has been found successful in cases which had resisted the influence of the latter preparation.

Number of Physicians and Pharmaciens in France.—In France there are 11,217 physicians, 7,221 officiers de santé, and 5,175 pharmaciens, about 1 medical attendant for every 1,040, and a pharmacien for every 6,914 of the population. There are nearly 600 towns or communes, with populations varying from 2,000 to 8,000 souls, which have neither physician nor pharmacien.

Tully's Materia and Pharmacology.—Dr. Tully's work, so far as it has yet proceeded, is occupied with generalities interesting to the physician rather than to the apothecary. Much that he says is open to criticism, much is contrary to received opinions, and, indeed, to well established facts, and the whole is enveloped in a strange and repulsive nomenclature, which, however, must be mastered to some extent, before we can arrive at the author's meaning. With all these drawbacks, we have no doubt that the work will contain much that is new and of real and permanent value. Dr. Tully does not travel in the beaten track; he is no mere retailer of other men's opinions, he has thought for himself, and, though he indulges largely in hypothesis and speculation, has likewise observed closely and acutely. We wait accordingly with great interest for that portion of the work which treats of the individual articles of the materia medica. With regard to the indigenous materia medica, of our own country in particular, we are persuaded Dr. Tully has much that is new and valuable to impart. From a notice of the publisher, we perceive that the publication of the first eight numbers is secured, but that the after continuation of the work will depend upon the success it meets with. We hope its success will be ample enough to render it remunerative, and we should look upon it as a national loss if the work should be stopped short of completion.

The Prescriber's Complete Hand-Book, *comprising the principles of the art of prescribing, materia medica coutaining all the principal medicines employed, and a concise sketch of pharmacy, by M. Trousseau, Professor of the Faculty of Medicine, Paris, and M. Reveil. Edited, with notes, by J. Birkbeck Nevins, M. D. London—Hyppolite Bailliere*, 219 *Regent street, and* 290 *Broadway, New York.* 18 *mo., pp.* 499.—If a great book is a great evil, much cannot be said for the small compends which so frequently issue from the press. They are condensed by the omission of all that is valuable, and hold out a promise of information which, when sought for, is found to be trivial and common-place. Such is by no means the case with the present volume; indeed the name of M. Trousseau is alone a sufficient guarantee for this. Designed mainly for medical students and practitioners, it gives a mass of information, admirably arranged, which will be of equal value to the apothecary. The book contains a short but excellent treatise on pharmacy, and, as the original is in French, it is of greater interest to our apothecaries, as affording a clear and succinct account of the preparations and modes of proceeding in France. The edition of M. Bailliere combines the advantages of good paper, admirable typography and moderate price. We could wish to see it in the hands of every apothecary and student of pharmacy throughout the country.

The American Journal of Pharmacy.—We had intended previously to have noticed the enlarged limits and improved appearance of the Philadelphia journal, but we hope it is not too late to congratulate our neighbors on the evidence it gives of past success and the hope it promises of increased usefulness. We wish them the success which is due to their enterprise.

NEW YORK

# JOURNAL OF PHARMACY.

MAY, 1853.

## ON QUINIDINE.

BY EDWARD N. KENT.

It has been recently asserted by M. Henry that quinidine is merely a hydrate of quinine, or quinine plus 2 atoms of water. This statement has been considered erroneous by other chemists, but no facts have been elicited which prove it to be so. From my own experiments on this subject, I am induced to believe that the two alkaloids are entirely dissimilar in their chemical composition.

Sulphate of quinine, dissolved in an aqueous solution of chlorine, and a few drops of ammonia added, furnishes a deep green color characteristic of quinine. Sulphate of quinidine, treated in the same manner, remains colorless if free from quinine.

Sulphate of quinine, dissolved in acetic acid, a few drops of tincture of iodine added, the mixture heated and allowed to cool, funishes a beautiful emerald green crystaline compound, called sulphate of iodo quinine by Dr. Herepath, its discoverer. Sulphate of quinidine, treated in the same manner, furnishes a *brown* precipitate.

The sulphate of quinine used for the above experiments was prepared by re-crystalizing the commercial salt. The sulphate of quinidine was prepared from a sample of pure quinidine, received from C. Zimmer, Frankfort-on-the-Maine. The first being a di-sulphate, and the second a neutral salt. The reaction with chlorine and ammonia being entirely independent of the acid or water of hydration, this test alone is sufficient to prove that quinidine is not a hydrate of quinine.

---

## APPLICATION OF THE DISPLACEMENT-METHOD IN PHARMACEUTICAL PRACTICE.

Herman Hendess, apothecary, at Sachsa, has prepared, by means of the displacement-method, a great number of extracts, tinctures, infusions, etc. For extracts, he found the method recommended by Bolle, of Angermünd, very satisfactory. He prepared by it the following extracts :—Extr. absinthii, bardanae, bistortae, cardui benedicti, cascarillae, centaurei minor, chamomillae, quassiae, chinae, dulcamarae stipitum, fumariae, graminis, ligni guaiaci, rubiae tinctor. marrubii, millefolii, quercus, ratanhiae, rad. glycyrrhizae, salicis, saponariae, secale cornuti aquos, sennae, simarubae, taraxaci, tormentillae, trifolii. The roots and bark were introduced into the apparatus in the form of coarse powder; herbs and flowers were put through a fine sieve. Extr. gentianae, rhei and scillae, on account of the large quantity of mucilaginous matter (Schleim) contained in these roots, cannot be so prepared, even when they are mixed in coarse powder with an equal quantity of sand, and introduced into the funnel, because the operation does not go on fast enough, and there is, therefore, danger, especially in summer, of the spoiling of the whole. The following table exhibits, comparatively, the quantities of extract obtained from some substances by the ordinary method of digestion and by the displacement-method:

| | By displacement. | By digestion. |
|---|---|---|
| 24 oz. rad. gramin | 11½ oz. extr | 11 oz. |
| 24 " cort. nuc. jugland immat. | 12 " " | 11⅛ " |
| 24 " " salicis | 6¼ " " | 4¼ " |
| 24 " " hb. cardui benedict | 9⅛ " " | 7 " |
| 24 " " rad. valerianae | 6¾ " " | 6 " |
| 24 " " hb. centaurei min | 7⅛ " " | 6¾ " |
| 24 " " folia trifolii aqu | 8½ " " | 7¼ " |

For narcotic extracts, the author prefers the method proposed by Scheidenmandel in Creuse. This method gave a great yield of extract. 1 lb. of fresh hb. hyoscyami yielded 2 oz. and 2 drachms of coarse powder, from which 7½ drachms of extract were obtained, whereas, by the ordinary method, one pound of fresh herb gives, on an average, only 4½ drachms extract.

Moreover, for aqueous, alcoholic and ethereal tinctures, the author found the displacement-method uniformly commendable. He prepared various tinctures, both by the ordinary method and by displacement, every other condition being equal, and, on comparing their specific gravities, he found them constantly higher in those made by displacement. Thus he found the specific gravity of

| | Prepared by digestion. | Prepared by displacement. |
|---|---|---|
| Tinc. chelidonii | 0.920 | 0.940 |
| " arnicae flor | 0.918 | 0.920 |
| " calami | 0.927 | 0.944 |
| " cascarillae | 0.904 | 0.952 |
| " digitalis | 0.920 | 0.940 |

Eight ounces of each of those tinctures were now evaporated to a moderate extract-consistence, and the residues weighed with the following results:

| | | By digestion. | By displacement. |
|---|---|---|---|
| Tinc. chelidonii | gave | 126 grains | ........220 grains. |
| " arnicae flor | " | 70 " | ........ 98 " |
| " calami | " | 88 " | ........160 " |
| " cascarillae | " | 128 " | ........160 " |
| " digitalis | " | 140 " | ........220 " |

For infusions, the author recommends the earthenware apparatus described by Schultz.—(*Archiv der Pharm.*, 1848, *Bd. II.*, *S.* 37.)

Finally, the displacement-method appears to be especially applicable for the preparation of *boiled oils*, because, in this case, no pressing out is necessary, and the oil is obtained at the same time ready filtered. As a displacement apparatus, the author uses, in many cases, a cylinder of tinned iron, the lower end of which is funnel-shaped. At the end of the cylindrical part, where the funnel is soldered on, a circular plate, perforated like a colander, is placed, upon which is laid filtering paper or flannel, according to the nature of the substance under preparation.—(*Archiv der Pharmacie CXXI.*, 30.)

H. W.

---

## PURIFICATION OF WHALE-OIL.

Saint-Simon-Sicard and Bonjour purify whale-oil by shaking it with three or four per cent. of potash or lime, and allowing it to settle. The purified oil separates itself from a thick mass which contains the impurities, such as blood, gelatine, etc.—(*Knop's Central-Blatt, August* 1852, *p.* 560.) H. W.

## LIQUOR FERRI ACETICI.

Bolle, apothecary, in Angermünd, has published a treatise upon liquor ferri acetici, in which he enumerates numerous casualities which have arisen from imperfections in this tincture, and, after mentioning various treatises, proposing improvements in its preparation, which have appeared hitherto, recounts some researches of his own, which had for their object the discussion of the following questions. What influence upon the permanence of this preparation have

(*a*) the kind of iron used in making it?

(*b*) the method of preparation of the acetic acid used?

(*c*) the relative proportions of oxide of iron and acetic acid?

(*d*) the temperature at which the oxide of iron is prepared?

(*e*) the degree of dilution of the liquor ferri acetici?

He obtained the following results:

(*a*) The greater or less purity of the iron employed does not appear to influence the decomposability of the preparation; for, although piano-forte wire is certainly a purer form of iron than iron-borings, yet the author found that a preparation made with the former actually decomposed sooner than one made with the latter.

(*b*) Bolle considers himself to have proved it probable that acetic acid, when it has been exposed to a high temperature, as when it is prepared from acetate of soda which has been fused, has undergone a certain modification, which he assimilates to the modifications which phosphoric acid, oil of turpentine, and other bodies are susceptible of; because, of all solutions of acetate of iron experimented upon by him, the decomposition began first in those made with acid derived from fused acetate of soda, while those in which the acid was derived from unfused acetate were much more permanent. The acetate of soda, in both cases, was made by the saturation of the same carbonate of soda by the same crude acetic acid.

[It is not necessary, however, granting the results of Bolle to be authentic, to suppose, with him, the important discovery of a new modification of acetic acid. It is more reasonable to suppose the presence in the acetic acid made from fused carbonate of soda, of some contamination, possibly sulphurous acid, which affects the stability of the medicinal preparation made therefrom.—H. W.]

(*c*) The decomposition of the iron solution is remarkably hastened by the presence of an excess of acetic acid.

(*d*) The author brings forward nothing of importance upon this point.

(*e*) The higher the specific gravity of the tincture, the longer it resists decomposition.—(*Archiv der Pharmacie*, 2 *R.*, *LXX.*, 264.) H. W.

---

## SYRUP OF PYROPHOSPHATE OF IRON.

BY E. SOUBEIRAN.

The pyrophosphate of iron and soda has been introduced into therapeutics, as having, among other special advantages, that of being easily taken by persons who cannot tolerate any other preparation of iron. I have had occasion to see two cases of this kind. The solution of pyrophosphate of iron, made after the following formula, was prescribed for them :

Dry per sulphate of iron..............6 grammes.
Crystallized pyrophosphate of soda....55 grammes.
Water............................q. s.

But this liquor has a salt, disagreeable taste ; to avoid which I have prepared the syrup after the formula I am about to give, and it has been taken without difficulty both by women and children.

I will first observe, that the pyrophosphate of soda is prepared by drying ordinary phosphate of soda, and fusing it at a red heat. The mass is re-dissolved by boiling water, filtered, and left to crystallize. A salt is obtained, whose formula is $2\ Na\ O + PO^5 + 10\ Aq$. It contains 40 per cent. of water of crystallization. It may be recognized by precipitating the salts of silver white, instead of yellow, like the ordinary phosphate of soda.

The pyrophosphate of iron corresponds to the preceding salt. Its formula is $2\ Fe^2\ O^3 + 3\ PO^5$. It is obtained by the double decomposition of the per sulphate of iron by pyrophosphate of soda. It is insoluble in water, but soluble in pyrophosphate of soda.

I now come to the syrup of pyrophosphate of iron:

Dry per sulphate of iron.........3 gram. 60 centig.
Water.......................60 gram.

Let it dissolve slowly, sometimes taking three or four days to it, or better still, let it dissolve in the vapor bath in a mattrass, or at a gentle heat.

In another vessel—

Crystallized pyrophosphate of soda........30 gram.
Pure water.............................220 gram.
Distilled mint water....................100 gram.

Dissolve them cold, or at a gentle heat. When the solution is quite cold, add to it the solution of the per sulphate of iron, and agitate them. At the moment of mixture, a precipitate is formed, which soon dissolves. Filter the liquor, and add:

Very white sugar...................590 grammes.

Dissolve it cold in a glass mattrass. The solution must be made either cold or, at least, at a temperature not over 50 degrees, otherwise the syrup would acquire a color of wine lees, which, at 70 or 80 degrees, would become very ark.

A spoonful (20 gram. of the syrup) contains 2 centigrammes of iron, in the condition of double pyrophosphate.

If the per sulphate of iron is not at hand, it may be prepared in a very short time in the following manner. For the above dose, or 1 kilogramme of syrup:

| | |
|---|---|
| Crystallized sulphate of iron | 5 gram. |
| Sulphuric acid | 1 gram. 60c. |
| Nitric acid | q. s. |

Put the sulphate in a capsule with a small quantity of water and sulphuric acid; warm it, and add nitric acid in small quantities, until no more nitrous vapors are disengaged; evaporate to dryness at a moderate heat; the product is neutral per sulphate of iron. By preparing a certain quantity beforehand, the trouble of repeating this operation at each manufacture of the syrup is avoided.—*Journ. de Pharm. et Chem., Jan.*, 1853.

---

## CHLORINE FUMIGATING-BALLS.

Sigl, apothecary in Munich, proposes to knead together with water the following substances, viz.:—Powdered common salt, copperas and potter's clay, of each 1½ lb., with 2 oz. manganese, and form the mass into balls of any desired size. These balls are applied for the purpose of fumigation, by throwing them upon hot coals, a slow evolution of chlorine being thus obtained.—(*Archiv der Pharmacie, CXXI.*, 76.)

H. W.

# FORMATION OF CARBONATE OF SODA ON A STOVE OF CAST IRON.

BY H. REINSCH.

A few months ago, I had a large stove of cast iron put up in my laboratory, of which the upper-plate, holding together the four walls, was luted with clay. The stove was not used for two weeks, and, therefore, no fire made in it. Already, on the eighth day, the joints on the plate were coated with a snow white mass, like wool, which appeared as extremely fine crystals, possessing an alkaline taste. This joint (about four yards round the stove) was coated, after two weeks, with a film of fine crystalline appearance, nearly half an inch broad and four-fifths of an inch thick, and was found after examination to be almost chemically pure carbonate of soda, containing much water of crystallization, and being very efflorescent, as soon as removed from the stove. Evidently this carbonate of soda was formed by galvanic action. The clay containing a salt of soda was decomposed by the electric current generated by the cast-iron plate and the British lustre spread over it. The soda (rather sodium ?) thus formed was converted into the carbonate by the oxygen and carbonic acid of the atmospheric air. After the fire of the stove had exsiccated the clay, no more carbonate of soda was formed.

This observation, although appearing slight, may be tried on a large scale, for other silicates will be decomposed as well as soda, which exists in the clay of silicate. I would merely mention of what consequence it were to obtain the potash in feldspar ; for I published already, eight years ago, that this mineral is decomposed by an electric current, and the experiment may readily be made with large batteries, constructed of cast iron plates, coated with British lustre, (graphites,) with the finely pulverized and acidulated feldspar placed between them. If we consider that feldspathic granite contains sometimes ten parts of potash in one hundred, we comprehend what immense quantities of potash could be obtained from these rocks, and how important a source of potash they might prove for soap, glass factories, agriculture, economy, etc., etc.

---

## PREPARATION OF SULPHATE OF ALUMINA.

The brothers Hurrier and Brunel, of Urcel, (Department of Aisne, France,) manufacture sulphate of alumina from ammonia-alum as follows:

The ammonia-alum is placed upon flat earthenware vessels in a drying-oven, to expel all its crystal-water. It is then pulverised and placed in a cast-iron cylinder, having at one end an iron cover, which may be luted on air tight. From the other end of this cylinder extends a cast-iron tube, connected with leaden pipes, which are full of holes, and lie horizontally in a wooden tank, lined with lead, which is filled with water to absorb the evolved gases. A safety tube is introduced to prevent the water from flowing back into the cylinder. A cherry-red heat is now applied, which decomposes the ammonia-alum, sulphate of alumina being left in the cylinder. The sulphite of alumina, which is one of the products of the decomposition, is used over again for making ammonia-alum, after having been converted into sulphate by oxydation in the air. The drying-oven lies over the oven in which the cast-iron cylinder is placed, and is heated by its waste heat.—(*Knop's Central-Blatt, August,* 1852, *p.* 544.) H. W.

# ON THE TESTS FOR THE CINCHONA-ALKALOIDS, KINOVIC ACID, KINIC ACID, AND OXIDIZED TANNIN (CINCHONA RED) IN CINCHONA BARKS.

BY DR. F. L. WINCKLER.

Of all long-known drugs none have in recent times so much engaged the attention of chemists as cinchona bark—the discovery of the various alkaloids contained in it having afforded a safe standard for the determination of its goodness.

This circumstance has been accompanied by a large number of results, which are of great importance in medical practice. It has removed the uncertainty of the notion of genuine and spurious barks, and made it possible to distinguish the former from the latter, and to determine their real value.

The excellent work of Von Bergen forms the foundation of our knowledge of the cinchona barks. Its theoretical part contains everything that could be obtained at the time of its appearance; but Von Bergen's account of the mercantile relations of this drug is of greater value, because nothing certain was known on this point before, and because for the medicinal use of barks an accurate knowledge of the material imported is certainly of greater importance than the origin of the barks. Notwithstanding all our present information, a long time must elapse before we can accurately arrange the barks imported into Europe, because, in consequence of the greatly increased consumption, for the purpose of obtaining the alkaloids, new sources are rendered necessary, and new districts in the native country are explored, by which, doubtless, new species of cinchona are discovered.

The correctness of this view is shown by the present occurrence of a considerable number of barks which were hitherto unknown; as, for example, the barks containing quinidine and paricine, and the numerous sorts of the so-called yellow barks; and it may without hesitation be asserted that these barks contain also a larger number of alkaloids than is known at present.

I have read with much interest Weddell's excellent work, from which Dr. Riegel, some time since, extracted (See Pharmaceutical Journal, vol. ix., p. 224) the information which is of most importance to the pharmaceutist. Although I am far from undervaluing the high merits of this distinguished traveller, the successor of Humboldt and Pöppig, I am, notwithstanding, of opinion that too great importance must not be attached to his researches. I consider that his proposal to determine the goodness of barks by their anatomical structure, has no greater value than as an application to botany generally, and to vegetable physiology in particular, for I have convinced myself, by numerous and most carefully performed experiments, that his assertion, that the shortly fibrous barks contain the largest proportion of alkaloid cannot be admitted, as its truth has been directly disproved. It is only applicable to calisaya bark, and even in that case has many exceptions. Were this alone not sufficient to raise doubts about the possibility of judging the goodness of barks by their structure, there is also another circumstance to be taken into consideration. The anatomical structure of bark is, as is well known, uninterruptedly progressive during vegetation; each stage offers a new formation, the bark of the trunk appears very different from that of the larger branches, and that of these varies again in its structure from the bark of the smaller branches. Lastly, we ought to examine the barks as Weddell did, in their fresh condition, in order to be enabled to judge of their structure. These views of Weddell's, however interesting they may be in other respects, are, I am convinced, of a very subordinate value for medical practice. We must, therefore, still follow the chemico-analytical route, if we wish to establish a scientific and safe classification of the cinchona barks.

Dr. Riegel was, no doubt, of the same opinion, when he appended to his extract from Weddell's work a synopsis of all the known methods of determining the proportion of alkaloids; and I am much surprised how he, under these circumstances, could express some doubts whether my experiments perfectly agreed with Weddell's statements about the origin of the barks, which was scarcely possible. All my experiments refer only to commercial barks, by the names under which they occur in commerce, and I have described their physical characters. Weddell, on the other hand, had quite another object in view, namely, the origin of the barks; and he made no comparative chemical investigations of them. Nevertheless, he, like his predecessors, has left us in uncertainty about the origin of many commercial barks; for I never can persuade myself that Loxa bark and the woody Carthagena bark are derived from the same mother-plant, Cinchona Condaminea; and every one who knows and has chemically examined both barks will perfectly agree with me.

We ought, therefore, while fully acknowledging Weddell's merits, not to overlook the difficulties of the subject. It would be unjust to expect that a traveller struggling with hardships of every kind should perform chemical experiments on the spot. This would be contrary to the purposes of so great an undertaking.

My object has hitherto been to arrange the commercial barks according to the specific proportion of alkaloid which they contain, as I have already done, in a small treatise.

There is, indeed, nothing that could materially obstruct such an arrangement, especially as by the discovery of the kinates we are enabled easily to distinguish similar spurious barks from genuine ones, whilst every uncertainty may be removed by one single experiment. Discrepancies like that which Riegel has noticed with regard to the chemical constitution of Pitaya or bicolorata bark, depend on the mistaking of one bark for another, which frequently arises from the employment of erroneous names. The bark which Peretti examined as cinchona bicolorata, cannot be identical with that whose alkaloid richness Muratori determined. According to Peretti, and his experiments agree with mine, the bark which he examined contained a peculiar, amorphous, uncrystallizable alkaloid (Peretti's *pittayin*) and is *decidedly no cinchona.*

As regards the testing of cinchona barks for the alkaloids, no notice has hitherto been taken of the proportion of kinovic acid, but as the very bitter taste of the spurious cinchona barks depends exclusively on this acid, and in some of the genuine barks kinovic acid is found, a mistake may be easily made by the taste. I have, for several years past, devised and employed a method by which not only the proportion of the alkaloid but also that of the kinovic acid may be quantitatively and qualitatively determined, whilst, at the same time, the proportion of both kinic acid and oxidized tannin (cinchona red) is indicated. So that all those constituents of the bark, which are of importance for medical practice, are determined.

The barks tested by this method yield, when employed for the manufacture of the alkaloid on a large scale, exactly the same quantity which they yield by the experiment, generally one-eighth to one-quarter per cent. more, the loss in working with large quantities being naturally less in proportion, and this, indeed, is the best proof of the efficiency of this method.

In the qualitative examination of cinchona barks, a number of tests have hitherto been employed, which have not only not aided this examination but have rendered it much more difficult.

The efficacy of the bark depends, as is well known, chiefly on the proportion of alkaloid, and of that of pure and oxidized cinchona-tannin. Of the kinovic acid, we only know that it does not act as a febrifuge. The medicinal virtues of kinic acid, or kinate of lime, have not yet been determined. We must, therefore, confine ourselves to the application of those tests by means of which these compounds can be detected in an infusion of bark, and their quantitative proportion at least approximatively determined. These are, as has been before stated in my monograph on genuine barks, as follows:

1. *Tannin*, for detecting the alkaloids. The more abundant the precipitate produced by this reagent in the aqueous filtered infusion, the more alkaloid do the barks contain.

2. *Chloride of iron* determines the proportion of oxidized tannin by the more or less intensely dark-grey coloration, which speedily becomes brown, and by the subsequent more or less abundant pulverulent precipitate of a dark, dirty, brownish-green color.

3. *Gelatine* (*solution of isinglass*), like chloride of iron, occasions the oxidized tannin to be precipitated. In the liquid filtered from the magma, the proportion of non-oxidized cinchona-tannin may be determined by iodic acid. The latter oxidizes the tannin, and causes the precipitation of a yellowish-brown powder; the mixture soon smells of iodine. The quantities of these two precipitates show the proportion of oxidized and of pure cinchona-tannin.

4. *Sulphate of copper* is perfectly indifferent to the aqueous infusion of bark, which contains no kinovic acid, but indicates the smallest proportion of this acid by a dirtyish green coloration of the mixture, which is speedily followed by a similarly colored fine powder, which is easily separated by the filter, and, after being washed, is distinctly recognized, by its very bitter and metallic taste, as kinovate of copper. The more abundant this precipitate, the greater is the proportion of kinovic acid. All other reagents hitherto employed can be absolutely dispensed with.

Of all the hitherto known methods for the quantitative determination of the alkaloids, I prefer the following:—If the quantity of bark at command be large, it is necessary, in the first place, to ascertain whether it consist of one or of several sorts. An experienced eye can readily determine this. The several sorts should be separated, and, for experiment, not too small a quantity selected from the entire mass of the coated and uncoated of the coarser and finer barks, taking of each sort according the various dimensions in which it is contained in the whole mass, about an equal weight. These pieces are to be finely powdered, and the residue mixed with the powder. Of this powder five hundred grains or one thousand grains are to be completely exhausted by digestion in the water-bath, with the necessary quantity of alcohol of eighty per cent. (I use six ounces of alcohol for one thousand grains bark); the cold tincture is to be strained through a thin but close piece of linen, the residue washed with alcohol and again digested, and completely exhausted with half the weight of the first employed quantity of alcohol. The residue which is now obtained to be once more exhausted by alcohol, then dried and preserved. (There is no occasion to spare the alcohol in this process, as the greater portion of it is recovered.) The united alcoholic tinctures are to be filtered and digested at the common temperature, with a mixture of equal parts by weight of recently prepared slacked lime and of crude well-burnt animal charcoal, of which in general half the weight of the employed bark is required. The mixture is to be frequently shaken, and the digestion continued until the supernatant liquid becomes perfectly decolorized. In the case of most of the genuine barks, this takes place in a short time; but the alcoholic tinctures of the spurious barks, which contain kinovic acid, as well as those which contain paracin, are very imperfectly decolorized by this process, a circumstance which serves to distinguish the paracin barks and spurious barks from the genuine ones.

The decolorized liquid is now to be removed from the residue, and the latter repeatedly shaken with small quantities of alcohol, washed on the filter with spirit of wine and dried. From the mixed filtered alcoholic tinctures the greater portion of the alcohol can be recovered by distillation in the water-bath. Beindorff's distillatory apparatus with Liebig's refrigerator is well adapted for this purpose—a similar and much cheaper apparatus can be constructed of tin. The whole quantity of alkaloid which was contained in the bark is now in the residue, and if the bark contained kinovic acid, in combination with the latter, and a peculiar fatty substance. Small proportions of oxidized tannin are frequently mechanically mixed with it. In order to purify the alkaloid of the latter, and to remove the kinovic acid and fatty matter, the residue is to be placed in a small evaporating basin, the distilling vessel is to be washed with a small quantity of water, slightly acidulated with sulphuric acid, and the solution added to the residue. A small excess of diluted sulphuric acid is to be dropped into this mixture, which is to be heated, and, when it again becomes cold, is to be filtered, and by this means the precipitated kinovic acid and fatty matter are removed and washed with distilled water. From the filtered acid solution the alkaloid is to be thrown down by a slight excess of ammonia; and the mixture evaporated by a slight heat to dryness. The sulphate of ammonia contained in the cold residue is to be removed by a small quantity of very cold water, and the residual alkaloid dried and weighed in this impure state; for the perfect purification of small quantities is attended with too great a loss to admit of the exact determination of the quantity of alkaloid contained in small quantities of bark. After having thus determined the weight of the alkaloid the further examination of it is proceeded with, the cinchonine and quinine are separated by ether, &c.

In order to determine the proportion of kinovic acid, dilute solution of ammonia is to be added to the yellowish, glutinous matter which adheres to the filter, and which is, for the most part, greasy to the touch. This takes up the kinovic acid, but not the fat. The solution is to be filtered, and to it a slight excess of muriatic acid added, to precipitate the kinovic acid, which is then to be collected on a filter. The well washed glutinous precipitate is to be removed whilst moist from the filter, and dried upon a watch-glass or porcelain capsule, and the weight of the thus obtained kinovic acid marked down. This, however, is only the larger portion of the quantity of kinovic acid actually obtained from the bark. A smaller portion of it is still contained, combined with lime, in the lime-residue which has been digested with the alcoholic tincture of bark. This kinovate of lime is very difficultly soluble in spirit of wine.

In order to obtain this smaller portion, the lime-residue, exhausted by alcohol, is to be dried and powdered, and then digested with cold distilled water. From the filtered liquid, which is almost as clear as water, the white and nearly pure kinovic acid is thrown down by a very slight excess of muriatic acid. It is then to be weighed, and the sum added to that before obtained. By the direct treatment of powdered bark with milk of lime, the whole quantity of kinovic acid can be extracted from the bark. Also for the quantitative determination of the acid it is advisable to weigh it in the imperfectly pure condition, the loss accompanying the purification being very considerable.

If the qualitative examination of the bark has shown that this substance contains none, or only a small proportion, of alkaloid, but a large quantity of kinovic acid, or the latter only, the bark is more appropriately first treated with diluted milk of lime, and the kinovic acid precipitated by muriatic acid, by which method the testing of the residue for a possibly slight proportion of alkaloid is considerably facilitated. The dry residue of lime is then exhausted by alcohol, like the powdered bark, &c. In this manner I obtained from sixteen ounces of bark, containing kinovic acid, one grain of cinchonine, besides a large quantity of kinovic acid. The last more important constituent of the bark, the kinic acid, is now easily obtained by exhausting the residue of the bark, which has been treated by alcohol, with cold distilled water, evaporating the filtered liquid and distilling it in a not too concentrated state with peroxide of manganese and moderately strong sulphuric acid; the least proportion of kinic acid in the liquid is soon indicated by the development and evolution of kinone, which takes place during this process; and the smallest quantity of the kinone, which is not distinctly perceptible by the smell, may be soon detected by the dark color, which the distillate assumes upon the addition of a few drops of a solution of ammonia.

This method of testing barks is distinguished from others by its great simplicity, by the correctness of the results, and by the possibility of detecting and quantitatively determining in one succession, and with the same material, all the more important constituents of the bark; I consider it as the best method known, not because it originates with me, but because it is adapted to the present stage of our knowledge of the chemical composition of cinchona barks, and *is practical.* It may be objected that it is rather troublesome, but this ought not to be of any consideration if we can be but sure of a correct result.

In conclusion, I must observe, that my method, though chiefly adapted for testing genuine barks, can be advantageously applied for examining new and apparently spurious barks. The occurring phenomena will then safely guide the experienced operator. With the barks containing paricine, the separation of the alkaloid is made very difficult, by its forming with the cinchona red, contained in the bark, compounds soluble in acids and alkalies, which can be decomposed only with great difficulty. I refer in this respect to my last treatise on the Production and the Chemical Condition of Paricine, in Buchner's *Repertorium.—Jahrbuch, f. Pharm.*, Bd. xxv., III., Sept., 1852, p. 129, *and Pharmaceutical Journal.*

---

## PURPLE INK FOR MARKING LINEN.

The portion of the linen which is to be marked is first wetted with a solution of 3 parts of carbonate of soda, and 3 parts of gum-arabic, in 12 parts of distilled water, dried and ironed. The writing is then made with a solution of 1 part of bichloride of platinum in 16 parts of distilled water, using of course a quill pen, and permitted to dry. After thoroughly drying, each character is brushed over with the feather of a goose-quill dipped into a solution of 1 part of protochloride of tin in 16 parts of distilled water.—(*Knop's Central-Blatt, September*, 1852, *p.* 608.) H. W.

# CORTEX *ALSTONIÆ SCHOLARIS.*

TO THE EDITOR OF THE PHARMACEUTICAL JOURNAL.

SIR—I have lately brought to Europe for distribution and trial, a medicine which, though in occasional use among the natives of some parts of India, has, to the best of my knowledge, never had a place in the general Pharmacopœia even of the Eastern physicians. In fact, it is a drug known only to the forest practitioners, who have a knowledge of the virtues of trees and herbs very far exceeding that possessed by the more civilized Indian native practitioners. These latter deal much more largely, and I may safely add much more destructively, in mineral remedies.

The medicine now under report is the bark of *Alstonia scholaris* R. Br., a great tree of the natural order *Apocyneæ*, found in the forests of Malabar, Canara, Soonda, and some other parts of India, and brother to the smaller *Alstonia venenata* R. Br., which (as the name imports) is very poisonous. It has obtained the trivial name *scholaris* from the fact of small planks of its finely-grained white wood being commonly used in some localities for the school-boards whereon the children trace their letters (with sand) as in the Lancastrian system, originally imported from the East. I had long known that the bark of the tree was occasionally used in bowel affections, but, from the suspiciously active family to which it belongs, I had dreaded to bring it into practical use, as my own opportunities for doing so were very limited, and I deemed it more than possible that its use in the hands of others might not be managed so cautiously as circumstances appeared to require.

Major Del'Hoste, of the Bombay army, had procured a quantity of the bark, and, having made a tincture from it, used it with some success in bowel complains, occasionally very prevalent in the extensive native establishments which he had under his control while constructing a new road in the south of India. When I visited the major in the course of a forest tour, I rejoiced to find that he had thus paved the way for a successful trial of the drug. I have since then repeatedly used it as a remedy in diarrhœa attended with tormina, and even with tenesmus, and I can safely say that in every case it has given relief to the symptoms. The relief has most gene rally been permanent, occasionally only temporary, and such as to require a repetition of the dose. My practical experience of its effects has not been sufficiently continuous to enable me to indicate the particular state of alvine or biliary secretion to which its use is most applicable. Points like these are for the determination of the clinical practitioner, having leisure and opportunity to record the results of hospital practice. It has also appeared to me to possess marked effects in promoting the expulsion of intestinal lumbrici. Of its effects in cholera, European or Asiatic, I have as yet only one case recorded, and that of the European form of the disease. The patient, a tailor, in Edinburgh, was treated solely with this medicine, and (as the accompanying letter testifies*) with the best effect. I send the

* The following is the letter referred to :—

"MY DEAR SIR—I cannot delay so long as till I see you, the pleasure of telling you about a very severe case of British cholera treated entirely with *Tinctura alstoniæ.* On Monday morning last a man was lying in a low house in Carruther's Close, having been in bed since the Friday, on which day he was seized with violent vomiting and purging, and when I saw him on the Monday he had taken nothing but a dose of castor oil, and had not tasted food since the Friday. He was very low and exhausted, with frequent clear watery evacuations, mixed with a quantity of clear mucus, showing the lining membrane of the bowels to be in a very irritable state. I immediately went up to Baillie Macfarlane's and got two ounces of *Tinct. alstoniæ*, and administered one teaspoonful, directing his wife to give him some toasted bread with hot water poured on it. In an hour and a quarter I called back; he had had three evacuations since I had seen him. I gave him another teaspoonful, and saw him an hour and a half afterwards, during which interval he had *no evacuation.* I made him some arrowroot with a little brandy in it, which he took, and it lay on his stomach, and, in half an hour, gave a third teaspoonful. He was now decidedly better, and felt inclined to sleep, so I left him. The next morning (Tuesday) better; had no stool since I saw him last, but much exhausted and sore all over. To-day he was up and at his work, which is a blessing, as he has a wife and five children depending on him. His name is Hugh Short, a tailor. Mr. Gibson will know who he is. The *Tinctura alstoniæ* seems, so far as I can judge, to be a fine aromatic astringent bitter, and the sooner it has a place in the Pharmacopœia of the Edinburgh College the bet-

case for your perusal. In the Central Hospital of Bombay it was tried in chronic diarrhœa, and the cases treated by means of it seemed to have an average of success about equal to those which were treated by other means. From this we may possibly infer that its use is less indicated in these chronic affections than in the sudden and more severe attacks attended by tormina. As I have now forwarded some for trial to Dr. Christison, of Edinburgh, to M. Guibourt, of Paris, to Mr. Quekett, of the College of Surgeons, to Mr. Macfarlane, druggist, Edinburgh, and to yourself, I indulge the hope that we may be able to have a good estimate of its value as a medicine in diarrhœa and in cholera, also as a vermifuge applicable to the destruction of lumbrici, which, from our experience in the East, we find to be almost invariably present in some visitations of epidemic cholera.

I have usually formed the tincture with ℥iij. of the bark, coarsely bruised, to a pint of proof spirit, and I have also occasionally given the powdered bark in a pill, combined with rhubarb, ipecacuanha and extract of gentian. The dose of the powder may vary from three to five grains.

I have the honor to be, Sir,
Your most obedient servant,
ALEXANDER GIBSON,
Surgeon Bombay Establishment.

*London*, 9*th Feb.*, 1853.

—*Pharmaceutical Journal*, *March*, 1853.

---

ter. I have no doubt that within twelve months it will be a known and *fashionable* medicine, for, strange to say, medicines have their fashions as well as ladies' dresses, and a new one is always in fashion; but I hope this will be something more, indeed a standard remedy in *all* bowel complaints, and be the means of doing away with pernicious treatment by means of drugs containing opium, substituting as it does a simple and uncomplicated medicine.

"I am, my dear Sir, most truly yours,

"*Willow Bank Newhaven*, *Nov.* 10, 1852. "WILLIAM GRAY.

"*To* DR. ALEXANDER GIBSON."

# USE OF COFFEE-LEAVES IN SUMATRA.

From the *Overland Singapore Free Press*, published Jan. 3, 1853, we extract the following letter, signed "*An old Sumatran*," upon the use of coffee-leaves for the preparation of a beverage in the island of Sumatra. We briefly alluded in the *Pharmaceutical Journal* for June, 1852, (Vol. xi., p. 578) to a project for employing coffee-leaves in this country as a substitute for tea:

"In the *Singapore Free Press* of the 17th September last, are extracts from the *Colombo Observer*, by which it appears a patent has been taken out by Dr. Gardner (known to us by his travels in South America*) for preparing the coffee-leaf in a manner to afford a beverage like tea, that is, by infusion, 'forming an agreeable, refreshing and nutritive article of diet.'

"It may be interesting to Dr. Gardner, his friends, and the public in general, to learn that an infusion of the coffee-leaf is an article of universal consumption amongst the natives of this part of Sumatra ; wherever coffee is grown, the leaf has become one of the very few necessaries of life which the natives regard as indispensable.

"The coffee plant in a congenial soil and climate exhibits great luxuriance in its foliage, throwing out abundance of suckers and lateral stems, especially when from any cause the main stem is thrown out of the perpendicular, to which it is very liable from its great superincumbent weight compared with the hold of its roots in the ground. The native planters, availing themselves of this propensity, often give the plant a considerable inclination, not only to increase the foliage, but to obtain new fruit-bearing stems when the old ones become unproductive. It is also found desirable to limit the height of

---

* It is Dr. John Gardner, of London, who exhibited prepared coffee-leaves at the Great Exhibition of 1851. Mr. George Gardner, late Superintendent of the Botanical Garden at Peradenia, Ceylon, and author of *Travels in the Interior of Brazil*, died in Ceylon, in March, 1849.—Ed. *Pharm. Journ.*

the plant by lopping off the top, to increase the produce and facilitate collecting it, and fresh sprouts in abundance are the certain consequence. These are so many causes of the development of a vegetation which becomes injurious to the quantity of the fruit or berry unless removed; and where this superabundant foliage can be converted into an article of consumption, as hitherto the case in Sumatra, the culture must become the more profitable, and it is clearly the interest of the planters of Ceylon to respond to the call of Dr. Gardner, and by supplying the leaf on reasonable terms, to assist in creating a demand for an article they have in abundance, and which for the want of that demand is of no value to them. It ought to be mentioned, also, that the leaves which become ripe and yellow on the tree and fall off in the course of nature, contain the largest portion of extract, and make the richest infusion; and I have no doubt, should the coffee-leaf ever come into general use, the ripe leaf will be collected with as much care as the ripe fruit.

"The mode of preparation by the natives is thus:—The ends of the branches and suckers with the leaves on, are taken from the tree, and broken into lengths of from twelve to eighteen inches. These are arranged in the split of a stick or small bamboo, side by side, forming a truss in such a manner that the leaves all appear on one side and the stalks on the other, the object of which is to secure equal roasting, the stalks being thus exposed to the fire together and the leaves together. The slit being tied up in two or three places, and a part of the stick or bamboo left as a handle, the truss is held over a fire without smoke, and kept moving about so as to roast the whole equally without burning, on the success of which operation the quality and flavor of the article much depends. When successfully roasted the raw vegetable taste is entirely dissipated, which is not the case if insufficiently done. When singed or overdone, the extract is destroyed and the aroma lost. When the fire is smoky, the flavor varies with the nature of the smoke. The stalks are roasted equally with the leaves, and are said to add fully as much to the strength of the infusion. By roasting, the whole becomes brittle, and is reduced to a coarse powder by rubbing between the hands. In this state it is ready for use, and the general mode of preparing the beverage is by infusion, as in the case of common tea.

"If the testimony of one who has been long personally accustomed to the use of an infusion of the coffee-leaf thus prepared can be of any avail in recommending the article to public notice, I freely offer mine in support of all that which Dr. Gardner's patent claims for it, viz., 'as forming an agreeable, refreshing and nutritive article of diet.' While I find the use of infusion of the *berry* for a few days invariably to produce on me, as on many others, the effects of nervousness and bilious obstruction, I drink a strong infusion of the *leaf* daily with evident benefit to my health and strength. As a restorative on exhaustion from the severities of labor or of the weather, from heat or cold, or long exposure to rain, I know nothing superior to it. It has also the advantage of being a powerful disinfectant, so far as neutralizing fœtidity goes, and a solvent of the viscid fluids which obstruct the circulation, often to the extent of becoming laxative if taken in extra quantity. Of its nutritive power, no proof can be stronger than that it suspends hunger and enables the laboring man to pursue his work for hours after he would be otherwise unable. That it would soon become a most valuable article of diet amongst the laboring classes, and on ship-board particularly, if once brought into use, there can be no doubt. The coffee-tree can be grown to advantage for the leaf in the lowlands of every tropical country where the soil is sufficiently fertile, whilst it requires soil and climate to produce the fruit.

"Nothing appears in the *Free Press* on the mode of its preparation by Dr. Gardner, but I should think if roasted and pulverized, and packed in air-tight cases like tea, it would retain its strength and bear transporting to every part of the world; and as it soon fixes itself more strongly than either tea or coffee in the taste, it would soon become a more absolute necessary of life than either of those articles. In fact, I am acquainted with no tropical production capable of being rendered so great a blessing to mankind as the coffee-leaf, and as it would tend materially to the desuetude of ardent spirits and strong drinks, its introduction ought to have the support of every friend to the moral and material welfare of society."

*Padang*, 12*th November*, 1852.

—*Pharmaceutical Journal*, *March*, 1853.

---

## ON A NEW SOURCE OF KINO.

BY ROBERT CHRISTISON, M. D., V. P. R. S. E.,
*Professor of Materia Medica in the University of Edinburgh.*

In a letter of the 20th of last July, from a merchant of Moulmein, Mr. R. S. Begbie, son of Dr. Begbie, of this city, I was informed that a species of kino—which seemed to him to present the physical and chemical properties of the commercial variety of that drug in the English home market, and which had been ascertained by a medical friend, at Moulmein, to possess also its medicinal virtues—might be largely obtained from a tree abounding in the adjacent provinces. Mr. Begbie added, that he believed "a small quantity had been sent some years ago to England; but as an article of export, generally, it has not yet been shipped." This notice was accompanied by a small specimen, which is now produced, and which is large enough to allow of its principal properties being accurately ascertained.

As the inquiries I have made lead me to suppose that the article in question is of a very fine kind, and that the fact of its production near Moulmein, and probably over a considerable part of the neighboring province of Pegue, is not hitherto known in Europe, I beg to present to the Pharmaceutical Society the following description of it, and the reasons which induce me to think that it is obtained from the identical tree which yields, in Malabar, the present commercial kino of European trade.

The small portion sent by Mr. Begbie consists partly of little angular fragments; but there are several larger masses which are portions of cylinders, about half an inch in diameter, apparently moulded by collecting the juice in reeds. These have externally a greyish, striated surface, most unlike that of the broken fragments of commercial kino. They are easily frangible; and the broken pieces have exactly the appearance of ordinary kino, except that they are even blacker, and more glassy by reflected light; and by transmitted light, though opaque when of very moderate thickness, they are of a splendid cherry-red color in very thin fragments. They are easily reduced to fine powder, which has a dark, dirty, lake tint. Their taste is very slightly bitter, and intensely astringent.

Cold water acts more quickly on this kino than on the kino of commerce, gradually dissolving a very large proportion of it, and forming a deep cherry-red astringent solution; and there is left a small proportion of greyish flocculent matter, which is slowly soluble, in a great measure, in boiling water, and which appears to be analogous to the insoluble variety of gum called bassorin. Boiling water dissolves this kino almost entirely, and the solution, when cold, continues nearly transparent for at least an hour; but afterwards it becomes slightly turbid, and a scanty, flocculent precipitate slowly subsides. Both the hot and cold solutions yield, when much diluted, a deep olive-green precipitate with the tincture of sesqui-chloride of iron; and when the solution is concentrated, a dirty grey precipitate is formed so abundantly that the whole fluid becomes a thick pulpy mass. A boiling solution in twenty-five parts of water forms with the iron test a pulp too thick to flow, which is one of the characters assigned in the Edinburgh Pharmacopœia to true officinal kino. But I find further that a solution in even seventy-five parts of cold water has a beautiful intense cherry-red color, and forms with sesqui-chloride of iron, in the course of an hour, a pulp so thick as to flow only sluggishly.

On comparing these characters with a fine specimen of kino of home trade, and also with a specimen collected in the neighborhood of Goomsoor, in Mysore, by Dr. Cleghorn, of the Madras Medical Service, when he was surgeon of the surveying corps in that country, I find that the last two are identical, with the single exception that Dr. Cleghorn's specimen is somewhat redder when seen in bulk, and that the Moulmein kino is blacker, more vitreous in lustre, rather more easily soluble in cold water, and with rather less flaky residue; and when the cold solution is diluted to the strength of one in seventy-five, it requires rather more sesqui-chloride of iron to throw down all its tannin, and consequently the precipitate forms with the water a somewhat firmer pulp.

The kino dissolves, with only a trace of flaky residue, in rectified spirit, which forms an intense cherry-red tincture, of very pure astringent taste. The quantity in my possession is scarcely sufficient to allow of a fuller examination of its chemical properties and composition. But its physical characters, the action of water, and the properties of the watery solution, even as I have shortly indicated them, are enough to prove that the Moulmein kino is identical in nature with the present kino of home trade, and in point of quality somewhat superior. I have no doubt, from its taste, and the action of the iron test, that an analysis will prove the presence of a larger proportion of tannin.

It does not absolutely follow, even from the exact correspondences now mentioned, that the Moulmein kino is derived from the same botanical source with the present officinal kino of Europe. The officinal sort has been accurately referred by the separate researches of Dr. Gibson, Dr. Pereira, and Dr. Royle, to the *Pterocarpus Marsupium* of Roxburgh, a fine forest tree abounding in the hills of Mysore and other parts of the Indian Peninsula. But the *Butea frondosa* also yields a fine kino, which I have shown in my Dispensatory to be scarcely distinguishable in chemical properties from the officinal kind.

Mr. Begbie, however, has fortunately supplied me with a description of the Moulmein tree, sufficient to identify it with the true kino tree of Mysore. "It is," says he, "one of the commonest trees in the adjoining provinces, and is called by the Burmese, *Padouk*. It grows to a great size and height. Immediately before the rainy season it is covered with long pendant yellow flowers, of an exeeedingly sweet odor, like that of jessamine. The tree flowers three times, at intervals of perhaps a week or ten days, each blow lasting about twenty-four hours. The wood is in color like mahogany, and exceedingly heavy. It is used in India for making gun-carriages; and at present we are preparing some for the London market, in execution of an order, I fancy, for the Royal artillery. It makes most beautiful furniture. The gum exudes slightly without incision; but on a cut being made into the tree, it bleeds freely." This description is not sufficiently botanical to enable me to determine the tree from its characters in botanical works. But on submitting Mr. Begbie's letter to Dr. Gibson, Conservator of the Forests of Bombay, who very lately visited Edinburgh, that gentleman at once recognized his old acquaintance of the Indian woods, the *Pterocarpus Marsupium*; which he was one of the first to discover to be the true source of kino, by observing that, when his companions, on a shooting party, cut their names into the bark of a tree beside which they had been resting, a red juice freely exuded, and concreted into a dark astringent gum, like the kino of commerce.

## UPON THE PASSAGE OF COLORING MATTER INTO THE URINE.

Kletzinsky has made researches upon the passage of the coloring matters of plants into the urine, with saffron and hematoxylin, and found that neither of them pass into the urine. The saffron-pigment or polychroite colors itself with nitric acid, at first red, then blueish, then green; with sulphuric acid, dark lilac; with baryta-water, red. In the urine of a person who has taken saffron, no polychroite can be discovered, although, on being mixed with concentrated sulphuric acid, it diffuses a strong smell of saffron. Neither do the fæces give any indication of the presence of the coloring matter.—(*Knop's Central-Blatt, September*, 1852, *p.* 623.)

H. W.

---

## DEATH OF JONATHAN PEREIRA, M. D., F. R. S., &c.

In all ages and in all conditions of society it has been customary, on the death of any distinguished individual, to commemorate the name of the deceased by recording the good deeds which in life rendered him illustrious. This has been done, not so much, perhaps, as a tribute of respect to the dead as an incentive to the practice of virtue by the living; and surely there is no character which presents so many opportunities for useful comment and example as that which, amidst the difficulties of circumstances, has triumphed over obscurity, and risen into honorable fame. This was the case with the late Dr. Pereira, whose determination of purpose and untiring industry enabled him to accomplish more in the space of one short life than is usually effected in that of many longer ones.

The subject of our present memoir was born in the parish of Shoreditch, in London, on the 22d of May, 1804. He received the rudiments of his education at some of the small schools in the neighborhood; and when he was about ten years of age he was placed under the tuition of a classical master of no ordinary attainments. This gentleman kept an academy at No. 10 Queen street, Finsbury, and Pereira remained with him for a period of four years, during which time he obtained the friendship of his preceptor, who was accustomed to speak of him as a boy of considerable merit. When he left school he manifested a strong desire to enter the medical profession; and accordingly, at the age of fifteen, or a little earlier, he was articled as an apprentice to Mr. Latham, an apothecary, of the City road. There he remained between two and three years, when his master became the subject of mental disease. This led to the breaking up of the practice and to the cancelling of Pereira's indentures. While he was with Mr. Latham he studied hard at his classics, and he drew a vocabulary of Latin terms for his guidance in dispensing.

At the close of the year 1821 he became a pupil at the General Dispensary in Aldersgate street, and he there attended the prelections of Dr. Clutterbuck on chemistry, materia medica, and practice of physic. He also availed himself of the lectures which were occasionally given by Dr. Birkbeck on natural philosophy, and by Dr. Lambe on botany. In the year following he entered to the surgical practice of Saint Bartholomew's Hospital. While thus engaged in the prosecution of his studies, a vacancy occurred in the office of apothecary at the Dispensary. This appointment he was anxious to secure for himself, but, as he was not yet qualified for it, it was necessary that he should proceed at once to the hall, and obtain its license: this he did on the 6th of March, 1823, when he was only eighteen years of age. In the same month he was appointed to the Dispensary, and we may date his illustrious career from that time. The salary at the Dispensary was not large—it was, in fact, only £120 per annum; and, with the view of increasing his income, he formed a class for private medical instruction. This he had but little difficulty in doing, as the lectures at the Dispensary were largely attended. His success in that undertaking was very great, and he thought it desirable to publish a few small books on the subjects in which he found his pupils most deficient. These were a translation of the "Pharmacopia" for 1824, with the chemical decompositions; the "*Selecta è Prescriptis*;" a manual for the use of students; and a "General Table of Atomic Numbers, with an Introduction to the Atomic Theory." These works were published in the course of the years 1824-5, 6 and 7; they had a very extensive sale, and two of them are in existence at the present time.

In the year 1825 he passed the College of Surgeons, and in the year following he succeeded Dr. Clutterbuck as a lecturer on chemistry. At that time he was only twenty-two years of age, but his appearance was commanding, and he, therefore, looked much older. His first lecture was given to a large class of pupils and friends. It was eminently successful, and he received the warm congratulations of his numerous admirers. Then, as ever afterwards, he sought to dazzle by the novelty of his facts and the profusion of his illustrations. His lecture-table was covered with specimens, and, among other things, he exhibited the new element, bromine, which Bolard, of Montpelier, had just then discovered.

In the course of a year or two after that time, he began to collect the facts for his "Materia Medica." He saw that the whole subject of pharmacology was involved in the greatest confusion, that its principles were misapprehended, and that its doctrines were founded in absurdity and conjecture. From this chaos and darkness he determined to relieve it. Accordingly, he commenced a diligent search for all the facts of the science; he studied the ancient fathers of physic, and made himself master of the literature of the subject, from the earliest period of history; he collected the works of English writers, and he undertook the study of French and German, in order that he might read those of the Continent. At that time he devoted his whole energies to the subject, and worked for about sixteen hours a day. He was accustomed to rise at six in the morning, and to read, with but little interruption, until twelve at night. This he continued to do for several years; and had he not been possessed of an iron constitution, of great physical endurance, and of a most determined purpose, he would unquestionably have sunk under it. As it was, the closeness of his application occasioned several slight attacks of epilepsy, and a frequent determination of blood to the head. After a short time he began to give lectures on materia medica, as well as on chemistry, at the Dispensary; and he must have been so completely engaged that he could not find leisure for original investigation. In fact, from the year 1827 until that of 1835, his name appears but once in the journals of the time. This occurred in 1829, when he published a short paper in the *London Medical and Physical Journal*, on the adulteration of hydriodate of potash.

In the year 1832 his affairs were in so prosperous a state that he ventured to leave the Dispensary, and to get married. He resigned his appointment in favor of his brother, and commenced practice as a surgeon in Aldersgate street. A reference to the *Lancet* of the time will show that he left the Dispensary about twelve months before the notorious quarrel occurred at that institution. It is probable that he foresaw the approaching storm, and retired from the falling house; but be that as it may, he had, in the year of his marriage, joined the new medical school in Aldersgate street; and in the year following he was elected to the Chair of Chemistry in the London Hospital. For a period of six years he lectured at both of these places on three subjects—namely, on Chemistry, Botany, and Materia Medica; and during the whole of each winter session he was accustomed to give two lectures daily. While he was at the Aldersgate Medical School he became very intimate with Dr. Cummin, who was then the editor of the late *Medical Gazette*, and in consequence of this and also of his great popularity as a teacher, he was engaged to publish his lectures on Materia Medica in that journal. They extended over a period of two years, viz., from 1835 to 1837, and amounted to seventy-four in number. There can be no doubt that they greatly added to his reputation; for we find that they were translated into the German, and re-published in India. In 1839, he re-produced them in another form—viz., in his "Elements of Materia Medica," and this work was so much appreciated that the whole of the first part was bought up long before the second was ready for delivery. A second edition was, therefore, immediately called for, and it appeared in the year 1842. Before this date, however, viz., in 1839, he had been chosen Examiner in Materia Medica in the University of London; and in 1841, he had been elected Assistant-Physician to the London Hospital. He took his degree at Erlangen, in 1840, and he obtained his license at the College of Physicians directly afterwards. About the same time he was invited by some of the authorities of Saint Bartholomew's Hospital to lecture at the medical school of that institution, and the arrangements for his so doing had been almost completed, for a syllabus of the course was actually published; but when it was notified to him that he would be required to give up his other appointments, he refused to relinquish his position at the London Hospital, at which institution he had experienced great kindness. He immediately afterwards, however, gave up the Aldersgate School.

In 1842, he gave two short courses of lectures at the rooms of the Pharmaceutical Society, and in the year following, he was appointed its first professor. During that year he published his work on Food and Diet, and he was elected on the Council of the Royal Society. By that time, his practice as a physician had become rather extensive, and as it was rapidly increasing, he determined to throw aside his more scientific pursuits Accordingly, in 1844, he resigned a part of the course of chemistry at the London Hospital into the hands of Dr. Letheby ; in 1845 he gave up a larger portion of it ; and in 1846 he relinquished it altogether. He continued, however, to lecture on Materia Medica at both the hospital and the Pharmaceutical Society, and there is no reason for believing that he contemplated any change in this matter until the new regulations of the Apothecaries' Society transferred his course to the summer session. This arrangement interfered with his usual habits, and also with his ideas of the importance of the subject, and, consequently, in 1850, he resigned his lectureship at the hospital, though he still continued to deliver a winter course at the Pharmaceutical Society. In 1845, he was elected a fellow of the College, and, in 1851, he became a full physician at the hospital. He had now reached the summit of his ambition: his reputation as an author was established, and the rewards of industry were falling thick about him. He was a fellow of many scientific societies, he was in constant communication with the learned of all countries, he was intimately connected with many of the greatest institutions of the metropolis, and was, in fact, their brightest ornament ; he had collected around him a large circle of friends and admirers, and he saw before him the prospect of wealth and happiness. In the midst of all this, however, he was stricken down, and that so suddenly that he had hardly time to take leave of those who were about him. He died on the 20th of January last, and within one week of health and hope he was placed in his last resting place. His funeral took place at Kensal Green on the Thursday following, in the presence of a large number of friends and pupils, who mourned in silent grief.

A retrospect of the labors of this distintinguished physician will show that he was a man of no ordinary capacity, that he was characterized by qualities which always ensure success. He had an unquenchable thirst for knowledge, an indefatigable spirit, unbounded industry, and a determination of purpose that was irresistible. Whatsoever he did he did well, and he, therefore, made his performances as valuable to others as they were creditable to himself. This is evidenced by the works to which we have alluded, for they have made for him the reputation he possessed, and have given to others the means of acquiring knowledge which is not to be found elsewhere. The great peculiarity of his efforts is, that he aimed more at bringing within our reach the treasures of other men's minds than of exposing those of his own. He has, indeed, been charged with want of originality, and, most certainly, if we estimate him by the value of his own independent researches, he is open to such a charge ; but it must also be admitted that it is an equally useful element of the human mind, that faculty which urges men to gather up the scattered facts of science, and to mould them into a shape that may be made available to all. This has our author accomplished, and the result of his labors will endure beyond the efforts of originality, for they will last through all time, as a monument of his industry.—*London Lancet*, Feb. 1853.

---

## NOTICE.

## AMERICAN PHARMACEUTICAL ASSOCIATION.

The annual meeting of the American Pharmaceutical Association will be held at Boston on the 24th of August, 1853. The object of the Association being the advancement of Pharmacy in the United States, it is desirable that a general interest in its favor should be created among the pharmaceutists and druggists. According to the requirement of the Constitution, the following conditions of membership are published, and an invitation is hereby extended to all who are eligible to membership, and who feel an interest in the Association, to attend the ensuing meeting :

" SECTION 2d, *Article 1st.*—All pharmaceutists who shall have attained the age of 21 years, whose character, morally and professionally, is fair, and who, after duly considering the obligations of the Constitution and Code of Ethics of this Association, are willing to subscribe to them, are eligible for membership.

" *Article 2d.*—The members shall consist of Delegates from regularly constituted Colleges of Pharmacy and Pharmaceutical Societies, who shall present properly authorized credentials, and of other reputable pharmaceutists, feeling an interest in the objects of the Association, who may not be so delegated, the latter being required to present a certificate signed by a majority of the delegates from places whence they come. If no such delegates are present at the meeting, they may, on obtaining the certificate of any three members of the Association, be admitted, provided they are introduced by the Committee on Credentials.

" *Article 5th.*—Every local Pharmaceutical Association is entitled to send five delegates." DANIEL B. SMYTH, President.

*Philadelphia, 4th mo. 11th*, 1853.

NEW YORK
# JOURNAL OF PHARMACY.

JUNE, 1853.

## ON THE COMPOSITION OF YEAST POWDER.

BY EDWARD N. KENT.

THE following analysis was instituted for the purpose of ascertaining the composition of the yeast-powders which are now extensively sold by grocers.

Mixed with water, effervescence is produced by liberation of *carbonic acid.* A portion remains undissolved by *cold* water, which, when heated, forms a clear gelatinous mass, which becomes blue with the iodine test, *starch.* The portion soluble in cold water gives precipitates with salts of lime, characteristic of *tartaric acid;* and with chloride of platina gives *potash.* A portion of the original powder heated to redness, and treated with burning alcohol, gives yellow and violet flame, indicating *soda* and potash.

A quantitative analysis of the yeast powder, gave the following results.

A portion treated with water, and the gas dried by chloride of calcium, gave ·085 carbonic acid.

A separate portion ignited, the residue treated with hydrochloric acid, and the alkaline chlorides thus formed separated by the double chloride of platina and sodium, gave ·137 potash, and ·096 soda.

Another portion treated with *cold* water gave ·227 starch.

The tartaric acid and water estimated as loss gave ·455. By

calculation as cream of tartar, this leaves ·045 water in combination with the soda.

The carbonic acid formed, is in larger proportion to the soda than exists in the neutral carbonate, and in less proportion than exists in the bicarbonate, from which I infer that an intermediate carbonate, which is sold under the name of soda-salæratus, is used for the preparation of yeast-powder.

The per centage composition of the powder is:

| | | |
|---|---|---|
| Carbonic acid.......... | ·085 | = 22·6, Soda-salæratus. |
| Soda.................. | ·096 | |
| Water................ | ·045 | |
| Potash ............... | ·137 | = 54·7 cream of tartar. |
| Tartaric acid and water . | ·410 | |
| Starch................ | ·227 | 22·7 starch. |
| | 1·000 | 100· |

SYNTHESIS.—Crystallized bitartrate of potash, powdered and sifted, is better than the same article which is sold in an impalpable powder, as cream of tartar, the latter being too fine, and onsequently the gas is liberated too rapidly when mixed with water. Corn starch is more palatable than that from wheat, and consequently is the best. These articles mixed with soda-salæratus, in the above proportions, gives yeast powder identical with the one analyzed.

---

## ON SYRUP OF IODIDE OF IRON AND MANGANESE.

BY WILLIAM PROCTER, JR.

THE attention of the medical profession has recently been awakened to the advantages to be derived from the use of the salts of iron and manganese in combination, when preparations of iron alone have heretofore been indicated. Among the compounds used by M. Petrequin, is a syrup of iodide of iron and manganese, but the method suggested for its preparation from the solid iodides, by M, Burin-Dubuisson, is too indefinite to be generally adopted, besides involving the necessity of pre-previously preparing and keeping the solid iodides. The following formula yields a preparation of the strength of the officinal syrupy solution of iodide of iron, and the manner of using it, and the doses are the same.

Take of iodide of potassium...............1000 grains.
proto-sulphato of iron (in crystals) .. 080 "
proto-sulphate of manganese " .. 210 "
iron filings (free from rust) ........ 100 "
white sugar (in coarse powder).....4800 "
distilled or boiled water, a sufficient quantity.

Triturate the sulphates and the iodides separately to powder, mix them with the iron filings, add half a fluid ounce of distilled water, and triturate to a uniform paste. After standing a few minutes, again add half a fluid ounce of distilled water, triturate and allow it to rest fifteen minutes. A third addition of water should now be made and mixed. The sugar should then be introduced into a bottle capable of holding a little more than twelve fluid ounces, and a small funnel, prepared with a moistened filter, inserted into its mouth. The magma of salts should then be carefully removed from the mortar to the filter, and when the dense solution has drained through, distilled or boiled water should be carefully poured on in small portions, until the solution of the iodides is displaced, and washed from the magma of crystals of sulphate of potash. Finally, finish the measure of twelve ounces, by adding boiled water, and agitate the bottle until the sugar is dissolved. The solution of the sugar may be facilitated, when desirable, by standing the bottle in warm water for a time, and then agitating.

Each fluid ounce of this syrup contains fifty grains of the mixed anhydrous iodides in the proportion of three parts of iodide of iron to one part of iodide of manganese, and the dose is from ten drops to half a fluid drachm.

*Remarks.*—Owing to the slight solubility of the resulting sulphate of potash, and the small quantity of water employed to effect the interchange of elements, but little of that salt is contained in the syrup. The object of the iron filings is to saturate any free iodine that may be eliminated during the exposure consequent on the gradual reaction of the salts. The use of either distilled, or cold recently boiled, water, is necessary to obviate the effect of air on the iodides. It is necessary to allow sufficient time for the complete decomposition of the sulphate of iron, else the syrup will be contaminated with it. The proper moment to lixiviate the sulphate is known by the cessation of the crystallization of the sulphate of potash. The bottle should be shaken from time to time during the filtration to protect the filtered solution, and the washing process should be stopped as soon as the sulphate ceases to have a well-marked taste of the iodides. Practically in this, as in all cases where syrups are made by agitation, and are not to be filtered, it is best to use pure lump sugar, and coarsely powder it for the occasion, as the commercial powdered sugar frequently contains dusty impurities. The preparation when finished has a very pale straw color; if the salts have not all been decomposed before the washing, the syrup will have a greenish color, and subsequently deposit crystals of sulphate of potash by standing.

—*American Journal of Pharmacy, May*, 1853.

---

## ON A SPECIES OF SMILAX, AND A NEW COMMERCIAl SORT OF SARSAPARILLA WHICH IS OBTAINED FROM IT.

BY ROBERT BENTLEY, F.L.S., ETC.

Professor of Botany, etc., to the Pharmaceutical Society.

The specimens which furnished the materials for the following paper were forwarded to me by Mr. Bell, who obtained them from the museum of the late Dr. Pereira. They consisted,

1st, of a portion of the stem of a species of smilax furnished with leaves and fruit, but there were no flowers; and, 2d, Of a bundle of Sarsaparilla root as imported, which was stated to be the root of the above species of smilax.

The history of the specimens is as follows:—The late Dr. Pereira received them from Mr. G. U. Skinner, one of the importers. They were collected in Guatemala, about ninety miles from the sea, in the province of Sacatepeques, by persons usually employed in the culture of cochineal, but who, through the failure of that crop last year, were glad to turn their attention to the other products of this region.

The first point to which I directed my attention was to determine, if possible, the specific name of the smilax under examination. This I found to be a matter of great difficulty, partly owing to the very imperfect manner in which the genus smilax has been described from the want of good specimens, and partly also from its extent (nearly 200 species being known to botanists. The difficulty was also increased in this case by the absence of flowers in the specimen. By referring, however, to Kunth's *Enumeratio Plantarum*, vol. v., p. 167, I at length found a description of a species of smilax, under the name of *smilax papyracea*, which corresponded in all the main points with the one I wished to determine. This species is thus described:—"Smilax papyracea, Poiret:—Caules angulati, sulcati, aculeati, glabri. Folia alterna, petiolata, ovali-lanceolata, acuta, basi rotundato-subtruncata, reticulato-trinervia, nervis venisque prominentibus, papyracea, viridia, utrinque glabra, 6-8 policaria longi, 2½ pollicaria lata. Petioli striati, pollicares. Reliqua ignota."

Four other descriptions are also given in the above work, under the name of smilax papyracea, described from specimens obtained from different sources; and a more detailed description by Grisebach may be seen in Endlicher and Martius's *Flora Braziliensis Fasciculus* 5 p. 5, where there is also a plate of the plant. As these descriptions all differ somewhat from one another in certain of their minor characters, and as in no case does it appear that the flowers or fruit were known to the describers, and as the specimen before me is therefore a more complete one in many respects than those previously noticed, I subjoin the description of it, as drawn up by myself:—Stem 4-angled, somewhat striated, smooth, furnished with scattered recurved prickles placed at the angles of the stem, the smaller branches being almost destitute of prickles. Leaves membraneous, scattered, alternate, ovate-oblong, ovate-elliptical or oblong, rounded at the base, or slightly cordate, acute, pointed, or occasionally rounded and mucronate, entire at the margins and somewhat wavy, glabrous, 5-nerved, reticulated, the three central nerves rather prominent, and leaving between them an oblong lanceolate space, the two lateral nerves indistinct, and passing close within the margins. Petiole about an inch long, without prickles, sheathing at the base, and furnished with two long spirally-twisted filiform tendrils, which are inserted into it at distances varying from two to four lines above its base. Leaves from four to six and a-half inches long, and from one to three inches broad. Peduncles axillary, without bracts, smooth, somewhat flattened, from one to four inches in length, bearing a roundish receptacle of about two lines broad, from which numerous pedicels (twenty to thirty) arise, arranged in a compact cluster. Pedicels smooth, from four to six lines long. No flowers. Fruit, a berry, about the size of a pea, red? two or three celled, two or three seeded. Seeds roundish, with a membranaceous testa, dark colored.

This plant has hitherto been found only at Cayenne, in French Guiana, and on the borders of the Amazon and its tributaries, in Brazil. The above specimen, therefore, if rightly referred to Smilax papyracea, will furnish a new locality for it, namely, Guatemala. I may add that I have searched in vain in the herbariums of the Linnæan Society and the British Museum, for any smilax resembling the present species. Through the kindness also of Sir William Hooker, I had an opportunity of examining his private herbarium, at Kew, but without success. Sir William Hooker pointed out one species to me, marked doubtfully as smilax cumanensis, Schlechtend; which certainly resembled mine remarkably in the texture and shape of the leaves, which were the only portion of the plant I took to Kew with me. Unfortunately there was no fruit on his specimen, and as the fruit of mine did not agree with the description of it as given by Schlechtendal, as well as differing also from the latter in some other particulars, it could not be the same plant, if this has been properly described.

The present specimen is, therefore, a very interesting one in many respects; in the first place, by furnishing us with a new locality for smilax papyracea; secondly, in being, probably, the only specimen of the plant in this country, and, indeed, the only one which has been described with regard to the flowers, stalks, and fruit, either here or abroad; and thirdly, in the fact, that smilax papyracea is now generally regarded in this country, on the authority of Martius and Riedel, as one of the sources from which the Brazilian sarsaparilla of commerce is obtained. Dr. Lindley, however, seems to doubt this fact, as he has not described the species at all in his *Medical and Economic Botany.*

Martius also states, with regard to the roots of smilax papyracea, that they abound more than any other species of smilax with Pariglin, or as it is now more generally called, Smilacin, and which is, probably, the chief active constituent of sarsaparilla, and hence, and also from the fact of Brazilian sarsaparilla having been, before the introduction of Jamaica sarsaparilla, the most esteemed kind in this country, we have *à priori* evidence, that the sarsaparilla root obtained in Guatemala, from probably the same plant, possesses also the medicinal properties usually considered to be possessed by it. The fact, however, of Brazilian sarsaparilla containing a larger amount of Smilacin than the other sorts, has not, I believe, been confirmed by the analyses of others.

Having now described the specimen of smilax somewhat in detail, on account of its great interest, we pass in the next place to the description of the bundle of sarsaparilla root which accompanied it, and from which it was stated to have been derived. The roots of which this is composed are unfolded, and tied together in the middle by means of a flexible monocotyledonous stem, resembling a species of sedge or rush, into a loose, somewhat cylindrical bundle. The bundle from which this description is taken is about two feet eight inches long, twelve inches in circumference, and weighs nearly two pounds. It is free from rhizome or chump. In the manner of packing, the only other commercial variety of sarsaparilla which it resembles is the Brazilian; thus it agrees with the latter in the roots being unfolded, and being free from rhizome or chump; and also in their being tied together into a somewhat cylindrical bundle or roll, by means of a flexible monocotyledonous stem. The rolls, however, of Brazilian sarsaparilla are of a much more compact nature, and the flexible monocotyledonous stem, called timbotitica, with which they are tied together, is not of the same nature as that which is used to tie up the bundle before us. Thus the timbotitica has a somewhat triangular shape, with three deep incisions into its interior, and a transverse section shows a very porous structure like a piece of cane; but the latter, although somewhat triangular in shape, is not of so firm a texture, has no incisions into its interior, and the transverse section does not present so porous a structure.

Externally the roots are much furrowed longitudinally, and are frequently swollen or gouty, resembling in these respects the Caraccas or gouty Vera Cruz sarsaparilla. They vary in color from a pale yellow to an orange red. All the roots are furnished, more or less, with branched rootlets or *beard.* Their average thickness is about that of a common writing quill, but they are frequently larger, and in some cases smaller. The cortical portion is very brittle, and is often cracked in an annular manner, and may be easily separated from the ligneous cord or meditullium beneath. When the roots are bruised or rubbed, a shower of white dust arises from them, which, when examined by the microscope, is found to be composed of starch granules, presenting generally the characters of those usually obtained from the root bark of the different commercial sorts of sarsaparilla, that is, the granules are frequently compound, consisting of from two to six, aggregated together, and when separate, they are seen to be of a small size, averaging the 2,000th of an inch in length, sometimes of an irregularly spherical or triangular shape, but more frequently, in consequence of their mutual pressure upon one another, they become more or less flattened at the base, so as to be mullar shaped, or in consequence of being pressed upon at more than one point, they present a dihedral or trihedral summit. The starch granules, however, of the root under examination present this peculiarity, that is, they have a very distinct hilum, which is generally cracked in a stellate manner, while the starch granules of the other commercial sorts of sarsaparilla, which resemble this in their amylaceous character, present a very indistinct hilum, or none at all, when viewed by ordinary light, although readily perceived by the aid of polarized light. This difference in the appearance of the starch granules is probably owing to some difference in the manner in which this sort of sarsaparilla has been prepared. The taste of the root is amylaceous, and perhaps slightly acrid, but it has no perceptible odor.

Upon making a transverse section, we find a thick cortical portion, which is generally colorless, but sometimes presenting a faint roseate or pinkish appearance. Within this cortex we find the ligneous cord, or meditullium. In thickness, the cortex is generally from one-half to one-third that of the meditullium.

When examined by the microscope, the cells of the inner cortical layers are found to contain bundles of acicular raphides, and a large number of the starch granules already described. The pith also is found commonly to contain a number of similar starch granules. The breadth of the pith is usually from one to one and a-half, or perhaps more, that of the woody zone. In this respect it resembles the Honduras sarsarparilla, and, according to Schleiden, also all those sorts of sarsaparilla which are obtained from Central America. The cells of the Liber, or, as it is called by Schleiden, the *nucleus sheath*, are elongated radially, or from within outwards, and have walls which are thicker on the inner than the outer side. In this respect, it resembles the South American and Mexican sarsaparillas, which Schleiden says always present this peculiarity. This microscopical appearance is remarkable, because, according to Schleiden, the Honduras and all the Central American sorts of sarsaparilla are characterized by having the cells of the nucleus sheath either square or somewhat elongated transversely, and all their walls of nearly equal thickness, and he believes that he can distinguish Central American from South American and Mexican sarsaparillas from the appearances thus presented, combined with the different relative proportions of the woody layer and the pith already alluded to. But, if this be true generally (which, so far as my experience goes, is not absolutely the case, having observed some sorts of Brazilian sarsaparilla in which the cells of the nucleus sheath were elongated somewhat in a direction from within outwards, and so far, therefore, agreeing generally with the anatomy of South American sarsaparillas, according to Schleiden, but yet had their outer and inner walls of nearly equal thickness, and thus agreeing with the Honduras variety), it is certainly not true in the present sort, for here we have a Central American sarsaparilla which agrees with Schleiden's arrangement generally as regards the relative proportions of pith and woody layer, but differs from it in the cells of the nucleus sheath being elongated from within outwards or radially, and having walls which are thicker on the inner than the outer side.

Having now generally described the external, internal, and microscopical characters of our specimen of sarsaparilla root, we have, in the next place, to notice briefly its chemical characteristics.

If we make a transverse section, and apply to it a drop of sulphuric acid, the woody zone is immediately changed to a dark red or nearly black color (owing to the action of the acid on the smilacin), while the pith and the inner cortical layers remain unaltered.

Again, if a decoction be made, it is seen to be much paler in color than that of Jamaica sarsaparilla, and if to it, when cold, a solution of iodine be added, it immediately becomes of a dark blue color, from the formation of iodide of starch. Again, if a strong decoction be poured into alcohol, a copious precipitate of starch is likewise produced. Again, if the extract prepared from this sort of sarsaparilla be rubbed up with water, it is not completely soluble, but it forms a turbid solution, which immediately becomes dark blue on the addition of tincture of iodine.

From the characters above given of our sarsaparilla root, and particularly in its thick, swollen, or gouty appearance; the large size and pale color of its cortical portion, as compared with the meditullium; the abundance of starch or meal contained in the cells of its inner cortical layers; and in its behavior generally with reagents, we have no difficulty in referring it at once to the mealy or amylaceous division of the sarsaparillas in the arrangement of the late Dr. Pereira. In this division we have described three commercial sorts of sarsaparilla, namely, the Honduras, the Caraccas, and the Brazilian. The question now arises, can our sort be referred to either of these? We think not, although, in some respects it has characters bearing resemblance to them all. Thus, it resembles the Brazilian, as we have seen, somewhat in its mode of packing. But it differs from it in the roots being generally larger; much more furrowed in a longitudinal direction externally; in being of a yellowish or orange red color, rather than the brownish or reddish-brown like it; and also in having generally more rootlets or beard. Anatomically, it approaches the Brazilian sort in the relative proportion of the cortex and meditullium, and also in the radial direction and other characters of the cells of the nucleus sheath; but it differs from it in the pith being smaller in proportion to the woody zone. Chemically, also, in the action of sulphuric acid on its transverse section, it precisely resembles the Brazilian sort, in the fact that the woody layer is changed to a dark red or nearly black color, while the pith and inner cortical layers are quite unaltered. This difference in the action of sulphuric acid on the woody layer, as compared with that on the pith and inner cortical layers, is, I think. not so strikingly the case in the other sorts of mealy sarsaparillas—at least, not in the Honduras—for, upon the addition of sulphuric acid to its transverse section, I have generally observed the inner cortical layers to become slightly reddened in addition to the change of color produced in the woody layer, as in the former instances. In the Caraccas sarsaparilla also, occasionally, we observe a somewhat similar alteration in the action of sulphuric acid on the inner cortical layers, but it is not so marked as in the Honduras kind. Caraccas sarsaparilla also, I find, has its pith generally more affected on the addition of sulphuric acid than the other mealy sarsaparillas. These few remarks, however, on the chemical action of sulphuric acid on the transverse sections of sarsaparilla require further examination; but still, as a general rule, I think they will be found correct.

The new sort of sarsaparilla differs altogether, in the manner in which it is packed, from the Caraccas and Honduras sorts. It resembles, however, the Honduras in thickness; also in the proportion borne by the pith to the woody zone; and also generally in the relative thickness of the cortex and meditullium. But it differs from it in commonly being marked externally by deeper longitudinal furrows; in its color; in having more rootlets or beard; in the direction and other characters of the cells of the nucleus sheath; and, as noticed above, also, in some degree, in the action of sulphuric acid on its transverse section.

To the Caraccas sort it bears some resemblance, in its thick, swollen, or gouty appearance; also somewhat in color; also in its presenting deep longitudinal furrows externally, and in the direction of the cells of the nucleus sheath. But it differs in having more radicles or beard; in the pith being smaller in proportion to the woody layer; perhaps, also, slightly, in the action of sulphuric acid on its transverse section; and generally in the cortical portion being smaller in proportion to the meditullium, and being less mealy.

From these remarks it may be seen that the new sort of sarsaparilla seems to resemble the Brazilian most in its internal structure and chemical characteristics, and the Caraccas sort most externally. The differences between it and the Brazilian are not greater than may be readily accounted for by differences of soil, climate, and mode of preparation; and there can, therefore, I think, be but little doubt that these two sorts may be produced by the same plant.

With regard to the therapeutical value of this sarsaparilla, I have but little hesitation in asserting that it is quite equal, if it be not superior to the other commercial mealy sorts. My opinion on this matter is founded in a great measure on some experiments made by Mr. Daniel Hanbury, with respect to the quantity of extract afforded by it, and the results of which he has kindly furnished me. Mr. Hanbury thus writes:—"My experiment as to the extract it would afford was made upon 12lbs. (avoirdupois), which having been treated in the usual way, that is, by repeated decoction and evaporation of the liquors, gave 2lbs. 11oz. (avoirdupois weight) of solid extract of good consistence." The yield, therefore, in this case, was about twenty-two per cent. Now, as the quantity of extract yielded by a given weight is usually considered as one of the tests of the goodness of sarsaparilla, this must be considered a most favorable result; for, according to the experiments of Mr. Battley, 5lbs. (troy) of Honduras sarsaparilla yielded 10½oz. of solid extract, or only about eighteen per cent. Again, according to the experiments of Hennell, 5lbs. of the root of Honduras sarsaparilla, of fine quality, yielded 1lb. of extract, or 20 per cent. The average yield of Honduras sarsaparilla, must be considered, therefore, as less than that of the present sample. Again, the average yield of extract by Caraccas and Brazilian sarsaparillas is probably somewhat less than Honduras. On the data furnished by yield of extract, therefore, the present sample must be taken as somewhat superior in quality to the other mealy sarsaparillas.

Now, as regards the *taste* of this sarsaparilla (another criterion of the value of different samples), I cannot distinguish any appreciable difference between this sort and the Honduras or other mealy sorts. No inference, one way or the other, can be drawn from this test, therefore. Again, the *beard* is usually considered as another criterion of excellence, and in this respect the present sample (as far as I can judge from the bundles I have seen), is superior, generally containing more beard than either of the other mealy sorts; and this is, no doubt, the reason why it yields more extract, as it has been generally observed that the beard yields a greater proportion of extract than the main root. As to the other criterion of goodness, namely, *color*, I do not think any positive inference can be drawn either way. On the above grounds, therefore, I think it must be admitted that the present sample is equal, if not superior, to Honduras, Caraccas, or Brazilian sarsaparillas.

Adding this new sort to the list of previously described mealy sarsaparillas, the division of these in the late Dr. Pereira's arrangement will now comprise four commercial sorts, namely, the Brazilian, the Caraccas, the Honduras, and the new sort, which I propose to call the Guatemala. Carrying out this arrangement, they may be subdivided thus:

A. Pith two to four times the breadth of the woody layer; cells of the nucleus sheath elongated radially, and having walls which are thicker on the inner than on the outer side.
  *a.* Pale, folded, often swollen or gouty roots, with the rhizomes or stems attached . . . . . . . . . . . . . 1. Caraccas.
  *b.* Reddish-brown, unfolded roots without rhizomes or stems attached, packed in rolls or cylindrical bundles 2. Brazilian.

B. Pith one to one and a-half times the breadth of the woody layer.
  *a.* Folded roots; cells of the nucleus sheath square or elongated transversely, and nearly equally thick on all sides . . . . . . . . . . . . . . . . . . . . . . . . . . . 3. Honduras.
  *b.* Unfolded roots without rhizome, packed in rolls or cylindrical bundles; cells of the nucleus sheath elongated radially, and having walls which are thicker on the inner than the outer side . . . . . . . . . 4. Guatemala.

In conclusion, I would throw out a suggestion, that as the distinctive characters between this new sort of sarsaparilla and the Honduras are by no means very remarkable, and as the plant which produces the latter is probably also a native of Guatemala, may not this also be derived from the same botanical source, namely, the smilax papyracea?—*Pharm. Journal, April*, 1853.

---

# PLAN OF PROTECTION

## SUGGESTED TO THE PHARMACEUTICAL BODY IN THE UNITED STATES,

BY MEANS OF A JOINT-STOCK CHEMICAL LABORATORY, FOR THE PREPARATION OF CHEMICALS AND OFFICINAL REMEDIES IN AN UNADULTERATED STATE, AT A REMUNERATING PRICE.

BY E. DUPUY, PHARM., N. Y.

---

THE injurious effects of adulterated medicines is well understood by all who have paid any attention to that serious subject. Although the attention of our legislatures has been attracted to it by occasional explosions of public opinion, and the general government has created offices of inspection, for the rejection of improper foreign drugs and chemicals, still we are very little better off than we were heretofore, because at home we have manufacturers who prefer disposing of their manufactured articles, at a price which shows on its face the impossibility of furnishing them unadulterated at the price at which even the wholesale druggist often disposes of them, after making his profit. The very convenient excuse is, that their goods would not be saleable at a higher price, or that it would ruin them to compete with other establishments, who have the reputation (although an unwarrantable one) of manufacturing pure articles, while they could not afford truly pure ones, at the same prices, with remunerative profit.

In my own store, I have received occasionally from respectable and trustworthy wholesale druggists chemical preparations, which, so far as they knew and believed, were pure; yet, on analysis, were found to be most grossly adulterated, for instance:

White oxide of zinc, containing but two-thirds of the oxide, to one-third of carbonate of lime.

Precipitated sulphur, containing ·44 hydrate of lime, to ·54 *sublimed* sulphur.

I know, also, from a reliable source, that some wholesale druggists are in the habit of bartering with manufacturing chemists, to add to the alkaloids most in use such a quantity of *mannite* as will bring the mixture (resembling greatly the pure article, at least so far as appearance and taste are concerned) to a price comparing favorably with that of other dealers. Such is the result of commerce in articles but little known to the public at large, and yet so useful to its suffering portion, when in the hands of parties losing sight of their responsibilities to their fellow-men and their Maker.

Must we, pharmaceutists, who wish to honor our profession, and be honored by it, allow ourselves to dispose at our counters, by prescriptions or otherwise, articles known to be impure? and yet, such is our dependence, that, as long as we cannot depend upon the sense of honor and high duty of manufacturers, we are in the absolute necessity of purifying ourselves our so-called pure chemicals, or of manufacturing them, at a cost of time, labor, and expense, which it is superfluous to expect to be seen performed by the great majority of our pharmaceutists.

But, if obstacles, insurmountable in practice, are to obstruct the path of individual pharmaceutists, though sincerely desirous to meet honorably the claims of their patrons, the physicians, and the public, there seems to be, however, open a mode of effecting the desired practical result by means of a joint-stock association. composed wholly of practising pharmaceutists and wholesale druggists, who would manufacture or purify, at a moderate yet remunerative price, all the officinal preparations which the pharmaceutist is in the habit of procuring from the manufacturing chemist, either directly, or by the agency of the wholesale druggist. A charter would be procured from the state legislature for the express purpose of manufacturing unadulterated chemicals and officinal preparations.

From the encouraging reception the plan has met with from competent parties, some of them ready to furnish, if necessary, one half of the requisite capital, so satisfied are they, both of the public utility of the enterprise, and of the remunerative influence of such an association, all that remains to do (which is, however, the most essential) is to bring it before the pharmaceutists of the United States, and receive from them such suggestions as will facilitate the accomplishment of so desirable a result.

---

## EMPLASTRUM EXTRACTI ACONITI RADICIS.

BY WILLIAM PROCTER, JR.

HAVING been requested by Dr. Francis Gurney Smith to prepare a plaster medicated with *aconitia*, the following formula was suggested by me, as being less expensive than one requiring the pure alkaloid, yet possessed of equal, if not superior efficiency, because the greater bulk of the extract would prevent the plaster from masking the power of the active ingredient, and its ready solubility more favorable to the influence of the remedy.

Take of aconite root, in coarse powder, four ounces.
" alcohol, sp. gr. 835, a sufficient quantity.
" adhesive plaster, three ounces and a-half.

Moisten the powdered aconite root with six ounces of alcohol, and permit it to macerate twenty-four hours; then put it in a small displacer, and when properly packed, pour on gradually sufficient alcohol to make a pint of tincture. Distil off three-fourths of the alcohol, evaporate the residue on a water-bath to a thick, syrupy consistence; then add the plaster previously liquefied, and stir constantly, until it is properly incorporated with the soft resinous extract, and cools. The resulting aconite plaster has a brown color and homogeneous consistence, and weighs about four ounces troy. This plaster should be spread in a thin stratum on skin or oiled silk, and may be used several times when its application has not been too long continued at first.

Dr. Smith has employed this plaster in several cases of neuralgia, especially about the head, and has obtained from it the well-marked effects of aconite; in some instances so decided as to require the removal of the plaster for a time. He has also used it in painful tumors of the breast, with much satisfaction.

---

## ON RACEMIC ACID.

The doubts which hitherto have existed relative to the formation of racemic acid have, at length, been completely removed by the recent researches of M. Pasteur.

It was somewhere about the year 1820, that M. Kestner, of Thann, in the department of Vosges, France, a manufacturer of tartaric acid, first noticed the existence of racemic acid; and having met with it whilst employing tartar, obtained from the grapes grown in his department, he came to the conlusion that it existed, ready formed, in the tartar thus obtained. Instead, however, of this acid continuing to appear as a regular product in his manufactory, M. Kestner found that, after a few years, it ceased to appear altogether. During the period in which racemic acid was obtained by him in the regular course of his manufacture, M. Kestner was in the habit of decomposing his crude tartars by means of carbonate of lime, using a large excess of sulphuric acid in the decomposition of the tartrate of lime, and passing a current of chlorine gas through the tartaric acid solution, for the purpose of removing its color. Subsequently, he modified his process of making tartaric acid, and was accustomed to decompose the tartar by caustic lime, using a slight excess only of sulphuric acid in the decomposition of the tartrate of lime, and omitting altogether the bleaching process.

It appears that Mr. White, of Glasgow, also a manufacturer of tartaric acid, had noticed in his manufactory a product differing from tartaric acid, and which he took to be racemic acid. In a letter to M. Pelouze, Mr. White stated also that the tartars he had been in the habit of employing, were imported from Naples, Sicily, and Oporto. M. Kestner, when informed of this circumstance by M. Pelouze, remembered that he had also used some tartars, the produce of Italy, at the time of his obtaining racemic acid. About the same time, also, it was found that large quantities of racemic acid were met with in commerce in England, although this product was quite unknown in the English manufactories of tartaric acid. On investigating the subject, it was found that this racemic acid came from some German manufacturers.

About the month of August last, M. Mitscherlich apprised M. Pasteur that M. Fikentscher, a skilful manufacturer in Saxony, prepared racemic acid, and had supplied him with some. In consequence of this information, M. Pasteur went to M. Fikentscher's manufactory, and learned from him that this acid was regularly produced in his manufactory, but that the quantity obtained had very much fallen off since his employment of tartars imported from Trieste. In fact, since M. Pasteur's visit, the quantity produced was so small as at last to be quite lost sight of altogether. In operating on Neapolitan tartars, the needle-shaped crystals of racemic acid were scarcely discernible, on account of the smallness of their quantity, amidst the large masses of tartaric acid contained in the crystallizing vessels. In addition, these small crystals of racemic acid did not make their appearance in the first crops of crystals, and in but small quantities in subsequent crystallizations; whence we see that this acid is but extremely little soluble in a concentrated solution of tartaric acid.

Knowing that M. Kestner formerly obtained racemic acid in such quantities as to be ablé to sell it by the hundred-weight, M. Pasteur was much surprised at the smallness of the quantity produced at M. Fikentscher's manufactory; it struck him, however, that the difference might be accounted for in the circumstance, that whilst M. Kestner employed the rough, unrefined tartars, M. Fikentscher used those which had been partially refined, and it appeared clear to M. Pasteur, that, if racemic acid existed, ready formed in the tartars, the principal portion of it would be remaining in the mother liquors of the refinery, whatever might be its condition in the crude tartar. The racemate of lime itself is, indeed, but little soluble in bitartrate of potash.

Having been informed by M. Fikentscher that there were extensive refineries of tartar at Trieste and at Venice, M. Pasteur started for those places, with a view to examine the mother-liquors of the refineries; but, whilst stopping at Vienna to visit some manufactories of tartaric acid, the question as to the origin of racemic acid became so clear to his mind, that he at once decided on considering is as a purely natural product. In the course of his visit to several tartaric acid manufactories, in company with M. Redtenbacher, he at first thought that no appearance of racemic acid presented itself, but on examining the different qualities of tartaric acid in the store of M. Nach, he soon recognized the small crystals of racemic acid present; the quantity, however, was so small that it took more than three hours to collect a few decigrammes. It has previously been supposed that, as M. Nach decomposed the tartrate of potash by means of sulphate of lime, these crystals were sulphate of potash. A circumstance, however, which militated against this supposition was, that it was only within about a year that these needle-shaped crystals had made their appearance in his manufactory, and that it was only during the last two years that M. Nach had employed the crude Austrian tartars. When partially refined tartars had been used, no racemic acid showed itself. Hence M. Pasteur concluded:—

1. That the crude Austrian tartars contain racemic acid ready formed; for it is evident that, if this acid were an artificial production, it would always make its appearance in the same manufactory, the mode of operating in which was not changed, but in which the quality only of the tartars used had varied.

2. That the crude Austrian tartars should contain this acid in less quantity than the crude Neapolitan tartars, since the latter, when partially refined, still furnish some racemic acid, and that, too, when the liquors are comparatively new.

Besides, as the mother liquors, remained upwards of one year, before giving indications of racemic acid, this acid does not appear until it has been accumulated by successive operations, which have gradually concentrated into a small compass the acid contained in a large quantity of tartar; the mother liquors of one being used in the treatment of new crude tartar. This result was confirmed by the fact, that in a manufactory which had been but a few months in work, no appearance of racemic acid had manifested itself, although crude Austrian tartars were employed. Lastly, the preceding conclusions were confirmed by facts of the same kind elicited in the manufactory of M. Seybel, in which the employment of partially refined tartars had for the last two or three years been discontinued, and last winter the small crystals of racemic acid made their appearance, which were at first supposed to have arisen from some impurity in the crude tartars employed.

It must be noticed that the tartars employed in M. Seybel's manufactory were obtained from Hungary and Styria, proving that the crude tartars of those countries contained racemic acid, as well as those of Austria and Naples.

On his return to France, M. Pasteur communicated these facts to M. Kestner, and assisted him in his endeavors to reproduce the mysterious acid which for thirty years had eluded his researches. For this purpose, M. Kestner has ordered crude Neapolitan tartars, and also some of the mother liquors of the tartar refineries evaporated to dryness, which he intends operating upon as crude tartars. In addition to this, M. Kestner has introduced into his regular course of manufacture the crude tartars of Tuscany, and has already, in the third crystallization, obtained racemic acid, thus furnishing a new proof that this acid is a natural product, and that the crude tartars of Italy do contain an appreciable quantity of it.

M. Redtenbacher has since written to M. Pasteur, to the effect that M. Seybel, on converting the mother liquors of his manufactory, which had been accumulating for three years, into tartrate of lime, had decomposed a portion of that salt, and that the acid liquor obtained yielded several kilogrammes of racemic acid. The quantity of liquor undergoing crystallization was about 1,400 kilogrammes (28 cwt.) This result coincides with that obtained by M. Kestner, whilst working up the mother liquors of an old manufactory, in which the tartars of Saintonge had been employed. These mother liquors had been purchased by M. Kestner, and having noticed the presence of racemic acid, he worked them up by themselves, converting them into tartrate of lime, and proceeding in the usual way to manufacture tartaric acid. The tartrate of lime thus obtained yielded about one per cent. of racemic acid. Hence, M. Kestner concludes that the tartars of France, at least certain parts, contain racemic acid, as well as those of Italy, Austria, and Hungary, and that this acid accumulates in the mother liquors of tartaric manufactories.

M. Kestner presented, through M. Biot, to the Paris Academy of Sciences, January 3, about nine pounds of the racemic acid so obtained, on which occasion the facts contained in this notice were communicated to the Academy.

In a notice of paratartaric (racemic) acid, which appeared in the *Pharmaceutical Journal*, of February, 1851, the author of the paper states, that "recent investigations have led to the conclusion, that most tartars contain a certain portion of this acid, which is lost in the process at present employed in the manufacture of tartaric acid. This fact may serve to account for the deficient results sometimes obtained."—*Ann. of Pharm*, Feb., 1853.

---

## OPIANINE.

BY M. HINTERBERGER.

THIS alkaloid exists in the opium of Egypt, and was discovered by M. Hinterberger, under the following circumstances:

M. Kugler, pharmaceutist at Vienna, in Austria, had occasion some years ago to treat large quantities of Egyptian opium, for the purpose of extracting the morphine. The infusion of opium was precipitated by ammonia, and the precipitate, first washed with water, then in cold alcohol, was dried and dissolved in boiling alcohol. The solution, decolored by animal charcoal, deposited, on cooling, crystals of morphine, which were mixed with a great quantity of other crystals, possessing the external character of narcotine. After a fresh solution in alcohol, the morphine remained in the mother liquor, and all the other crystals separated from the liquor. M. Hinterberger having had occasion to examine these crystals, proved that they constituted a new alkaloid. He has given this alkaloid the name of *opianine.*

Opianine crystallizes in long, colorless, transparent, and brilliant needles. Precipitated by ammonia from its solutions, it constitutes a fine white powder. It is inodorous, and its alcoholic solution possesses a powerful and persistent bitter taste. It is insoluble in water, and dissolves only in a great quantity of boiling alcohol, from which it separates completely by cooling. The alcoholic solution possesses a powerful alkaline reaction. The solutions of the salts of opianine are precipitated by the fixed and volatile alkalis in white flakes. With the chlorides of platinum and mercury, this base forms double combinations. Concentrated sulphuric acid does not affect it, and nitric acid dissolves it of a yellow color. Sulphuric acid containing nitric acid colors it of a blood red, but this color soon passes to a light yellow. It contains:—

| | Experiments. | | | | |
|---|---|---|---|---|---|
| | I. | II. | III. | | Theory. |
| Carbon ..... | 62·99 | „ | „ | $C^{66}$ | 63·06 |
| Hydrogen... | 5·698 | „ | „ | $H^{36}$ | 5·73 |
| Nitrogen.... | „ | 4·12 | 4.411 | $N^{2}$ | 4·45 |
| Oxygen..... | „ | „ | „ | $O^{21}$ | 26·76 |
| | | | | | 100·00 |

Its composition is consequently expressed by the formula—

$$C^{66}\ H^{36}\ N^{2}\ O^{21}$$

When to an alcoholic solution of hydro-chlorate of opianine is added an aqueous solution of bichloride of mercury, there is formed a voluminous white precipitate. It may be obtained crystallized by dissolving it, after drying, in a mixture of 2 volumes of alcohol, and 1 volume of concentrated hydrochloric acid, and adding distilled water to this liquor by degrees, until the cloudiness which appears becomes permanent. By a gentle heat the cloudiness disappears, and, at the end of twenty-four hours it deposits groups of concentric needles, which contain:

| | Experiment. | | Theory. |
|---|---|---|---|
| Carbon ........ | 49·14 | $C^{66}$ | 49·50 |
| Hydrogen ..... | 4·608 | $H^{37}$ | 4·63 |
| Nitrogen ...... | „ | $N^{2}$ | 3·50 |
| Oxygen ....... | „ | $O^{21}$ | 21·00 |
| Mercury ....... | 12·28 | Hg | 12·50 |
| Chlorine ....... | 9·310 | $Cl^{2}$ | 8·87 |
| | | | 100·00 |

Their composition is consequently expressed by the formula

$$C^{66}\ H^{36}\ N^{2}\ O^{21}\ H\ Cl\ Hg\ Cl$$

*Action of Opianine on the Animal Economy.*—According to the experiments of M. Hinterberger, opianine is a narcotic much resembling morphine. Two cats which were poisoned, one by 0.145 gr. of morphine, the other by the same dose of opianine, exhibited the same symptoms of prostration. This dose was not, however, sufficient to kill them.

---

# AN INQUIRY INTO THE ACTION OF THE ANTHELMINTICS.

BY DR. KÜCHENMEISTER, OF ZITTAU.

Dr. Küchenmeister has examined the various vermifuges, by immersing the living intestinal worms of fowls, cats, and dogs in albumen, at a temperature exceeding 77° Fahr., and adding the anthelmintics in the form of infusion or of powder. In some cases, a mixture of warm milk and water was substituted for the albumen. The experiments were not continued for more than from forty to forty-eight hours, if the worm had not been killed before the expiration of that time. Dr. Küchenmeister made use of electricity as the most delicate re-agent for proving the occurrence of the death of the worms. In the first place, electricity cannot be considered as a vermifuge. The author subjected a female *Heterakis vescicularis*, taken from a partridge that had been killed, to the action of a rotatory apparatus, which was kept up with longer or shorter intervals during an entire day. The animal was not destroyed by the experiment. He next tried the remedies employed for the removal of tæniæ, and first tested kousso in the following manner:—A living *Tænia crassicolis*, procured from a cat, was placed at four o'clock in a mixture of albumen and dolichos pruriens. The worm appeared to be perfectly well in this mixture, and at two o'clock on the following afternoon exhibited the most vigorous movements. The tænia was now transferred to a vessel containing a mixture of infusion of kousso and some of the infused as well as some of the fresh powder with albumen. The temperature of the mixture was 30° R. (99·5° F.) On its introduction, the worm quickly extended itself; after some time it was found to be dead, its color having changed to a dirty reddish-yellow. Two *Tæniæ serratæ* were placed at about half-past one in the afternoon in a mixture of albumen and kousso; at two o'clock they were dying, and at three completely dead. Two *Tæniæ serratæ* from the same dog were brought in contact with kousso and milk at half-past one in the afternoon, and at two o'clock were dead.

Two *Tæniæ serratæ* were placed at half-past one in the afternoon in albumen, mixed with decoction of pomegranate root, and with some of the powdered root: they died in three hours. Two others were placed in milk mixed with the decoction only: they died in three and a-half hours.

A *Tænia crassicolis* was put into a mixture of albumen with ethereal extract of male fern: it died gradually in three hours and three quarters. A number of *Tæniæ cucumerinæ* were placed in a mixture of albumen and oil of turpentine: they were dead in an hour and a quarter.

A number of the same were put into a mixture of albumen and castor-oil. They appeared lively at first, but were dead in seven hours. Similar worms were put into a salad, composed of pieces of unwatered herring, boiled potatoes, large pieces of onion and garlic, albumen, vinegar, and a large quantity of oil. They died in eight hours. Lastly, the author tested the vermifuge powers of the brown oxide of copper: fifteen grains were administered in the course of four days to a strong cat. When the body was opened, the entire intestinal canal was found to be full of fluid, yellow, flakey fæces, the intestine was softened and denuded of epithelium, especially at the termination of the ileum, where the adjoining Peyer's glands were much swollen, particularly in two situations, one of which was an inch and a-half long, by one-third of an inch broad; the other was nearly circular, and its diameter one-third of an inch. The cat had been purged. The tænia and ascarides it contained were lively. It would hence appear that this substance is both inefficacious as a vermifuge and dangerous to the system. The following are the results of the above experiments:—

In milk boiled with kousso, tæniæ died in half an hour.

In a mixture of oil of turpentine and albumen, in one hour to one and a-quarter.

In decoction of kousso with albumen, in one and a-half to three hours.

In decoction of pomegranate root with milk, in from three to three and a-half hours.

In decoction of pomegranate root with albumen, in three hours.

In ethereal extract of male fern with albumen, in three and a-half to four hours.

In castor oil with albumen, in eight hours.

In salmagundi, with garlic and onions, in eight hours.

Kousso would therefore seem to be the most efficacious remedy against tæniæ. When pomegranate bark and male fern-root fail, their failure may be owing to the habit of administering a laxative in from four to six hours after the exhibition of the vermifuge, by which the latter may be carried beyond the worm. With regard to pomegranate root, it must be observed, that in large doses it occasions diarrhœa. The same remark applies to castor oil. The author also alludes to cold water, strawberries, dolichos pruriens, and filings of tin. When tæniæ are placed in water containing ice, they are instantly benumbed, and if allowed to remain in it, they will always be found, at the end of ten hours, to be quite dead. Strawberries may be useful as a mild remedy in cases of tapeworm; if large quantities of them be taken on an empty stomach, entire portions of the worm will often be passed. Dolichos pruriens, with which the author tried many experiments, appears to possess no power of destroying worms. The author has also minutely studied the medicines recommended for the removal of round worms. In albumen, these worms behave as the tæniæ; in water, at about 77° F., they live for some days, but swell, stiffen, become longer, thicker, and more sluggish; they lose their power of suction, and their motions become slow and only partial,—they resemble leeches which have gorged themselves. In general, however, the males and young neutrals resist the effects of water longer than the mature, impregnated, egg-bearing females, which become quite rigid and inflexible, and swell considerably. Milk and whey affect the worms like water. The following are the medicines, the effects of which were tested:

1. Camphor. An ascaris lived from eighteen to twenty hours in albumen into which some camphor had been introduced. 2. A mixture of oil of turpentine and albumen killed some ascarides which were placed in it from two and a-half to six hours. 3. Ascarides lived forty hours in albumen and wormseed, whether the latter was employed in the form of powder or infusion. 4. Some ascarides were placed in albumen mixed with santonine; they did not die in it, nor did they die in a watery infusion of santonine. When santonine was dissolved in oil, especially in castor-oil, and mixed with albumen and ascarides, the latter died in ten minutes. An injection of santonine and castor-oil was thrown up the rectum of a cat, and produced numerous motions containing dead worms; and on killing the cat, the entire of the lower portion of the intestinal canal, was ascertained to be free from worms, while four were found near the stomach, rigid and extended, and retaining but little life. A *Tænia crassicolis*, however, was found in the intestines, and appeared to be quite uninjured and very lively. 5. A mixture of albumen and aniseed, with a strong infusion of the latter killed the worms in about twenty-four hours. 6. Parsley mixed with albumen, killed ascarides very slowly. 7. Flour of mustard and albumen destroyed them in about four hours. 8. In rue the worms lived upwards of twenty-four hours.

9. The same was the case with millefoil. In contact with tansy, valerian, and millefoil, great numbers of them lived for twenty-four hours. With onions and garlic, they perished in from ten to fifteen hours. A decoction of cloves, with or without albumen, killed them in twelve hours. In an infusion of ginger, with or without albumen, they lived about twenty-four hours. Petroleum, mixed with albumen, killed them in less than six hours, as did also oil of cajeput and albumen.

A series of vermifuges taken from the class of balsamics, was tried in like manner, namely, assafœtida, ammoniacum, balsam of Peru, extract of juniper, and Venice turpentine. In all these the worms lived more than twenty-four hours. Of the class of empyreumatics (brenzlichen stoffe) the following were tried:—Oleum chaberti [a mixture of four parts of oil of turpentine, and one of the animal oil of Dippel], oil of amber, castor oil, tar-water, creasote, wood-vinegar, and wood-soot. In these, for the most part, the worms lived twenty-four to forty-eight hours, except the wood-vinegar, in which they lived rather more than twelve, and creasote, in which they died within two hours. Of bitters the author tried aloes, gamboge, ox-gall, wormwood, myrrh, gentian, quassia, hops, bitter orange, and acorus calamus; in all these the ascarides lived from twenty-four to forty hours. Of astringents, pure tannic acid, pomegranate root, kousso, extract of walnuts, cinchona bark and quina, elm bark, willow-bark, and the flowers and stalk of meadow-sweet, oak-bark, dragon's blood, catechu, and kino. In these the worms died in from twenty-four to thirty hours, with but two exceptions, namely, tincture of galls and pomegranate root, both of which killed them in the space of eleven hours. Of saline preparations, sulphate of soda, chloride of sodium, and the roe of the herring were tried. In the first the worms died in from fifteen to eighteen hours; in the second, in from two to six; and in the roe of the herring, in four hours. The following metallic poisons were experimented on: Arsenic, calomel, corrosive sublimate, and the salts of tin, of lead, and of copper. Corrosive sublimate alone destroyed the worms in so short a time as two hours; all the other metallic salts required a much longer period. From these experiments it would appear, that santonine, mixed with oil, is the most powerful vermifuge, then chloride of sodium, the roe of the herring, garlic, onions, &c. The author advises that santonine should be given as a vermifuge, mixed with oil, in the proportion of from two to five grains to an ounce of castor-oil. This solution should be given in the doses of a tea-spoonful, until the effect is produced. As auxiliary treatment, chloride of sodium, herring-brine, mustard, onions, and garlic, may be employed.—*Froriep's Tagsberichte uber die Fortschritte der Natur- und Heilkunde.* Pharmakologie, Band 1, *p.* 317.

---

M. MOUCHON states, that by combining 48 grammes of syrup of orgeat, or syrup of milk, with 16 grammes of castor oil and but 20 centigrammes of calcined magnesia, we may obtain a syrup of castor oil for young children, which purges in a dose of from 30 to 60 grammes, without possessing the slightest unpleasant taste. It may be rendered more pleasant by the addition of a drop of the essence of peppermint, lemon, bitter almonds, &c. —*L'Abeille Medicale.*

---

# EDITORIAL.

## MEMOIR OF M. ORFILA.

IN our last number we published some account of the life and labors of Dr. Pereira. The death of the great English pharmacologist has been speedily followed by that of one who in a somewhat different sphere had attained a still higher and wider-spread reputation. Orfila was born at Mahon, in Minorca, on the 24th of April, 1787. He was intended by his friends for the naval service, but, after a short trial, he gave up the sea, and, in 1804, sought a more congenial pursuit in the university of Valencia. He early applied himself to chemistry, and so distinguished himself, that, in 1807, he was sent, at their own expense, by the Junta of Barcelona, to Paris, to acquire in that great capital a knowledge of his favorite studies which could not be afforded him in his native country. The invasion of Spain by Bonaparte, soon deprived Orfila of the pecuniary assistance thus afforded. Fortunately, a member of his own family, settled in France, agreed to make him an annual allowance until he had finished his studies, and obtained the doctorate. Years afterward, at a time when the acceptance of his proposal would have entailed great personal sacrifice, with a gratitude that does him honor, Orfila offered to return to Spain, and enter into the service of the Junta; the unfortunate position of the country, however, prevented the acceptance of his offer.

On his graduation, Orfila supported himself by private teaching, giving lectures on chemistry and forensic medicine, while he devoted his leisure to researches on the means of detecting poisons, not only when in a state of simple solution in water, but when mixed with various organic matters. He thus early laid the foundation of his future eminence.

Orfila was soon elected a member of the Institute. In 1816, he was appointed one of the physicians of Louis XVIII. In 1819, he was elected Professor of Forensic Medicine. In 1823, he was chosen Professor of Medical Chemistry.

In his new situations, the interest which he was enabled to impart to his subject, his happy delivery, and the profusion, the appropriateness, and the clearness of his illustrations, soon gathered around him a numerous auditory. He soon became one of the most popular lecturers in Paris, and the doors of his lecture-room were besieged by crowds of students long before they were opened. He devoted himself assiduously to the study of toxicology, and his authority on this point was soon universally acknowledged. Cases from all parts of France were referred to him for examination. One of the most important of his discoveries was the detection of poison in the tissues of the body itself. He not only prevented crime by rendering its detection comparatively certain and easy, but often saved the innocent from unjust punishment, by proving the non-existence of poisoning in cases in which, on insufficient grounds, it had been suspected.

On the accession of Louis Philippe, in 1830, Orfila became Dean of the Faculty of Medicine, and soon afterwards member of the Council General of Hospitals, and of the Council of Public Instruction, and he was made successively, Chevalier, Officer, and Commander of the Legion of Honor. In all these appointments he sustained his high reputation, and was the originator of numerous reforms and improvements. Among others, a new botanical garden, and the Orfila Museum, attest his zeal and munificence.

Orfila now was at the height of prosperity—wealthy, courted, in high office, his time filled by important duties and scientific studies. The revolution of 1848 deprived him of all his appointments except his professorship, which could not be taken from him. He seems to have felt the blow acutely, and it is said to have embittered the last years of his life. Other misfortunes weighed upon him. His son, long subject to epilepsy, became impaired in intellect, and had finally to be placed in a *maison de santé*. His death, however, was unexpected. Soon after announcing the magnificent bequests which were recounted in a former number, at a time when it was still a matter of consideration how the physicians of Paris should best show their sense of his noble liberality, he was attacked with pneumonia, and expired on the 12th of March, only eight days after he had appeared in the lecture-room.

M. Orfila has left distinct works on forensic medicine, on medical chemistry, and on toxicology. The 5th and last edition of his *Elements of Toxicology*, in two thick octavos, was published last year. Besides these, he is the author of a great number of papers and reports, on subjects relating to medical jurisprudence.

*The Pocket Formulary and Synopsis of the British and Foreign Pharmacopœias: comprising standard and approved Formulæ for the Preparations and Compounds employed in Medical Practice.* By Henry Beasley. 1st American, from the last London edition, improved and enlarged. Philadelphia, Lindsay and Blakiston, 1852. *pp.* 443.

*The Druggist's general Receipt Book: Comprising a copious Veterinary Formulary and Table of Veterinary Materia Medica, numerous Receipts in Patent and Proprietary Medicines, Druggists' Nostrums, &c.; Perfumery and Cosmetics, Beverages, Dietetic Articles, and Condiments; Trade Chemicals, &c. With an Appendix of useful Tables.* By Henry Beasley. Second American, from the last London edition, corrected and enlarged. Philadelphia, Lindsay and Blakiston, 1853. *pp.* 472.

We have placed these two books, by the same author and from the same publishers together, though they have objects entirely dissimilar. The first, as its title expresses, is a digest of the American, British, and foreign Pharmacopœia, together with numerous formulæ, derived from the special pharmacopœias of various hospitals, and from the works of practitioners of eminence. It seems exceedingly well arranged, and contains a large amount of valuable information, which cannot readily be found elsewhere, compressed into so small a space. If, as it deserves, the book should reach a second edition, we would recommend the publishers to enlarge the table of synonyms. It is not every one who would be able to discover the "Poudre du frère Cosme," under the head of "Pulvis Escharoticus Arsenicalis."

The second work is intended more especially for the druggist. Its title sufficiently announces its contents, and if carefully and well prepared, as we have good reason to believe it is, it cannot fail to be generally useful.

---

*The Action of Medicines in the System; or, On the Mode in which Therapeutic Agents introduced into the Stomach, produce their peculiar Effects on the Animal Economy*, being the prize essay to which the Medical Society of London awarded the Fothergillian gold medal for MDCCCLII. By Frederick William Headland, B. A., M. R. C. S., etc. Philadelphia, Lindsay and Blakiston, 1853. 8vo., *pp.* 560.

Mr. Headland's book is a full and clear exposition of the doctrines which have now begun to prevail, in regard to the manner in which medicines produce their physiological and therapeutic effects. It is well and carefully written, and deserves to be carefully studied.

---

*A Treatise on General Pathology.* By Dr. J. Henlé, Professor of Anatomy and Physiology, in Heidelberg. Translated from the German by Henry C. Preston. A. M., M. D. Philadelphia, Lindsay and Blakiston, 1853. 8vo., *pp.* 391.

The subject of Dr. Henlé's work does not come within the purpose of this journal, but the work itself reflects credit on the enterprizing publisher, and cannot fail to be useful and acceptable to the medical profession. The translation is by Dr. Preston, of Providence, R. I.

NEW YORK

# JOURNAL OF PHARMACY.

JULY, 1853.

## OTTO OF ROSES:

### WHERE PRODUCED—THE QUANTITY MADE—USED IN SNUFF—LANGUAGE OF FLOWERS.

THE truthfulness of accounts by travellers in foreign countries of the customs, manners, products, politics etc., is as much dependent upon the company they fall in with and the acquaintances they make, as upon their own observations.

The writer of the following letter has evidently fallen into good hands. He has consulted those who know and who have not labored to deceive.—Our readers will perceive that his account of the production of oil of Roses confirms in the main the account given in the letter which was published in No. 2, Vol. 1, of this Journal.

The statements set forth in the present communication, though generally accurate contain some errors which we now propose to set forth.

The centre of production is the town or small district of "Kissanlik" and not "Hasanlik" as here spelt, probably a typographical error.

An error also occurs in the account of the weights—Nine of

the Turkish drachms or metical here called weigh one ounce avoirdupois.

The Geranium oil is now almost exclusively the substance used for the adulteration of Rose oil.—The peculiar property which the latter has of becoming concrete in a crystalline form in moderately cold weather is not sensibly injured by the addition of 50 per cent of Geranium oil showing that this property does not indicate purity.

The statements that a variation in adulteration of 2 per cent can be detected by the Constantinople dealers by the smell is a hard story to believe—I have no faith that any mortal nose can discriminate in a variation of 10 per cent.

The writer has paid considerable attention to the detection of adulteration in this article but has arrived at no satisfactory result. It is a misfortune that no accurate test either chemical or mechanical is known to exist, as it is well known that the nose is a very unreliable instrument; but so it is, may we hope for a better and that science will soon throw light on the subject.

---

THE "spicy East," "the perfumed gales of Araby" "redolent of odors as an oriental bride"—these common phrases indicate our usual associations with the East. It is true that the Orientals love perfumes, and perhaps have a religious regard for them, because Mohammed loved them excessively, and praised the use of them. But, instead of depending on Eastern resources, the Constantinopolitans are equally the purchasers with ourselves of the essences and pomades of Paris. When the emporiums of commerce for the Western barbarians of Europe were in the East, they of course received their perfumes from thence; but the source from whence sweet-scented odors is derived is the wide, wide world, and no longer the indefinite East. Even the queen of aromas, otto of roses, so far as used in Europe and America, is nearly all of it raised in Europe. The word "otto" is more properly written "attar," which simply means perfume, and the substance itself, as used in Turkey is usually called Oil of Roses.

The time has been when Tunis used to furnish the finest otto of roses known in Europe: at present not an ounce is exported from there. Mecco, Aleppo, and Damascus have been said to yield it in abundance; but now all these places, including Tunis, are supplied from the market of Constantinple. Ghazipore, in India, on the Ganges, and not in

> "the Vale of Cashmere,
> With its roses the brightest the world ever gave,"

still prepares a rich and extremely dear oil, but it is never exported thence to England. It is almost entirely consumed among the people there on festival occasions. Its price also is enormous, said to be one hundred dollars an ounce.

The centre of production in Turkey in Europe for the oil of roses which is exported is in a small district called Hassanlik, in Bulgaria. Hassanlik is a shire-town, about 200 miles northwest of Constantinople, and gives its name to a district of thirty-six villages, which is devoted mainly to the cultivation of the rose. Though the villages are all situated on a plain on elevated ground, yet as the plain is protected by high mountains, the climate of the region is very moderate. The inhabitants are all of the Bulgarian Sclavonic race, in part Mussulmans, and in part Christians. The rose which they cultivate for the sake of the leaves is the red *Centifolia*,

> "The flowret of a hundred leaves,"

and is planted in the open fields with the same profusion as corn or potatoes with us The roses are in full bloom by the month of May, and before the second week in June, the harvest of leaves has been completed, and nothing is done in collecting them at any other time. During the season of flowering, the whole country for miles beyond the district is redolent with the odor of roses. The digging and pruning of the bushes, collecting the leaves, the process of distillation, and the manufacture of vessels to hold the oil, occupy the people nearly the whole of their time.

In distilling the oil, the usual process for extracting volatile or essential oils is pursued. The rose leaves, while fresh, are placed in the alembic, and fresh water is poured upon them. The water which comes over is successively distilled, and finally, the oil, being the lightest, rises to the top, and is skimmed off. The oil is limpid, but with a tinge of orange color. It is said to take three hundred thousand roses to yield an ounce of oil. It is brought to Constantinople in flat-sided, round-edged tinned copper vessels, each hermetically closed, and sealed with the maker's name. These cases vary in size from those capable of holding an ounce to those which hold seven pounds, or even more. At Constantinople, after passing into other hands, it is put up in gilt bottles, which preserve the antique form of two hundred years back, and are manufactured in Bohemia expressly for the purpose.

The quantity of otto of roses produced in any one year varies like that of most productions of the soil. In the year 1837, a very good one, the district yielded 4,465 pounds. In the worst years they do not obtain more than 1,500 pounds, and an ordinary year's amount of production may be estimated at something less than 3,000 pounds. The weight employed in buying and selling it is a peculiar one, the *metical*, which is just a drachm and a half, and nine drachms make a Troy ounce. The fair price of the veritable pure otto is about 65 cents the *metical*, or $6 an ounce, equal to $72 a pound. Consequently, one of those copper cases may be worth $500, and the oil is worth five to seven times its weight in silver. The price of the oil commonly to be found may not be more than $4 or $5 an ounce; but as the amount exported is nearly doubled by mixing with foreign oils, the value of the trade in otto of roses to Turkey, may annually be about $400,000.

The oil that was formerly mixed with otto of roses was sandal wood oil, which is worth only $5 or $6 a pound. In the mass it has little or no smell, but when diffused, its odor is very agreeable. It is much less liquid and flowing than the oil of roses, and adheres a long time to the hand. Within comparatively a few years, a new oil has been introduced to dilute oil of roses, and render it less overpowering. It is called by the Arabs, who bring it from Mecca, *ittri shahi*, which means "shepherd's perfume," and by another name is called shepherd's crook, or crane's bill. This is a kind of geranium, the odor of the oil of which very nearly resembles the odor of the leaf of the pennyroyal geranium much more than it does the odor of the flower called with us crane's bill. The Arabs say that they make this oil among themselves, and they sell it as low as $2 a pound, or one thirty-sixth of the price of the otto of rose. Its odor in the mass is extremely agreeable, and produces none of the oppressive and even nauseating effects upon some constitutions that oil of roses does. Both on account of its cheapness, a certain similarity of odor, its likeness in color and weight with otto of roses, no other oil combines so many qualities to render it appropriate to mix with it and reduce its strength. In the common oil of roses found in the shops there is probably fifty per cent. of foreign oils; and on account of the diffusibility of aroma, it will bear to receive, without any perceivable depreciation (in the opinion of ordinary judges) of its virtues and character, even eighty per cent. of foreign oils, especially of the oil of geranium, if it has been cleanly washed in water, and well bleached in the sun.

The reduction of its strength by mixture begins at Hasanlik. The people there are probably ready to supply nearly as much as there is a profitable demand for. The oil of geranium is sometimes poured upon the leaves and distilled over with the liquor of the roses. A suitable quantity of oil of geranium to suit the necessary profits of the seller and the price the buyer is willing to pay, is also added previous to exportation; and large quantities of the same oil are exported to foreign lands, and may serve to adapt the quality of otto of roses to the exigencies of purchasers. It is a proof of the progress of refinement and luxury, and of the prosperity of America, that the highest-priced and therefore the purest of otto of rose is more and more sought for from Turkey.

There are individuals in Constantinople whose profession it is to examine and test for the merchants the quality of otto of roses, and they will readily divide the samples offered to them into five or six qualities, almost entirely by the sense of smell, and they are the persons who most successfully perform the manipulations necessary in mixing. It is said, they never fail of coming within two per cent. of the amount of foreign oil existing in any specimen offered to them to examine. The common test among all classes engaged in the trade is to moisten a piece of white paper with oil of roses, and, if it is pure, it will entirely evaporate, leaving not a trace upon the paper, but yet a very marked perfume. If it is a mixed oil, it will, on the contrary, leave a stain upon the paper, but no odor.

The usual appearance of otto of roses is here sufficiently well known by all but the greenhorns. They, however, are always numerous enough to induce the Jews of Smyrna and Constantinople to prepare, in exchange for people's money, the meanest compound of scented grease and oils, and they waylay sea captains and travellers, in the streets, and induce them to buy, at prices not much below common otto of roses, numerous bottles full of something resembling rather spermaceti and oil, as choice presents for their wives and friends. Occasionally such persons go home with most fabulous stories of the cheapness of oil of roses. One afternoon last year, an American traveller returned to his hotel from an excursion in the bazaar of Constantinople, and exultingly showed to his fellow travellers a precious speculation he had made in otto of roses. He had bought six ounces, in as many bottles, for five dollars a bottle. An intelligent companion soon convinced him that he had obtained nothing but six bottles of olive oil scented with rose, and in a natural fit of indignation and mortification, he opened the window, and threw bottle after bottle on the pavement of the street below. As otto of roses is an oil, many seem to suppose that the more oily it is the better the otto, even if it is as unctuous as bear's grease.

America is probably a larger consumer of otto than any

country of the same amount of population, but no indication can be found in this of the strong attachment the ladies may have for costly aromas. For one pound of otto of roses that is sold to the perfumer, a hundred pounds are sold to the snuff manufacturers, to scent therewith their best snuffs.

The water that has been employed in the process of distillation to obtain the oil of roses, furnishes what is called rose water. It is brought abundantly to the city in barrels, like wine, and sold about as cheap, costing not more than eight or ten cents a quart. Constant use is made of it on festival occasions in the Greek and Armenian churches, and it is also sprinkled on guests, as a token of welcome, by the members of a family.

In concluding this long talk about the rose, I cannot help adding that the signification of the thought or idea spoken by the rose, in the Eastern language of flowers, is not a whit more intensive than that of many more common plants and flowers. Perceval has said:

"In Eastern lands they talk in flowers,
And tell in a garden their loves and cares;
Each flower that in their gardens blow,
A strange and mystic language bears."

But the poetry of the language of flowers, in Turkey at least, reduces itself to the merest play or puns upon words. Thus, as pomegranate in Turkish is *nar*, and, as *nar* means "fire," so if a pomegranate is sent with other flowers to one's beloved, it expresses the fire that burns in your breast, albeit the pomegranate is one of the most cooling fruits we have. The kind of language of love that the rose speaks is also derived from the sound of its name in Turkish, which is *gul*, and which at the same time means "laugh," or "be pleased." And hence, a present of a rose to your *inamorata* is an invitation to her to be pleased with the love you bear her.—*Correspondence of the "New York Daily Times."*

*For the N. Y. Journal of Pharmacy.*

# LETTER FROM DR. GUTHRIE.

DEAR SIR:

As time slips away and the indications of Summer remind me of the fact that only about three months will elapse before the annual meeting of the American Pharmaceutical Association, an oft entertained purpose, kept down by the press of business hitherto, of calling attention to the important questions to come before that meeting, induces me again to address you.

Aside from the questions that were so ably discussed at Philadelphia last year, and upon which I trust the committees will make full, able and complete reports, there are others of quite as much importance that will merit our attention.

I have myself two or three propositions which I intend to bring before the association, and that Druggists and Apothecaries may have time to think upon them, and improve them as I know they can, I will state this long in advance.

1st. In regard to Druggists and Drug stores, for retail of medicine, I propose to recommend each state and legislature to pass an act requiring every such store to have in their employ, either as principal or assistant, a regularly educated graduate of medicine or pharmacy.

2nd. In regard to *Patent Medicines*, I propose to recommend each state to require every person offering for sale any patent or secret medicine, designed and recommended for exhibition as a remedial agent, to file in the proper office of each state wherein such remedy is offered, a full and complete formula of such remedy, and that under oath, moreover such person so offering goods for sale, on agency, or otherwise, shall obtain from the proper authority, of such county, a general or special license; allowing such agent or proprietor only such privileges as other pedlars enjoy.

3rd. I propose that Druggists, as a body, or at least the members of the A.P. Asso. pledge themselves to require of every agent or proprietor of patent medicines, offering them such goods for sale, the full formula of such preparations—and decline to give the sanction of their name, and the influence of their houses in bringing into notice and giving character to any secret remedy, unless such request is complied with.

Something of this kind is required, and the reasons for offering these suggestions, is to bring the matter before our brethern of the profession of pharmacy now, so that any improvements may be suggested, and reasons for and against, be brought forward on the 24th day of August next, at our meeting in Boston.

Yours, &c.

C. B. GUTHRIE.

Memphis, May, 20th 1853.

---

## ON A SUBSTITUTE FOR LAUDANUM.

BY DAVID STEWART, M. D., OF BALTIMORE.

Believing that the product of the following formula has a peculiar value as a therapeutic agent apart from its excellence as a *definite* compound, and its pharmaceutic value; I have taken the liberty to request the National Medical Association to substitute it for Mc Munn's Elixir of opium, and other nostrums that are used as substitutes for the officinal anodyne preparations, and if it deserves the superiority we have attributed to it, to give it a place in the Pharmacopœia.

The National Pharmacopœia does not recognize any preparation of opium of definite strength, except the solution of morphia—and the increasing and extensive substitution of other formulæ (for the officinal) by the most learned and judicious members of the faculty, shows clearly that some improvement is demanded or other preparation required. For we can hardly suppose that the mystery thrown around a nostrum and its high price would tempt the notice of so many of the profession.

Take of opium, two ounces or one thousand grains ; lime (an hydrous), half an ounce, = ℥ ; water, twelve ounces, = ℥ xij ; alcohol, one pint, or a sufficiency ; muriate of ammonia, five grains.

Shake the lime, and make a "milk" with two ounces of water, in a porcelain dish or an enamelled iron vessel. Combine the opium with four ounces of water, by levigating it in a mortar of porcelain, until it is throughly divided ; separate the infusion from the dregs of the opium, by means of a muslin cloth, and wash the dregs by repeated affusions of boiling water. Boil the solution of opium with the milk of lime for a few moments ; filter while hot, through a "plain filter ;" wash the magma with a few ounces of lime water until the filtrate measures (10) ten ounces ; separate one ounce of the filtrate ; concentrate it to about half an ounce ; add the five grains of muriate of ammonia ; boil for a few moments ; collect the morphia that is deposited after twelve hours, and if it weighs (6) six grains, add nine ounces of alcohol to the nine ounces of the remaining filtrate, or a sufficient quantity, so that each ounce may contain (3) grains of morphia.

The above formula produces a tincture resembling the laudanum of the pharmacopœia in color, taste, and smell,—it differs from a simple solution of morphia in possessing all of the volatile narcotic principles of opium, and does not require more than two hours manipulation during an interval of one day: while that of the pharmacopœia requires two weeks, and when completed exactly in accordance with the formula, may vary in strength from one to four grains of morphia per ounce, (as the best varieties of opium vary in this proportion.)

It will be noticed that our process is based on the facts—that morphia and the volatile narcotic principles of opium are soluble in lime water, and that codeia and narcotine, are insoluble in this menstruum. We know that those who have the most experience in the use of opium prefer the volatile principles (or smoke it); and as many patients cannot use codeia and narcotine in their natural combinations, it is to these facts we owe the preparations of Sydenham, Battely, &c., also the black drops, morphia, &c. And as the successful treatment of most cases is more intimately connected with the comfort of the patient and tranquility of the nervous system than any other condition; every judicious and humane practitioner will attach more importance to means of this class than any other.

Respectfully,

DAVID STEWART,
77 N. Eutaw street,
Baltimore, Maryland.

29th April, 1853.

---

## PHARMACEUTICAL NOTICES

BY F. MAYER.

*German and American Pharmacy.*

After having previously spoken of Pharmacy in general, I now proceed to treat of its special departments, and in the first place to a review of the officinal preparations, (verrathigen-arzneimittel) the acids, ethers, plasters, tinctures, essences, syrups &c. One would fancy, since in Germany everything must be prepared strictly according to the Pharmocopœia, this could be done quickly and readily, but this is not so, on the contrary, since Germany is divided and split up into so many different states, each of which must have its own pharmacopœia, and avail itself as little as possible of that of its neighbors, the confusion there is greater than in other countries.

To the acids belong first the medicated vinegars, and of these there were formerly an immense number in the pharmaceutical hand-books. The acid employed was sometimes simple distilled wine vinegar. Since the quick vinegar manufacture from corn spirits has become common throughout Germany, by which a good vinegar which contains about 18 per cent acetic acid, of which an ounce will saturate about a dram and a half of carbonate of soda, can be had at a very low price, the wine vinegar manufacture has received a great blow. Instead of diluting such a vinegar, commonly termed double vinegar, (doppelessig) with simple water, a corresponding quantity of wine is added in preference, by which an excellent wine vinegar is obtained, which improves in strength by keeping. It will immediately be seen that such a vinegar, thus diluted with wine instead of water, however excellent for all ordinary purposes, may be too vinous for medicinal use. When the vinegar is prepared by diluting it with equal parts of wine and water, little objection can be made, since even ordinary wine vinegar, although the quantity of wine will be exceedingly small, will generally contain some which has not undergone decomposition.

Of the medicated vinegars, (Aceta medicata.) there are still employed, acetum aromaticum, prepared from aromatic herbs, with a greater or less quantity of spirits of wine, and raw or distilled vinegar. Instead of this preparation an acidum aceticum aromaticum is often used, made from sweet smelling oils and acetic acid.

Acetum Lavandulæ, Rosæ and a few other aromatic vinegars may be passed over as more or less insignificant. Acetum Rubi Idaei is best made with syrupus Rubi Idaei and wine vinegar. Acetum Scilliticum by a solution of extractum scillae, spirituoso-aquosum, in diluted wine vinegar.

I may mention here that in many of the old handbooks an

acetum saturni is spoken of, which has also received the half modernized name of acetum plumbicum, and is the well known solution of the basic acetate of lead in water. In this country the name, by means of the ordinary abbreviation might lead to a mistake on the part of the apothecary, since acet. plumbi, represents alike acetas plumbi, sugar of lead and the so called acetum plumbicum.

The aceta medicata are for the most part popular preparations and their preparation cannot on this account be subjected readily to rational improvement, yet it would be preferable to mix a vinegar of a known strength and as pure as possible, or formic acid with good etherial oils.

Of the ACIDS of course little is to be said.

*Acidum aceticum.* The best mode of preparation appears to be the decomposition of dry acetate of soda, by means of sulphuric acid. When we employ the sulphuric acid as a simple hydrate in the proportion of two equivalents to one equivalent of acetate of soda, and then carefully distil by means of an oil bath, we readily obtain a perfectly pure glacial acetic acid.

When we do not desire to obtain glacial-acetic acid, the preparation of which is somewhat expensive, but only a good acetic acid such as is commonly officinal, I prefer in all cases the decomposition of the acetate of lime by means of muriatic acid to that of acetate of lead.

*Acidum Benzoicum* is in Germany, still in very general use. Lately they have returned for its preparation to what is termed employed, acetum aromaticum—prepared from aromatic herbs, the dry way, [via sicca] which for a long time was deserted for the moist method. To speak my own mind plainly and wholly upon the matter I look upon this dry method as trifling and prefer obtaining the acid by boiling gum benzoin with caustic lime and afterwards precipitating by means of muriatic acid to all other methods.

*Acidum Boracicum* has in Germany few uses. In France it is employed for the preparation of Tartarus boraxatus. Its preparation by the decomposition of purified biborate of soda, by muriatic acid seems to me to give the most satisfactory results.

*Acidum Carbonicum.* This excellent medicine is very little employed in the German shops, when we except its preparation extempore as in the Potio Riverii and in effervescing powders. The acid springs of Germany give it to the public in a form so well liked and in such quantity, that its artificial preparation as carbonic acid wateris less a necessity than in other countries.

*Acidum Citricum* is an article of commerce and seldom prepared by the apothecary. When we reflect that the juice of unripe grapes contains this acid, while when ripe they contain scarce any but tartaric acid, one might suppose for medicinal use, this latter was a riper product of organic chemistry than the former.

*Acidum Formicum* is not officinal, though for the preparation of scents it is far preferable to vinegar.

*Acidicum Gallicum vel Gallarum* is seldom used by the physician and then mainly in combination with bases as quinine. There is so much regarding the preparation and relations of this acid, particularly the part, which from late researches sugar plays in its formation,which is still unknown, that it offers a wide field for the practical observer.

*Acidum Hydrochloricum.* This acid has been so thoroughly investigated in all its aspects that I have no remark to make upon it except to notice the confusion created by the varying strength which is directed by the numerous pharmacopœias in Germany, the acid differing from 1.10 sp. gr. as diluted to 1,33 and 1.60 as strong.

I had never occasion in Germany to meet with a hydrochloric acid at once so strong and so free from impurity as I can obtain here in commerce. I was acquainted in Germany with a colleague who was also an examiner, and who always held it for an important point when he entered the shop of another to ascertain if the hydrochloric acid was entirely free from chlorine, in fact as common and important an impurity as conversely the presence of muriatic acid in chlorine water, which often brought my friend to the verge of despair.

# ON THE EMPLOYMENT OF THE ALBUMINATE OF IRON AND SODA AS A THERAPEUTIC AGENT, IN VARIOUS CASES IN WHICH FERRUGINOUS PREPARATIONS ARE INDICATED.

BY ANGELICO FABBRI, PHARMACEUTICAL CHEMIST AT GUBBIO.

Simple contact, at the ordinary temperature of the atmosphere, of white of egg with a salt of iron and soda, is capable of instantly producing a soluble albuminate of iron and soda, or an albumin-ferrate of the alkaline base. The chemical combination of this compound is such, that it is not altered by the yellow ferrocyanide of potassium the most delicate test of the salts of iron unless a few drops of acid, as for example the hydrochloric, be previously added to the soluble albuminate, thus proving that this decomposition cannot be effected by the agency of the alkalies, but only by some acids, since the potassium of the cyanide is not able to displace the oxide of iron, becoming oxidized at its expense, and setting the metal free, as occurs with the other ferruginous preparations. Considering that we find in the blood, albumen soda in excess, and iron, and having shown how these three bodies, by simple direct contact, form a soluble salt, the chemical combination of which is so powerful that it is not destroyed by the most delicate re-agents, may we not fairly infer that the iron exists in the blood as an albuminate of iron and soda; and would it not therefore, be reasonable to administer iron in the various diseases in which it is prescribed, principally in reference to the state of the sanguineous system, in the form of albuminate, as that in which nature itself has placed it within our organism,—one of the products, so to speak, on which our life depends. When I read in works of chemistry that the yellow ferrocyanide of potassium is not capable of demonstrating the presence of iron in the blood, until a stream of chlorine has first been passed through the latter to destroy its coloring matter, I am confirmed in the opinion that the iron exists in that fluid as an albuminate of iron and soda, because this salt, requiring the addition of an acid to render it capable of detection by the cyanide, is supplied with it by the chlorine, which in destroying the organic coloring matter, becomes converted into hydrochloric acid by uniting with their hydrogen. Physicians have been long puzzled, and are still at a loss, how to administer iron, a most valuable remedy, in the manner most suitable to the internal organism; hence the great number of preparations of this metal. Some object to its saline combination with mineral acids, on the ground that these are inorganic, and they prefer giving it in the metallic or oxidized state, leaving to the acids of the stomach to form with it compounds which may be carried into the circulation. Others, unwilling to run the risk of having the greater part of the iron—little, or not at all acted upon—expelled with the fœces, prescribe it in the saline state, but combined with organic vegetable acids; hence we have the malate, tannate, citrate, &c., of iron. Others still more scrupulous, wish to have it united to acids of an animal nature, and prefer the lactate, the cyanide &c., and I, going still farther, would recommend its employment in the state of albuminate of iron and soda, requesting physicians to take into consideration what I have advanced, and to ascertain if practice will in this instance corroborate theory.

In preparing the albuminate of iron and soda, I employ the following process. Take 112 grains of caustic soda, and 104 of sulphate of iron. Having dissolved both in a sufficient quantity of distilled water, let the solutions be poured on the whites of four eggs previously beaten up; let all now be shaken together and poured upon a filter to separate the hydrated oxide of iron which has precipitated, since all the iron is not in this case converted into albuminate. To the filtered liquid, which now contains, in addition to the albuminate, sulphate of soda formed by the decomposition of sulphate of iron by the soda present in excess, lime water is to be added, to decompose the sulphate of soda, by which an insoluble sulphate of lime is precipitated; to separate the latter, the mixture is to be again filtered, and as the filtered fluid will now contain an excess of lime it is to be subjected to the action of a stream of carbonic acid, care being taken to avoid using an excess of the latter; and again filtered to get rid of the insoluble carbonate of lime thus formed. The filtered fluid is now to be allowed to evaporate in a wide shallow vessel, and with the aid of the heat of a stove, until it is reduced to a pint. A clear orange yellow, slightly saltish, chalybeate solution is thus obtained, which, as already mentioned, does not give a precipitate with ferrocyanide of potassium without the previous addition of an acid. Each ounce of this liquid contains approximatively four grains of the albuminate plus an excess of albumen and soda, as may be seen by referring to the process employed, the solution consequently has a slightly alkaline re-action. It is desirable that the soda should thus be present in excess, in order that the compound shall be conformable to the state in which it exists in the blood, where we find the albumen rendered alkaline by an excess of soda. This albuminate of iron and soda is represented by the following formula $C^{130} H^{50} O^{10} + HO + Fe^2 O^3 + Na O \pm 2 HO =$ $AL\ Fe^2 O^3 + 2 HO$ water. As the albumen loses a portion of its nitrogen in order to be converted into albuminic acid, we must suppose that a portion of the soda by its presence determines the formation of a fatty matter at the expense of other principles of the same albumen, and then becomes saponified. I have given the formula of the albuminate of iron and soda above, neglecting the excess of albumen, which, though united to the liquid, perhaps with some other soluble salts of the albumen of the egg, (chlorides) I do not consider to form part of the saline compound, which may be obtained in radiated crystals by evaporating the solution to dryness.—*Bulletine della Scienze Mediche di Bologna*, Nov. and Dec., 1852, p. 385. *Dublin Quarterly Journal of Medical Science*, May 1853.

## CULTIVATION OF INDIGO IN CAUCASUS.

In the Russian province of Caucasus, the plant *polygonum tinctorium* has been cultivated since the year 1835. The Russian government has bestowed much attention upon the cultivation of the plant, and large quantities of the seed have been obtained and placed in the hands of a citizen, named Pepinoff, who perfectly succeeded in cultivating the plant, but does not seem to have had the chemical knowledge necessary to the preparation of the indigo. An individual denominated Tumadoff was thereupon despatched to India to learn the method of preparing the color from the plant, who returned in 1848, after the death of Pepinoff, bringing with him 30 kilogrammes (about 66 lbs.) of the seed; and forthwith proceeded to the cultivation of the plant at Elizavetpol, in Georgia. Before the culture had made any important progress however, Tumadoff also died, and the indefatigable Russian Government committed the enterprise to another person named Antonoff. In the mean time, information was obtained from an Indian dervise, who sojourned for some weeks at Elizavetpol, which led to the successful preparation of the Indigo. In the years 1847 and 1848 were obtained about 17 lbs. of indigo, which sold for from 1½ to 2 silver rubles ($1,12 to $1,50) per pound. This Indian indigo plant grows at Elizavetpol only to the height of one foot or eighteen inches; the Chinese plant grows 4 or 4½ feet high.

So far, the culture was merely a garden experiment, and the product of no commercial importance, but in the year 1851 the merchants of Moscow contributed the sum of 5000 silver rubles to make the experiment on a large scale. They expect this year to obtain a yield of 60 to 80 *puds* (2160 to 2880 lbs.) The product of indigo in the neighborhood of Elizavetpol is estimated to be 7 *puds* per *hectare* (equivalent to 102 lbs. per acre), 8 kilogrammes of seed being sown upon a hectare (7.14 lbs per acre.)

Elizavetpol and Poti upon the Black sea, are the most favorable places yet found for the growth of the plant, these two localities combining the qualifications of abundant *moisture* and *heat.* The following is the process followed in Caucasus to obtain the indigo from the plant.

At the proper time, that is, as soon as the first leaves appear, the plants are cut, placed in a stone reservoir containing water, and allowed to remain therein for 8 or 10 days. The water, upon which small bubbles of a coppery appearance form, is then drawn off into two lower basins and allowed to stand for three hours. The liquid is then beaten with large wooden ladles for an hour and a half or two hours, to force the air into it. This is of course for the purpose of oxydizing the white indigo and converting it into blue indigo. The color now begins to precipitate, and after standing at rest for about two hours, all the indigo contained in the liquid is found deposited upon the bottom of the vat in small grains. After drawing off the water, the indigo, which is in the form of a fluid paste, is carefully collected, and allowed to dry in the air to some extent, before it is submitted to the final operation, which is as follows. A coarse cotton cloth is spread over the dried mass, upon which cloth is sprinkled an alkaline liquid made from the ashes of the willow or some other soft wood, which alkaline liquid "has the property of absorbing a portion of the indigo and making it light." This sprinkling operation is repeated every half hour, and when the indigo has lost one-tenth of its weight, it is considered to be finished. The more weight it loses during this operation, the better the indigo is, and upon the success of this last operation depends the whole result of the manufacture. To the use of this process in Caucasus is due the production of a light and fine grained indigo, which approaches in quality to the best Indian samples.—*Dyngler's Polyt. Jour.* CXXVI, 304.

[Is it not exceedingly probable that it may be found possible for us to cultivate the *polygonum*; or some other of the plants which produce indigo at some points in our southern states? If the U. S. Government would take the same interest in such matters as that of Russia, or if the merchants of one of our southern cities would follow the example of the merchants of

Moscow, we should not long be dependant upon foreign countries for a supply of this costly and valuable color. No fear need be entertained of failure in the preparation of the color from the plant. This is merely a simple chemical problem, all the conditions of which are familiarly known. The function of the alkali used in the above very imperfect process practised in Caucasus, on which so much stress is laid, is undoubtedly merely to separate the *indigo-brown* with which the crude indigo is always more or less contaminated; indigo-brown having the property of forming a soluble compound with potash, which *indigo-blue* has not.]

H. W.

---

## UPON QUINIDINE.

Bussy and Guibourt have investigated the relations of quinidine to quinine with a view to the possibility of substituting quinidine for quinine in medicine. Their conclusion is, that the two differ entirely, both in their chemical and physical properties.

(1) Quinine separates from its aqueous-alcoholic solution in the form of a syrup, which on drying in the air remains transparent. Spread out in thin layers upon glass it becomes opaque, while the mass assumes a crystalline structure. In the first condition, the quinine appears to contain 3 equivalents, or 14. 29 per cent. of water; in the second condition but one equivalent, or 5. 26 per cent. on the supposition that its formula is $C^{20} A^{12} NO^{2}$.

Quinidine, on the other hand, separates from its aqueous-alcoholic and alcoholic solutions in crystals, the primary form of which is the right rectangular or rhombic prism. The secondary forms which occur are the rectangular octohedron, the rhombic octohedron (very similar to those of sulphur,) the right rhombic and rectangular prisms. The crystals lose no water at 212° F.

(2) Quinine dissolves easily in ether and alcohol. Quinidine requires 140 to 150 parts of ether, 45 parts of absolute alcohol, 105 parts of alcohol of 90 per cent., and 3.7 parts of boiling absolute alcohol.

(3) The crystalized sulphate of quinine dissolves in 57 parts of absolute alcohol and in 63 parts of alcohol of 90 per cent. The sulphate of quinidine dissolves in 30—32 parts of absolute alcohol, and in 7 of alcohol of 90 per cent. The sulphate of quinine dissolves in 256 parts of cold water and 24 of boiling water. The sulphate of quinidine in 73 of cold and 4.20 of boiling water according to Howard, but according to Leers in 16 of cold, and 130 of hot water.

(4) The oxalate of quinine is wholly insoluble, the oxalate of quinidine soluble and crystalizable.—*Jour. de Pharm. et de Chimie*, 3 Sec. XXII, p. 401. H. W.

---

## ON THE SUBSTITUTION OF THE CARBONATE FOR THE OXIDE OF SILVER IN COMMERCE.

BY MR. JOHN BORLAND.

At the present time, when attention is so properly directed to the detection and exposure of adulterations and impurities in many substances used in dietetics and medicine, I beg to be allowed to draw attention to the existence of a fraud which appears to me to be very generally practised with a medicine that is now come into extensive use as a tonic in dyspepsia and other complaints of the digestive organs. I allude to the substitution of carbonate of silver for oxide of silver.

I have carefully examined several specimens, all purchased from different respectable wholesale druggists in London, and have found that each of them, besides being contaminated with the oxides of copper, lead and iron, contained a large proportion of carbonic acid, and effervesced strongly when thrown into diluted nitric acid.

As none of the specimens was wholly soluble in liquor of ammonia, but contained a considerable quantity of some substance insoluble in this menstruum, I was led to suppose that the evolution of the carbonic acid might be due to the presence of some earthy or alkaline carbonate that had been added by way of adulteration. This, however, after close examination, I found not to be the case, so that the effervescence could not be accounted for in any other way than by supposing the carbonic acid to be combined with the oxide of silver.

That it was carbonic acid I satisfied myself by holding a watch-glass moistened with lime water above the eervescing solution, when a thin whitish film of carbonate of lime was visibly and quickly formed. I also passed the acid into a solution of pure caustic potass, and, on afterwards testing the solution found it to contain *carbonate* of potass.

In the preparation of this sophisticated article, the manufacturer, I suspect, has employed a solution of the carbonate of some one of the fixed alkalies in place of its caustic solution, to precipitate the oxide of silver.

The product yielded by this process is consequently greater, as it contains the additional weight of the carbonic acid with which it is combined—a sum which is easily calculated if we consider how much the equivalent weight of the carbonate of silver, which is 138, exceeds that of the oxide, which is 116.

The manufacturer who disposes of this at the price of the pure oxide is thus enabled to realize, besides the legitimate profit due to him as maker of the article, an *additional profit* of a sum equal to the commercial value of about 2½ ozs. of oxide of silver on every 16 ozs. that he sells.

This pecuniary point of the subject should, however, be only of very secondary importance to the dispensing Chemist, whose duty it is *not* to pry into the profits of the manufacturer, but above all to endeavor to serve his customers with a genuine article, and faithfully to carry out the intentions and wishes of the physician who may prescribe for them. Neither of these objects is effected by the dispensing of this or any other adulterated medicine.

In illustration of the difference between the two substances, I shall suppose that a patient receives from his physician a prescription for one dozen of pills, each of which is to contain one grain of oxide of silver. The prescription is with all confidence placed in the hands of the Chemist, to be carefully and properly made up; and the Chemist, either through the cupidity and dishonesty of himself or the manufacturer, or it may be through his own ignorance of, and inattention to the quality of the article supplied to him, in this case by using the carbonate, makes up the pills with only ten grains of oxide of silver in place of twelve grains.

The difference, it may be said, is not great; but whether it be trifling and insignificant or not, it is no extenuation or palliation of the culpability attending the substitution of one medicine for another.

The Chemist who is so coolly indifferent as to whether or not he sells a genuine or an adulterated article, will, with equal levity of feeling, be careless whether the impure medicine be one that is potent in its effects, or one that is capable of producing little or no appreciable influence on the living organism.

The process of qualitative analysis which I pursued for detecting the presence of the oxides of copper, lead, and iron, has nothing of novelty in it, and therefore need not be described. I may, however, remark that from several experiments which I made, I have reason to think that the carbonate of silver contains a small quantity of water, it may be from not having been properly dried after being washed, or from its being combined with it constitutionally as a *hydrate*.

This additional impurity, together with those already referred to, make the the difference between the oxide and carbonate greater than it really appears to be, from a mere comparison of their respective equivalent weights.

*Princes street, Kilmarnock, March* 22, 1853.

Dr. Hunter Lane wished to observe, with reference to the communication before the Meeting, that the occurrence of such cases as that alluded to, could not fail to raise in the minds of physicians a feeling of mistrust of the accuracy with which their prescriptions are dispensed, when taken to Chemists who are unknown to them; and this, he believed, was the principal cause of the practice, which the physician was sometimes driven to, of recommending a Chemist in whom he could place confidence. Instances had frequently come under his notice, in which substitutions of a more serious character than that mentioned in the paper, had been practised by the dispensers of medicines; and he trusted, as indeed he believed, that the Pharmaceutical Society would exert a beneficial influence in inducing among Pharmaceutical Chemists a more faithful discharge of their duties, from which would result a better understanding and mutual confidence between them and the members of the medical profession.

Mr. Waugh, while he was ready to admit that there might be some grounds for the observations which had been made, thought that physicians ought to be very careful how they passed judgment on Chemists in any particular cases, for he had reason to believe that injustice was sometimes done in this way. He mentioned a case which came under his own immediate observation, in which a physician had condemned a quantity of sulphate of quinine as impure, because it was not soluble in a small quantity of sherry wine, and had recommended the customer to return it, and go to another Chemist in whom he said he could feel confidence. This physician was subsequently convinced that it was not the medicine, but his chemistry, that was at fault; but such an occurrence might cause serious and unmerited injury to the Chemist, especially if he was a young man, or recently established.

Mr. Allchin thought, with reference to the case alluded to in the paper, that the presence of carbonic acid was probably accidental rather than intentional, having been caused by the use, in its preparation, of a caustic alkali, not wholly free from carbonic acid. The statement would have been more satisfactory, if a quantitative analysis had been made.

Mr. Redwood agreed with Mr. Allchin, that the carbonic acid should have been quantitatively determined. As, however, the author of the paper had sent two specimens of the "oxide of silver" alluded to, he had just examined them with an acid, and found the effervescence to be much greater than could be accounted for in the way mentioned by Mr. Allchin. He was aware that oxide of silver was sometimes sold at a price below that at which it could be made if pure.

Mr. T. B. Groves said he had recently seen some pills composed of oxide of silver and extract of hop, which, after having been kept for some time, had swelled up and become very spongy, as if some gas had been disengaged. He was unable at the time to account for this result, but he now thought it most probable that oxide of silver, such as that described in the paper, had been used; and that reduction of the oxide having taken place, the carbonic acid had been liberated.

Mr. Lofts had known pills, containing one grain each of oxide of silver, to produce salivation; from which he inferred that oxide of silver was sometimes adulterated with oxide of mercury.

Mr. Morson said that a case of that kind had occurred some time ago at one of the hospitals, when it was found that black oxide of mercury had been sold for oxide of silver.

# ON THE FERMENTATION OF CITRIC ACID.

BY J. PERSONNE.

The makers of citric acid have long been acquainted with the fact, that the impure citrate of lime cannot be kept for any time, without undergoing total decomposition. It has likewise been observed, that carbonic acid is one of the products of this decomposition, and remains combined with the lime, but beyond this nothing was known of its nature. The author has investigated the subject, and finds that the change is a true fermentation, consisting in the partition of the citric acid into acetic, butyric, and carbonic acids.

When clear lemon-juice is saturated with lime in a vessel to which a gas discharge-tube can be adapted, and kept at a temperature between 86° and 95° Fah., an evolution of gas commences at the end of forty-eight hours, and continues until the citrate of lime is entirely decomposed. The unstrained juice is decomposed more rapidly. Pure citric acid is decomposed still more rapidly, when mixed with citrate of lime and yeast.

The liquor in which the decomposition of the citric acid takes place gradually, assumes the odour peculiar to the butyric fermentation, and disengages a mixture of carbonic acid and hydrogen, the relative proportion of these gases varying throughout the process.

The acids contained in the soluble lime salts obtained by evaporation, and combined with the oxide of silver, proved to be butyric and acetic acid; the silver salts yielding respectively 56.13 and 62.75, 62.60, 62.86 per cent of silver. The calculated per centages of silver for these salts are 54 and 64.

The author separated the acids by fractional distillation, and at the same time endeavored to ascertain whether the butyro-acetic acid, assumed by Nickles to be a product of the fermentation of tartaric acid, was formed. The acids were combined with soda, and again separated by phosphoric acid, after which they furnished silver salts, with per centages of silver corresponding with theory. He therefore considers the decomposition to be as follows:

$$4\ (C^{12}\ H^{5}\ O^{11}\ 3\ HO)\ +\ 4\ HO = 3\ (C^{4}\ H^{4}\ O^{4})\ +\ 2\ (C^{8}\ H^{8}\ O^{4})\ +\ 20\ CO^{2} \bowtie H^{8}).$$

It is possible that lactic acid is formed in the first instance, for:

$$4\ \ (C^{12}\ H^{5}\ O^{11}\ 3\ HO) \bowtie 4\ HO = 3\ (C^{4}\ H^{4}\ O^{4} \bowtie 4\ \ (C^{6}\ H^{6}\ O^{6} \bowtie 12\ CO^{2},)$$

and is afterwards decomposed, yielding the butyric acid, carbonic acid, and hydrogen—

$$4\ (C^{6}\ H^{6}\ O^{6}) = 2\ (C^{8}\ H^{8}\ O^{4}) \bowtie 8\ CO^{2} \bowtie H^{8}.$$—*Comtes Rendus.* from *Chem. Gaz.*, March 15.

---

## ON THE ADULTERATION OF PERU BALSAM.

BY G. L. ULEX.

Among the substances fraudulently mixed with Peru balsam, castor oil, and copaiba balsam, are the most difficult to detect. The author recommends the following method:—Ten drops of Peru balsam are mixed in a watch-glass with twenty drops of concentrated sulphuric acid, and then diluted with water. If the balsam is pure, a brittle resin is thus obtained, but when adulterated with castor oil and similar substances, this residue is proportionably soft. Sulphurous acid is likewise disengaged, which is not the case when the adulterating substance is copaiba balsam.

Considerable variations in the specific gravity of Peru balsam must not be altogether overlooked. It usually varies between 1.14 and 1.16, and when adulterated with as much as 25 per cent. of castor oil, it is much lower.

To detect copaiba balsam, the substance is to be heated in a small tube retort, until a few drops of a yellow oily liquid have passed over, which takes place at a temperature of 374° Fahr. This distillate is acid, and soon deposits crystals of cinnamic acid. If the balsam used was pure, it solidifies completely; but when adulterated with copaiba, the crystals float in copaiba oil. The distillate is then to be saturated with caustic potash, and the solution of cinnamate removed by means of blotting paper. The drops of oil which are then left mix quietly with iodine if the balsam was pure, but cause an immediate explosion if copaiba was present in it.—*Archiv. der Pharmacie, January,* 1853.

---

## UPON THE TANNATE AND GALLATE OF QUININE.

Lintner has been induced, by a suggestion of Buchner, since deceased, to make some investigation of the tannate of quinine, recently introduced as a remedy, with reference to the question whether a somewhat impure tannate, prepared simply by precipitation of the extract of the bark with tannic acid, would have the same therapeutical value as the pure salt.

Coarsely pulverized Peruvian bark was treated with six times its weight of ordinary distilled vinegar, and after 24 hours digestion, boiled for some time, strained, the residue again boiled with half the quantity of vinegar, and the resulting liquids, after complete cooling, filtered. To the filtrate was added freshly-prepared clear infusion of gall-nuts, as long as a precipitate was produced. The precipitate was collected, well washed, and dried. Five grammes of four different kinds of cinchona treated in this way gave the following results:

| | | | | | | |
|---|---|---|---|---|---|---|
| Cinchona regia gave | 0.134 | tannate | of quin., | or | 2-68 | per cent. |
| Cinchona huamalis | 0.108 | " | " | | 2.16 | " |
| Cinchona flava | 0.089 | " | " | | 1.78 | " |
| Cinchona fusca | 0.071 | " | " | | 1.42 | " |

The product of the last kind consisted, however, more or less of tannate of *cinchonine*.

The tannate of quinine is almost wholly insoluble in water, and possesses, therefore, scarcely any taste, which makes it a remedy easily taken. If it is left in contact with water for a long time it is gradually changed into soluble *gallate* of quinine.

Perhaps, when taken into the stomach it is also converted in the same way into gallate by the digestion, which may contribute much to the good operation of this remedy.

The gallate of quinine prepared by the saturation of a solution of pure gallic acid with pure quinine is soluble in water and alcohol, and possesses, therefore, the same bitter taste as the sulphate of quinine. By evaporation of its alcoholic solution it is obtained in wart-like aggregations. When moistened with water it appears to be gradually decomposed in the air.—(*Knop's Central-Blatt*, April, 1853, p. 238.)

H. W.

---

# EDITORIAL.

We give below the circular of the Secretary of the Treasury in relation to the manner in which the Drug Inspection Law is to be construed. It will be seen that the admission of all the more valuable of the New Grenada barks is provided for, while only the inferior Carthagena barks are excluded. The standard assumed in the case of the drugs specified is a high and good one. In drawing up the circular, we believe the Secretary has availed himself chiefly of the advice of Dr. Bailey, of this city:

## TO PREVENT THE IMPORTATION OF ADULTERATED DRUGS AND MEDICINES.

### TO COLLECTORS AND OTHER OFFICERS OF THE CUSTOMS, UNDER THE ACT OF 26TH JUNE, 1848.

Treasury Department, June 4, 1853.

It being represented to this Department, that much embarrassment has been experienced by officers of the customs, at some of the ports of the United States, in reference to the provisions of the act of 26th June, 1848, " to prevent the importation of adulterated and spurious drugs and medicines," it is deemed expedient, with a view to avoid future difficulties arising from misconstructions of the law, and to secure uniformity of practice at the several ports in carrying out its provisions with precision and efficiency, to furnish you with the additional instructions which follow, explanatory and in modification of the circular instructions addressed to you by the Department on the 8th of July, 1848.

To avoid the recurrence of a difference of opinion between the officers of the customs as to what particular articles of commerce should be considered drugs and medicines, and as such subject to special examination by the special examiner of drugs and medicines, it is thought proper to state that, in conformity with the evident spirit and intent of the law, it is required that all articles of merchandise used wholly or in part as medicine, and found described as such in the standard works specially referred to in the act, must be considered drugs and medicines, and that all invoices, therefore, of such articles, in whole or in part, must be submitted to the examination of the special examiner of drugs and medicines, before they can be permitted to pass the custom-house.

In the examination on entry of any medicinal preparation, the said special examiner is to unite with the appraiser.

With a view to afford a reliable guide to the examiner of drugs and medicines, as well as to the analytical chemist, on appeal, in ascertaining the admissibility of such articles under the provisions of law, founded on their purity and strength, the following list is given of some of the principal articles, with the result of special tests agreeing with the standard authorities referred to in the law, all of which articles are to be entitled to entry when ascertained by analysis to be composed as noted, viz. :—

Aloes, when affording 80 per cent. of pure aloetic extractive.

Assafœtida, when affording 50 per cent. of its peculiar bitter resin, and
" " " 3 per cent of volatile oil.

Bark, Cinchona, when affording one per cent. of pure quinine, whether called Peruvian, Calasaya, Arica, Carthagena, Maracaibo, Santa Martha, Bogota, or under whatever name, or from whatever place; or

Bark, Cinchona, when affording two per cent. of the several natural alkaloids combined, as quinine cinchonine, quinine aricene, &c., the barks of such strength being admissible as safe and proper for medicine, and useful for chemical manufacturing purposes.

| | | | | |
|---|---|---|---|---|
| Benzoin, | when affording | 80 | per cent. | of resin, or |
| " | " | 12 | " | of benzoic acid. |
| Colocynth | " | 12 | " | of colocynthin. |
| Elaterium | " | 30 | " | of elaterin. |
| Galbanum, | when affording | 60 | " | of resin. |
| " | " | 19 | " | of gum; and |
| " | " | 6 | " | of volatile oil. |
| Gamboge | " | 70 | " | of pure gamboge. |
| resin, and | | | | |
| Gamboge, | " | 20 | " | of gum. |
| Guiacum, | " | 80 | " | of pure guiac. |
| resin. | | | | |
| Gum ammoniac, | " | 70 | " | of resin, and |
| " | " | 18 | " | of gum. |

Jalap, when affording 11 per cent. of pure jalap resin, whether in root or in powder.

| | | | | |
|---|---|---|---|---|
| Manna, | when affording | 37 | per cent | of pure mannite. |
| Myrrh, | " | 30 | " | of pure myrrh resin. |
| and | | | | |
| Myrrh | " | 50 | " | of gum. |
| Opium | " | 9 | " | of pure morphine. |
| Rhubarb | " | 40 | " | of soluble matter, whether in root or powder. None admissible but the article known as East India, Turkey, or Russian rhubarb. |

Segapenum, 50 per cent. of resin.

Segapenum, 30 per cent. of gum, and

Segapenum, 3 per cent. of volatile oil.

Scammony, 70 per cent. of pure scammony resin.

Senna, 28 per cent. of soluble matter.

All medicinal leaves, flowers, barks, roots, extracts, &c., not herein specified, must be, when imported, in perfect condition, and of as recent collection and preparation as practicable.

All pharmaceutical and chemical preparations, whether crystalized or otherwise, used in medicine, must be found on examination to be pure, and of proper consistence and strength, as well as of perfect manufacture, conformably with the formulas contained in the standard authorities named in the act, and must in no instance contain over three per cent. of excess of moisture, or water of crystalization.

Essential or volatile oils, as well as expressed oils used in medicine, must be pure, and conform to the standards of specific gravity noted and declared in the dispensatories mentioned in the act.

"Patent or secret medicines" are by law subject to the same examination, and disposition after examination, as other medical preparations, and cannot be permitted to pass the Custom House for consumption, but must be rejected and condemned, unless the special examiner be satisfied, after due investigation, that they are fit and safe to be used for medicinal purposes.

The appeal from the report of the special examiner of drugs and medicines, provided for in the act, must be made by the owner or consignee within ten days after the said report; and in case of such appeal the analysis made by the analytical chemist is expected to be full and in detail, setting forth clearly and accurately the name, quantity, and quality of the several component parts of the article in question, to be reported to the collector under oath or affirmation.

On such report being made, a copy of the same will be immediately furnished by the collector to the special examiner of drugs and medicines, who, if the report be in conflict with his return made to the collector, and he have cause to believe that the appeal and analytical examination have not been conducted in strict conformity with the law, may enter his protest, in writing, against the reception and adoption by the collector of such report and analysis, until a reasonable time be allowed him for the preparation of his views in the case, and their submission to this department for its consideration.

JAMES GUTHRIE,
Secretary of the Treasury.

---

## DELEGATES TO THE AMERICAN PHARMACEUTICAL ASSOCIATION.

At a meeting of the Massachusetts College of Pharmacy, held June 2,

Daniel Henchman, Wm. A. Brewer,
Thomas Restiaux, H. W. Lincoln,
T. Larkin Turner,

were elected Delegates to the Pharmaceutical Association.

---

At a meeting of the College of Pharmacy, held Tuesday, June 28, for appointing Delegates to the National Pharmaceutical Association, to be held at Boston on the 24th of August next, the following gentlemen were appointed:

Geo. D. Coggeshall, J. S. Aspinwall,
T. B. Merrick, Eugene Dupuy,
J. Gridley.

F. A. HEGEMAN, Sec.

# NEW YORK

# JOURNAL OF PHARMCY.

AUGUST, 1853.


## NOTES IN PHARMACY.

BY BENJAMIN CANAVAN.

No. 7.

GUARANA VEL PAULLINIA.—A specimen of this article, brought from Brazil, was presented to me by Dr. Brownlee, of the United States Navy, the history of the use of which by the natives of the country where it is manufactured and used, suggests its importance and superiority as a dietetic, where it may be desirable to combine highly nutritive properties with astringency, containing, as it is said to do, a larger proportion of *caffein*, or as it is in this instance called *guaranin*, ascertained to be identical substances than coffee or tea themselves, united with tannic acid. It is described as being prepared from the seeds of a tree, *Paullinia Dorbilis*, from which it has one of its names. The seeds are beaten into a pulp with water, and formed into lengthened conoidal ended masses, some two inches or so in circumference, and dried in the sun, to a very hard consistence. When wanted for use it is scraped off and added to the food as a condiment, or prepared with warm water and sweetened, is used as a beverage like tea or coffee, and is employed as a preventive or antidote to bowel complaints, so apt to occur in warm climates or seasons. It appears to be worthy of a trial for that purpose, or as a remedial agent conjoined with other treatment, and it would be desirable to have it imported in sufficient quantity to allow its therapeutic or prophylactic properties to be tested.

COOK'S PILLS.—Adjoined is a formula for those pills which I do not find in any published formulary I am acquainted with. They are much used, and seem to be a peculiarly appropriate purgative, in the south-western States, and are frequently asked for by travellers from thence. I quote from memory, never having made or seen any written formula, but have frequently prepared them, and believe the proportions to be sufficiently accurate.

℞ Hydrarg. Submur.
Pulv. Rhei.
— Aloes aa ʒ ss.
M. fiat massa quam divide in pil. no. xxiv.

ETHER CHLORIC.—The discrepancy in the strength of this ether, as generally manufactured, may be avoided by the apothecary, its necessary characteristic being its solubility in water, by bringing the concentrated ether as generally to be had, which is insoluble and sinks heavily to the bottom in water, to the necessary point by dilution with alcohol.

PSEUDO ALKALOIDS.—A class of articles bearing the technology applied to the proximate principles, has been somewhat extensively used in certain extra professional quarters not at all amenable to the objection of "old fogeyism," and is attempted to be introduced more generally. They are not at all what their absurdly assumed nomenclature would indicate, and are liable even to be confounded with the proper article, or it with them, and thus lead to confusion and error. I have reference to the articles misnomed *Podophyllin*, *Jalapin*, and so forth, which are strictly and merely *precipitated resins*, not *alkaloids*, being prepared from alcoholic solutions or tinctures, by precipitating them with water. The process in itself is not undeserving of attention as being an apt mode of separating the active resinous elements of some medicinal agents, and obtaining thereby their active properties in a concentrated form, and is preferable to the mode of solution and evaporation, avoiding the volatilizing effects of the heat necessary to the process of evaporation.

SOLUTIO CITRATIS MAGNESIÆ.—Some trouble is experienced from the insoluble deposit which takes place in this preparation very soon after being bottled, diminishing its strength in a material degree; to avoid which I prepare it as follows:

℞ Acid Citric, ℥ vj.
Magnes. Carb., ℥ iij.
Syrup Acid Citric, ℥ xij.
Aqua, oiij. et ℥ xij.
M. ft. solutio.

As fit solutio of this, when wanted for use, 6 oz. are taken, and 40 grains of carb. magnesio added to it, suspended in sufficient water to fill an ordinary citrate of magnesia bottle or to make about 10 ozs.; this first solution does not deposit on standing, and the balance of the magnesia to be added being greater than ordinary more fully ærates the solution.

APOTHECARIES' COMPANY.—Credit is due to Mr. Dupuy for having opened this subject, which has long occupied my own thoughts, and frequently been a topic of conversation with others; but it appeared always that, in order to prevent effectually the abuses which were meant to be corrected, and to which such a concern itself would be liable to, equally with individual enterprises,—for the number of persons is never a guarantee of integrity,—and might even tend to the perversion into a monopoly of evil practices the very means which were intended to counteract them—an essential principle should be, that it would be in no sense a *money making concern*, which would be also necessary to insure that *prestige* which such an institution should possess, and which should be its chief object to attain. This may and does seem impracticable, but it is the safety valve of such an enterprise; and there is surely public spirit enough amongst the different branches of the medical profession to furnish the means, without loss to themselves,—as full interest but no more should be paid on the capital,—to protect the public and themselves from the evils sought to be avoided; or if means could not be obtained by subscription, what reason is there to suppose the Legislature would refuse to loan a portion of some public fund for such a purpose? Such an institution as here contemplated would be, indeed, a novelty, and one worthy of the age and country, and would command the respect of the civilized world.

---

# ON THE OIL OF HOPS.

BY DR. RUDOLPH WAGNER.

THE ethereal oil of the female flowers of the hop plant (*Humulus lupulus*) is quite unknown with regard to its technical importance. A superficial examination by Payen and Chevallier has been a source of innumerable errors with reference to the properties of oil of hops. It has been believed, in consequence of this examination, that the oil resembled oils of mustard, assafœtida, &c., and belonged to the ethereal oils containing sulphur; that it dissolved largely in water, and on this account preserved the beer, and that it acted partly as the narcotic ingredient of beer and of hops.

The following research, conducted by me with oil carefully prepared by Hertel, shows that the deductions of Payen and Chevallier are incorrect. The oil was distilled from fresh hops with water, and constituted about eight per cent. of the hops, which were dried in the air. It was of a clear brownish-yellow color, possessed a strong odour of hops, and had a slightly bitter taste analogous to thyme and origanum. Its specific gravity was ,908 at 61 Fahr. It scarcely reddened litmus paper, which, when moistened with the oil and exposed to the atmosphere for a considerable time, assumed a decided red color. A small quantity shaken with water dissolved in such a small degree that the water only had the odour of the oil. It requires more than 600 times its weight of water for its solution.

It was examined for the purpose of ascertaining whether it contained sulphur, but with a negative result. The oil rendered anhydrous by distillation over fused chloride of calcium, evaporates partly at a temperature below the boiling point of water. It begins to boil at 257°, the boiling point then rises to 347°, where it remains stationary for some time, and at which nearly one-sixth of the oil distils over. The first distillate (A) was colorless, clear as water, and possessed a slight odour of hops, but more resembled rosemary. The portion (B) passing over between 347° and 437°, and constituting one-half of the oil, was also very clear, and had the odour of the crude oil. That which passed over between 437° and 455° was colored yellowish. The residue in the retort, about one-sixth of the oil, was brownish, and like turpentine. It is, therefore, evident that oil of hops is a mixture of oils. The crude oil did not give, with an ammoniacal solution of silver, a metallic mirror. It is not, therefore, an aldehyde. When mixed with an alcoholic solution of potash the oil becomes brown, and by distillation the mixture affords alcohol and an oil with the odour of rosemary. After the greatest part of the oil and spirit has distilled over, a violent evolution of gas ensues, probably hydrogen, and carbonate of potash remains, mixed with a potash salt of a volatile fatty acid. The odour which the acid evolves when set free from the potash with diluted sulphuric acid, leads to the conclusion that this acid is a mixture of caprylic and pelargonic acids.

The oil which passed over during this reaction, and resembles the previously mentioned one (A), boils between 347° and 356°, and has the formula $C^5 H^4$. It, therefore, belongs to the large class of camphenes.

The portion B of the crude oil was subjected to fractional distillation, and the part which passed over at 410°, during which the thermometer was constant for a short time, consisted of $C^{20} H^{18} O^2$. This oxygenated oil is in the crude oil undergoing continuous oxidation, and dries, when exposed in a watch glass to the air, at last to a gummy mass.

This oil is isomeric with Borneo camphor, oils of cajeput and bergamot, and with the aldehyde of campholic acid $C H^{18} O^4$.

I have made, in conjunction with Dr. Bibra, researches on animals to ascertain whether the oil of hops has a narcotic action, and find that it has no such action.—*Journal für Pracktische Chemie and Annals of Pharmacy.*

---

## DETECTION OF QUININE IN THE URINE.

Dr. Viale states that tannic acid is a very safe reagent for the detection of quinine in the urine. He has used it for this purpose in the medical clinique at Rome, by the advice of Professor Latini, and announces that in any quantity of urine from three ounces up to three pounds, from seven hours to two days after the administration of the quinine, even after the administration merely of decoction of cinchona bark, the quinine can be detected. The precipitate is very slight and white, with a greenish tinge.

All the urines examined by Viale were distinctly acid, the quinine existing probably in the form of sulphate. The precipitate obtained always gave the greenish tinge with chlorine and ammonia.—(*Journal de Pharm. et de Chim.*, 3 Sec., XXII., 303.)

H. W.

# ON THE CONSTITUTION AND PREPARATION OF THE ETHEREAL OILS.

BY DR. CHARLES LÖWIG.

All plants, and parts of plants, which are distinguished by a strong odour are indebted for this odour to peculiar odorous compounds, which, on account of their physical properties and resemblances, are termed volatile or ethereal oils. They are allied, in many respects, to the compounds of the benzid and spiroyl groups, which bear the name of empyreumatic oils, because they are mostly the products of dry distillation. Many bodies which may be considered, in regard to their sources and their physical properties, as essential oils, must, on account of their chemical relations to other substances, be described independently, as oil of rue, oil of bitter almonds, oil of cinnamon, cinnamine, spiroylous acid, oil of gaultheria procumbens, &c., and only those will be spoken of here which, in reference to their composition and chemical analogies, stand in unequal relation, like the compounds of the above groups, whether they exist already formed in plants and animals, or are produced artificially by dry distillation, by fermentation, or other influences. The ethereal oils are most widely diffused in the vegetable kingdom. Many plants contain the same oil in all their parts; others have different oils in their roots, leaves, flowers, and fruit, as is manifest by the various odours of the oils.

Most volatile oils are obtained by distillation of plants, or portions of plants, with water. It is probable that many volatile oils are first formed by action of water on peculiar compounds existing in plants, through a process of fermentation analogous to that by which oil of bitter almonds is produced from amygdaline. Although the boiling points of all volatile oils are higher than that of water, nevertheless they distil over by reason of the general property of volatile bodies to evaporate under their boiling points with the vapor of water which is saturated with their vapors. As the volatile oils are not insoluble in water, the precaution must be observed in their preparation that the quantity of water which passes over with the oil is not so great that all the oil remains dissolved in it. By the use of tall and small distillatory apparatus, this result can be partly prevented, and also partly by the elevation of the boiling point of the water through the addition of common salt. The greatest quantity of ethereal oils is obtained by conducting compressed steam through the vegetable material. Many plants contain so little oil that the same water must be several times distilled from a fresh quantity of the substance before the oil separates (Cohobation). When the vegetable substance is rich in volatile oil, it can be procured by expression; thus the oils of lemon and orange are obtained from the peel of the fresh fruit. Oftentimes mixtures of essential oils with resins exude partly *per se*, and partly after incisions made, from different plants, which are termed natural balsams. When these balsams are distilled with water, their resins remain behind, while their volatile oils volatilize (turpentine, copaiba balsam).

The volatile oils, as they are obtained from plants by simple distillation with water, are almost always mixtures of two, and often of three, different oils, of which the more volatile are free from oxygen, and the less volatile contain that element. When the crude oil is subjected to distillation, the oxygenated portion goes over last. The first portions, however, which distil over are, as will be readily comprehended, always mixtures of oxygenated with non-oxygenated oils, and the complete separation of these oils can only be accomplished by chemically acting bodies. If such a mixture is distilled over fused caustic potash, the oxygenated oil remains behind, however, generally decomposed, while the non-oxygenated passes over. The latter are mostly represented by the formula $C^{10} H^{8} = C^{20} H^{16}$, and are termed terebenes, or camphenes.

The volatile oils are only soluble in small quantity in water, but the oxygenated are taken up in greater proportion than the non-oxygenated oils. Their watery solutions possess the odours of the oils. They are usually obtained by distilling the vegetable substance with so much water, that the oil, which passes over with aqueous vapor, remains dissolved in the condensed water (*aquæ distillatæ* of pharmaceutists). With anhydrous alcohol the ethereal oils mix in all proportions; and alcohol, which contains water, dissolves less oil the weaker it is (the use of essential oils in perfumery). The ethereal oils are dissolved largely by ether, and are completely mixable with fatty oils (adulteration of volatile oils with anhydrous alcohol and fixed oils).—*Annals of Pharmacy, June*, 1853.

---

## PENCILS FOR WRITING UPON GLASS.

Brunnquell prepares pencils with which he writes labels, etc., very conveniently, immediately, upon the glass of bottles, in the following manner:

Four parts of spermaceti, (or stearine,) three parts of tallow, and two parts of wax are meted together in a small dish, and then six parts of minium and one part of potash stirred in. The mass is heated for half an hour, and then poured into glass tubes of the size of a lead pencil. After quick cooling they are easily removed from the tubes, and then form pencils, by means of which dry and clean glass may be written upon in a very satisfactory manner.—(*Dingl. Polyt. Journ.*, CXXVII., 236.)

H. W.

# ON THE USE OF THE ALCOHOLIC EXTRACT AND THE TINCTURE OF THE SEEDS OF THE ŒNANTHE PHELLANDRIUM.

BY DR. TURNBULL, OF LIVERPOOL.

Having found the tincture, and also the alcoholic extract made from the seeds of this plant, of great service in relieving the cough and other pectoral symptoms in almost every case of consumption in which I have prescribed them, I wish to direct the attention of the profession to their medicinal properties, feeling assured that they will be found a valuable addition to our ordinary means of treating this disease. On referring to Dr. Woodville's *Medical Botany*, I find it stated that the seeds, when taken in large doses, produce a remarkable sensation of weight in the head, accompanied with giddiness, intoxication, &c.; and that, therefore, they may be deemed capable of proving an active medicine; also that, distilled with water, they yield an essential oil of a pale yellow color, and of a strong penetrating smell; and that one pound of the seeds affords nearly two ounces of spirituous extract, of which nearly three drachms consist of resin. He also quotes some ancient authorities to prove their good effects in several diseases, more particularly those of the bladder, also in asthma and consumption. Stephenson and Churchill, in their work on Medical Botany, make the following observations on their properties and uses:—"The seeds of phellandrium aquaticum are carminative, narcotic, and diuretic. They have been much recommended on the continent in pulmonary consumption; and many cases are recorded in which the disease, if not cured, was evidently relieved by them." Also, "the seeds were employed by the ancients in calculous complaints; and have been highly extolled by Heister, Ernsling, and others among the moderns, as possessing valuable diuretic, antiseptic, and expectorant properties." Sir Alexander Crichton, in his work on consumption, strongly recommended the seeds in the dose of from a scruple to a drachm to relieve the cough in this disease. My first trials of the remedy were made with the powdered seeds, given as he had recommended. When used in this way, I found so little effect from them that I was at first disposed to think that their virtues had been exaggerated; and it was only after giving a strong tincture prepared from the seeds that I became convinced of their efficacy. I have since used an alcoholic extract,* which may be given in the form of a pill, and is more suitable than the tincture in those cases where we wish to avoid the stimulating effects of the rectified spirit, with which it is necessary that the tincture should be prepared.

In examining my notes of cases, I find that the effects of the tincture, and of the extract of phellandrium, have been carefully observed and recorded in ten cases of consumption under my care in the Royal Infirmary. It was given only in those where the cough was complained of as being troublesome; in all of them it was more or less decidedly relieved, and in some, more than by any medicine which had been previously given. In almost all the cases the expectoration was rendered easier, and the quantity was in several materially lessened, as occurs not unfrequently where other resinous or balsamic expectorants are taken. In some instances the patients, after using the phellandrium, slept better at night; but, beyond this, I have not been able to observe any narcotic effect. In a case of emphysema of the lungs, with chronic bronchitis, I also used the phellandrium with advantage.

My experience, then, of the phellandrium gives me confidence in recommending it as a safe and valuable remedy, de-

* I am indebted to J. B. Edwards, Ph. D., Chemist, Berry-street, Liverpool, for the preparation of this extract.

serving of more attention in the treatment of consumption than it has hitherto received; and I feel also satisfied that the tincture and alcoholic extract are preparations by which we are enabled to obtain from them, with more certainty and power, the whole of their beneficial properties.—*Pharmaceutical Journal, June,* 1853.

---

## ON PHARMACEUTICAL PREPARATIONS OF ŒNANTHE PHELLANDRIUM AND ŒNANTHE CROCATA.

BY J. B. EDWARDS, PH.D., LIVERPOOL.

At the request of Dr. Turnbull, I have prepared for the use of the Liverpool Royal Infirmary various preparations of the above drugs. Having exhibited the powdered seed, an aqueous extract, and a weak tincture of phellandrium, with little effect, Dr. Turnbull required a more active preparation, and found that the essence and the alcoholic extract prepared as below prove very valuable and active remedies in the relief of consumption and bronchitis.

### ESSENCE OF PHELLANDRIUM.

Seeds of phellandrium, well bruised, 16 ozs.

Rectified spirit q. s. to displace by percolation f ℥ xxxij.

f ℥ j. is equal to ʒ ss. of the seeds, and the dose is from f ʒ ss. to f ʒ j.

### ALCOHOLIC EXTRACT OF PHELLANDRIUM.

Seeds of phellandrium, bruised, 16 ozs.

Rectified spirit, Oiij.

Displace by percolation, and distil Oijss. of spirit, evaporate the remainder to the consistence of an extract. Product 1½ oz. to 1¾ oz. Dose from gr. iij. to gr. v.

These preparations are both approved by Dr. Turnbull, who, in many cases, prefers the latter given in the form of a pill.

The preparations of œnanthe crocata were obtained from the fresh root by maceration in the cold, the starch being separated. These from the taste and smell appear to be very active preparations, but they have not yet been freely exhibited.

### ACETIC EXTRACT OF ŒNANTHE CROCATA.

Two pounds of fresh root digested in distilled vinegar, strained and evaporated, yielded 2½ ozs. of strong extract.

### ALCOHOLIC EXTRACT OF ŒNANTHE CROCATA.

Two pounds of fresh root digested in rectified spirit, and the dregs percolated, the spirit distilled, and the extract evaporated, yielded 2¼ ozs. of alcoholic extract.—*Pharmaceutical Journal, June*, 1853.

---

## ADULTERATION OF TOLU BALSAM.

BY G. L. ULEX.

Pure tolu balsam, heated in sulphuric acid, dissolves without any disengagement of sulphurous acid, yielding a cherry-red liquid. When, however, colophony, with which it is frequently adulterated, is present, the substance blackens, swells up, and discharges much sulphurous acid.—*Archiv. de Pharmacie, January*, 1853.

## ON THE PREPARATION OF TANNIC ACID.

On testing the method prescribed in the Prussian Pharmacopœia, for the preparation of tannic acid, Sandrock finds that it does not fulfil the desired object. In directing that water should be added to the ether employed, the authors of the Pharmacopœia would appear to have aimed at an approximation to the method originally adopted by Pelouze, in which crude ether was used; and to have assumed that when watery ether is used, the lower layer of the percolated liquid is a solution of tannic acid in water. However, Mohr found that this is not the case, but that the lower layer is a solution of tannic acid in ether; and Sandrock has obtained the same result on repeating his experiments. The addition of water to the ether is, therefore, useless, and moreover injurious, for the solution of tannic acid in ether is so thick that the percolation goes on very slowly, and sometimes stops altogether. The use of pure ether is open to the same objection.

The extraction of the tannic acid from galls may, on the contrary, be effected with ease by crude ether, on account of the small quantity of alcohol which it contains. The alcohol facilitates the percolation by rendering the solution of tannic acid less viscid.

Instead of crude ether a mixture of sixteen parts ether and one part alcohol may be used with equally satisfactory results. The percolated liquid separates into two layers. The lower one containing the tannic acid may easily be separated, and yields a perfectly pure product on evaporation. The upper layer contains the gallic acid, coloring matter, and some tannic acid.

When a mixture of eight parts ether and one part alcohol is employed, the percolate still separates into two layers, but the lower one is smaller than when the proportion of alcohol is less, and the upper layer contains a considerably larger quantity of tannic acid.

Finally, when a mixture of four parts ether and one part alcohol is employed, the percolate does not separate into two layers, and it is difficult to separate the tannic acid from the impurities with which it is mixed.

By means of the above process a much larger product of tannic acid may be obtained than with either pure or watery ether. The tannic acid remaining in the upper layer may likewise be obtained by evaporating the liquid to dryness, treating the residue with pure ether, until the lower of the two layers into which the liquid separates no longer presents a green color. It is then separated, filtered, if necessary a little alcohol added, and evaporated.

The process recommended by Mohr, of treating the galls with a mixture of alcohol and ether in equal volumes, then evaporating the percolate which does not separate into layers, and regarding the residue as tannic acid, is altogether inadmissible, inasmuch as it gives a very impure product.—*Archiv. der Pharmacie*, December, 1852, *and Pharmaceutical Journal.*

---

## ON THE CINCHONAS, AND THE QUESTIONS WHICH, IN THE PRESENT STATE OF SCIENCE AND COMMERCE ARE MORE IMMEDIATELY CONNECTED WITH THEM.

BY MM. A. DELONDRE AND BOUCHARDAT.

### *Rolled Cinchona Calisaya.*

Very thick epidermis, rough, uneven, marked at distances with annular fissures, and, in the intermediate space, with transverse and longitudinal cracks, more or less close to each other, often anastomosed, of a silvery or greyish white. Internal face, purely fibrous, of a yellow fawn, even texture; very clear transverse fracture, externally very resinous, with short fibres internally.

These barks are produced, as we have before observed, by the branches of the tree whose trunk gives the flat bark. Less alkaloid is procured from them than from the former, and, in accordance with the size of the bark, the produce varies from 15 to 20 grammes of sulphate of quinine, and from 8 to 10 grammes of sulphate of cinchonine per kilogramme.

### *Cinchona Carabaya.*

This bark comes from the province of Carabaya, by Arequipa, to the ports of Islay, and sometimes of Arica; the thickness is from 2 to 3 millimetres in the bulk of the serons, which are, the same as the above, of the weight of 72 to 75 kilogrammes.

The internal surface is of a very even texture, but very brown, and often contorted by dessiccation. The external surface, instead of longitudinal ridges, is covered with small, almost black points, which are formed by the adherence of the epidermis, and sometimes in slanting ridges. The transverse fracture is clear, fibrous within, with a resinous layer outside. It sometimes comes in very small pieces, producing scarcely 12 grammes of sulphate of quinine; but when the thickness we have mentioned is taken as the average, 15 to 18 grammes of sulphate of quinine, and 4 to 5 grammes of sulphate of cinchonine may be obtained.

### *Columbian Cinchonas.*

The cinchona pitaya, which M. O. Henri has proved to be so rich in febrifuge alkaloids, has more especially retained the name of Columbian cinchona.

What is to be understood by Columbian cinchonas? It is evident that so general a term can have no precise meaning. Carthagena is a port of New Granada; all the cinchonas which bear the name of Cathagena cinchonas are, therefore, Columbian cinchonas, for New Granada is a portion of Columbia. All the cinchonas which Mutis has discovered in New Granada are likewise Columbian cinchonas.

*Cinchonas known in Commerce as Carthagena Cinchonas.*

There are several species found in the forests of New Granada, and sent to Europe from the ports of Carthagena, Saint Martha, and Maracaybo, in serons of from 50 to 55 kilogrammes.

We owe the discovery of all these cinchonas to Senor Mutis, a Spanish medical man.

We cannot read the following lines in M. Guibourt's *Histoire Naturelle des Drogues Simples*, without astonishment :

" A man who has acquired a great reputation as the discoverer of cinchonas, but who has only helped to fill the history of these barks with confusion and obscurity, is Mutis, a Spanish botanist, who started in 1760 for New Granada,* where he remained, and whom the desire of making a reputation at the expense of the Flora of Peru, has caused to commit errors which are found in all recently published works on this subject. To justify this *severe judgment*, it will suffice for me to say that Mutis, who could not help knowing the real Peruvian cinchonas, has given their names to quite different and *almost valueless* barks, growing at Santa Fe. Thus his vaunted *orange cinchona* is only a very fibrous kind of Calisaya of very bad quality. His *red cinchona*, the bark of his *cinchona oblongifolia*, is only the *bad bark*, since named *cinchona nova*. His *yellow cinchona*, different from that of La Condamine, and produced by his *cinchona cordifolia*, is what we now call *cinchona Carthagena*."

After this violent diatribe against the eminent man, whose great merit was recognised by all his contemporaries, we turn with pleasure to the striking justice which Linnæus renders to Mutis : *Nomen immutabile quod nulla œtas unquam delebit!*

* He died there in 1808.

We may also cite the testimony of those celebrated men Humboldt and Bonpland, who went through the same forests after him, and have confirmed all his observations, whose truth is even more strongly shown when we consider the richness in alkaloids which characterises the cinchonas of New Granada.

Yes! the name of Mutis is as imperishable for his discoveries of cinchonas, as the names of Pelletier and Caventou are for the discovery of the sulphate of quinine.

*Orange Yellow Cinchona of Mutis.*

On the internal surface this bark is of a rather red orange yellow; the thickness is from 2 to 8 millimetres on the average of the serons, the texture is uniform, like the cinchona calisaya, but not so close, and with longer fibres. The external surface is nearly smooth, and of a redder yellow than the inside, sometimes marked transversely with whitish traces of the very thin epidermis which was on it. Transverse fracture, woody internally, and suberous externally. A fresh bitterness, similar to that of the calisaya, slightly styptic, very persistant and rather aromatic. The barks which are thinner and almost always rolled, found in the serons mixed with the larger barks, differ neither in bitterness or color; but if treated separately, less alkaloid will be obtained.

The whole together produces 15 to 16 grammes of sulphate of quinine, and from 6 to 8 grammes of sulphate of cinchonine per kilogramme: 1 gramme of these sulphates gives the same quantity of bitannate as those of calisaya with tannin or an infusion of nut galls.

M. Delondre sent a very large sample to M. Guibourt some months ago; that he might convince himself by his own analysis of the error into which he had fallen respecting this cinchona.

*Yellow Cinchona of Mutis.*

This cinchona presents at the first view the same characters as the preceding, but the internal color is of a yellow ochre color, the texture is less united, and sometimes with rather deep longitudinal furrows, especially the larger barks. The surface is more or less wrinkled, of a duller yellow, with more whitish traces of epidermis, and in some places with crusts, which are easily removed, and which leave deep hollows.

The bitter is slightly acid and more styptic than that of the orange yellow. The product is from 12 to 14 grammes of sulphate of quinine, and from 5 to 6 grammes of sulphate of cinchonine per kilogramme.

According to M. Delondre's experiments, the peculiar crystallization to which he, in conjunction with M. O. Henri, gave in 1833, the name of quinidine is obtained with greater ease from this sulphate of quinine than from others, although in mall quantity; this substance has been again examined of late, notwithstanding the observations published by them in 1831, to prove that this crystallisation is due to a state of hydration of the quinine.

*Red Cinchona of Mutis.*

The barks of this cinchona are from 2 to 15 millimetres in thickness in the bulk of the serons. Internally, the color is of a reddish brown, the texture is very close, with some deep longitudinal furrows in the thick barks. The exterior is of a lighter red, even and spongy, covered in some places with a light epidermis, of a dull white, very adherent, and in some parts with crusts, which are easily detached, and leave deep hollows, as in the preceding cinchona. Transverse fracture, slightly rose-colored, with fine fibres internally and suberous externally. The bitterness developes itself easily and is persistant, but without the slightly aromatic taste peculiar to the orange yellow.

The internal surface of the young barks which are rolled does not differ in color; the texture is finer and the exterior more rugged, and sometimes in ridges.

This is the cinchona which comes over in the smallest quantity from New Granada. From 12 to 14 grammes of sulphate of quinine, and from 6 to 7 grammes of sulphate of cinchonine may be extracted from it. The same results are obtained by tannin and nut galls as from the other species. The sulphate of quinine produced from this cinchona furnishes with greater ease and quantity, according to the experiments of M. Delondre, the peculiar crystallization which he considers a special state of sulphate of quinine.

According to the experiments of MM. Delondre and Henri, this sulphate of quinine is completely soluble in 60 parts of sulphuric ether and 60 parts of ammonia for one part, by the old process of M. Liebig. Whereas the sulphate of quinine proceeding from the cinchonas calisaya, carabaya, and orange yellow of Mutis, are completely soluble in 8 parts of ether and 2 parts of ammonia, using the modification of the same process proposed by MM. Bussy and Guibourt in the *Journal de Pharmacie*, December, 1852.

One gramme of sulphate of quinine in these last conditions was dissolved in alcohol at 36°, with heat and filtered, 2 grammes of ammonia were then added, it was then mixed with pure water until *lactescence* was produced; crystallisation had commenced at the close of thirty-six hours, and had not become very distinct for several days. The sulphate proceeding from the yellow and red cinchonas of Mutis, treated in the same manner, furnished this crystallisation after some hours repose, under the form of small laminæ.

The difference of these sulphates, then, consists, according to MM. Delondre and Henri, in the greater or less promptitude with which this peculiar crystallisation is formed.

M. Delondre insists on these details because it was on the occasion of having to manufacture a lot of two hundred serons of this cinchona that the conflict between quinine and quinidine aròse, which has been already mentioned.

M. Bussy wished him to recall his old labors with M. Ossian Henri, so as to give value to this product as a substitute for sulphate of quinine, and, perhaps, he said, as preferable in some cases. Notwithstanding this proof of his affection for him, M. Delondre persisted in his conviction that there was nothing either new or useful in the results which he had just obtained, for if the peculiar crystallisation (called *quinidine*) were to be separated, the prices would be exorbitant. The surest and most economical substitute for sulphate of quinine is cinchonine, which is naturally united to quinine in all cinchonas, and which is only separated from it by the chemical operations. Moreover, its sulphate is worth 5 francs for 30 grammes, whereas the price of sulphate of quinine is from 14 to 15 francs; and for more than a century those cinchonas have been preferred which contain chiefly cinchonine.

M. Delondre has likewise given a large sample of this red cinchona to MM. Bussy and Guibourt, because it has been hitherto but little known, and is still very rare.

It is difficult to appreciate the value of this cinchona, for in the works on this subject it is confounded with the bark, improperly called *china nova*, and which is not a cinchona at all, as we shall prove hereafter.—*Repertoire de Pharmacie*, March, 1853.

---

## ON THE COVERING OF MEDICINAL SUBSTANCES.

BY M. CALLOUD, OF CHAMBERY.

Some years since an improvement in the distribution of certain officinal preparations was introduced into pharmacy, which obtained from physicians the encouragement which it well merited—I speak of covering medicinal substances. Without injury to the essential therapeutical properties of the preparation, it has the advantage of rendering the act of swallowing it easy and agreeable to the patient, preserving it from the deteriorating influence of the air, from atmospheric hygrometricity and from variations of temperature.

This improvement has been well tried with certain preparations whose disagreeable odor and flavor often caused them to be rejected by the patient; we can now ensure the easy administration of balsam of copaiba, cod and skate liver oil, &c., by means of gelatinous capsules. This manufacture has obtained the greatest success, and is become an important source of profit to several manufacturers who have secured a legal monopoly of it for a certain number of years. But what cannot justly be done in an identical manner, because of the rights of property, may be permitted as an additional improvement; moreover, art is liable to extension, and where there are opportunities of making inventions, they ought to be multiplied and spread all over the world. Whence it follows that art has no respect or limited dominion; there always remains at its disposal an immense number of variations; consequently, without in any way touching on the monopolised methods of manufacture, I shall present some means of covering medicinal substances.

I shall now consider the value of the covering substances which may be useful, both in a physiological and pharmaceutical point of view.

The speculative question of covering medicines depends on these two essential points: the preservation of medicinal substance in its normal conditions, and the agreeable distribution of the medicine in whatever form it may be given.

The practical question depends on the ease of its production and the greatest economy of time.

As ferruginous preparations may very usefully guide any physiological investigations, in their action on the economy, by their preservation of their chemical state in the first degree of oxidation, a condition which renders them so appropriate as absorbants of acid in the digestive organs, and so valuable as absorbents of an injurious excess of oxygen when dissolved in the blood; therefore, these ferruginous preparations should particularly employ the attention of practitioners. We must add that in the first degree of oxidation, preparations of iron have an atramentary taste which is very unpleasant; and we may observe that their physiological value is in the direct ratio of the disagreeableness of their taste. It appears as if it were decreed that life should always be purchased by sacrifices, trouble and pain; but if this is a natural law, so it is likewise intended that science and art should bend their energies to oppose and to overcome it.

To appreciate this fact it will be sufficient to recall to mind the cruel torture of surgical operations before the discovery of the wonderful properties of the vapor of ether and chloroform. Now those cruel operations, formerly rendered so frightful by such distressing circumstances, are performed as if by enchantment, and without pain to the patient. In fact, it is the same with the effects of remedies in cases of internal disease; if their efficiency is assured, it is in a greater or less degree at the price of a disagreeable taste.

It is with a view of avoiding the convulsive movements which are the consequence of a natural repugnance that the practical utility of coverings has been admitted.

Air and heat coming in contact, simultaneously, with the preparations of the protoxide of iron readily caused their superoxidation, especially with those of the carbonated or ioduretted type. M. Blancard's process for ioduretted pills has already fixed the attention of practitioners; it is very satisfactory for its purposes. I have endeavored to find an easy, and in every respect a satisfactory process for covering pills of the carbonated type.

After having tried powdered gum, starch, and sugar as coating agents, I found that using them either alone or mixed did not answer the purpose in every respect.

Hygrometricity was soon apparent on the surface with sugar and gum, which are both hygroscopic substances; and this deliquesence proceeds either from the air or state of the pillular substance enclosed, which is never dry, but of a soft consistence. By dessication in dry air the covering cracks and leaves fissures in the surface of the pills, which render the medicinal substance accessible to the external influence, which it is important to avoid. As for starch, it does not form an elastic covering capable of intercepting the access of air; this can only be ensured by rolling the pills several times in it, so as to give them several layers, which would increase their size, another defect as much to be regretted as the other.

I then tried the dried mucilage of linseed prepared with sugar, and I at length arrived at a satisfactory result.

I operated as follows:

℞ Linseed............................1 part
White sugar......................3 "
Spring water......................q.s.

After having obtained a thick mucilage of linseed, by a careful decoction, I added the sugar, then stirred the whole over a fire until concentrated, and then continued the evaporation to dessication, either in the sand bath or a stove.

By this manipulation, the sugar, being perfectly mixed with a mucilaginous substance which is very slightly hygrometric, is not so likely to attract humidity, and may, when once reduced to powder, be useful for covering medicinal substances in a pillular form. The operation is easily and quickly performed. The pills are moistened with water, either simple or aromatised, and then rolled, in the ordinary manner, in this sweetened linseed, thoroughly dried, and reduced to impalpable powder.

This method of covering, used cold, is what I have employed for pills whose principal ingredient is carbonate of protoxide of iron. It evidently may be applied to many other preparations according to the inclination of the practitioner.

Garot's process of a gelatinous covering may be very usefully applied to many preparations which unite a disagreeable odor to an unpleasant taste. In this latter case, it conceals the odor peculiar to certain remedies better than the process I have just described. Thus the pillular preparations of assafœtida, valerian, castoreum, &c., are completely concealed by a gelatinous covering. Those pillular preparations with resinoid bases may likewise be subjected to this treatment, which are liable to be injured and assume a streaky angular appearance under the variable influence of temperature, such as pills containing gum ammoniacum, and the resins of jalap and scammony. In a gelatinous covering these pills perfectly retain their globular form. By coloring the solution of gelatine with carmine we can give to these pills the agreeable appearance of hawthorn berries or gooseberries.

One other process appears to me to deserve the attention of medical men, that is the employment of butter of cacao as a covering, as uniting in itself many valuable conditions for carrying a medicine into very delicate parts, as in cases of gastritis, gastralagia, and neuropathy. Thus it often happens that taking quinine in complicated intermittent cases produced acute pains in the gastric regions. The pectoral and softening influence of cacao is well known. The idea of using it as a covering of pills has struck me. The operation is very simple: the pills when prepared are steeped in butter of cacao, melted in a sand bath; they are then removed with a perforated ladle, then rolled in powdered sugar prepared on purpose. Sugar of milk is preferable, for, being less soluble than cane sugar, it ensures the covering against removal during its transit through the first passages.

The various methods of covering have been repeatedly tried, and I have used them for the exact pillular preparations which I have just mentioned: I can, consequently, recommend them to the attention of the pharmaceutist and physician.—*Journal de Pharmacie et de Chimie*, April, 1853.

# ON PILLS OF SULPHATE OF QUINIA.

BY EDWARD PARRISH.

Although it is not always left to the discretion of the apothecary what excipients to employ in compounding prescriptions, yet he should be so familiar with the subject as to be able to advise and instruct medical men in regard to those which are really most advantageous in the case of each of the leading remedies extemporaneously prescribed. There are few intelligent apothecaries who have not a salutary influence in modifying the views of neighboring practitioners in regard to the art of prescribing, and none who have not frequent occasion to exercise their own judgment, not only in the selection of excipients, but in other practical points in extemporaneous pharmacy.

There is, I believe, no medicine so frequently prescribed in the pillular form as the sulphate of quinia, and, perhaps, none in making which into pills there is so great a diversity of practice. The following substances are much employed as excipients for this object:—Gum arabic, simple syrup, syrup of gum arabic, honey, molasses, conserve of roses, crumb of bread, flour, and simple water; and besides these, tannic acid, extract of cinchona, and various tonic, astringent, and narcotic extracts, which assist, or in some way modify, the effect of the alkaloid to meet particular indications in disease.

Most pharmaceutists and medical practitioners have, no doubt, a preference for one or other of these, and, as is well known, there are in standard works several formulæ indicating similar preferences.

Dr. Pereira directs the pills to be made with conserve of roses, and in the three formulæ given in the Pharmacopée Universelle, crumb of bread, honey, and conserve of roses are directed. Dorvault directs in L'Officine, for disulphate, the extract of wormwood; for the acid sulphate, conserve of roses. The pills are not officinal in either of the British Pharmacopœias. In our own officinal directions, in the edition of 1850, gum arabic and honey are prescribed, while in that of 1840, gum arabic and syrup were the excipients.

The use of gum arabic and syrup was abandoned on account of the pills becoming insoluble by keeping. Gum arabic and honey used together are probably less objectionable. The omission of the gum entirely is, perhaps, an improvement, honey answering the purpose alone. As quinine is now more frequently prescribed in 2, 3 and 5 grain doses than in the 1 grain dose that used to be given, it is a desideratum to use an excipient which will produce the smallest possible increase of bulk at the same time that it gives a plastic mass.

The following formula is, I think, preferable to those in which gum arabic is employed, as well for the diminutive size as for the increased solubility of the pills:

Take of sulphate of quinia..........12 grains.
Powdered tragacanth.........1 grain.

Triturate the powders thoroughly together, and add sufficient water to form a plastic mass. Divide this into the required number of pills. Made in this way a three grain pill is not inconveniently large.

The use of simple water as an excipient is, I am told, common in domestic practice in the Southern States. The mass produced in this way possesses too little adhesiveness to render it satisfactory. Tannic acid has been used of late with a view of diminishing the intense bitterness of the quinine, but has not found favor generally, as far as my observation has extended. How far the known insolubility of the tannate of quinia in water should operate against this combination is a question for the therapeutist. Conserve of roses, in addition to its bulk, may be objectionable in this as in some other cases, on the score of containing tannic acid, which it does when made from Rosa gallica.

The following formula I have used for several years with

great satisfaction to myself and to those physicians who have prescribed it. It was first suggested by a southern *medical student:*

Take of sulphate of quinia..........20 grains.
Aromatic sulphuric acid......15 drops.

Drop the acid into the sulphate of quinia on a tile or slab, and triturate with a spatula until it assumes a pillular consistence; then divide into the required number of pills. Made in this way, a five grain pill is not inconveniently large.

Although the ingredients when mixed form a fluid, they soon thicken into a paste, and finally become quite solid, and so adhesive as to be readily divided and rolled into pills; care must be taken not to allow the mass to become too dry and brittle before dividing it, as it is liable to do if allowed to remain too long.

In this form, a portion of the disulphate being converted into the soluble neutral sulphate, the preparation more nearly resembles the solutions in composition, and is believed to be more rapid and certain in its action.

When it is desired to incorporate other substances in powder with the quinine thus prepared, they should be added to the mass when it is just so soft that, upon their addition, it will immediately assume the proper consistence.

It is not, however, advisable to employ this process when any considerable quantity of other ingredients are prescribed with the quinine, unless a little syrup of honey is also added to prevent the too rapid hardening and consequent crumbling of the mass.—*American Journal of Pharmacy, July,* 1853.

---

## ANALYSIS OF A NOSTRUM.

Winckler has analyzed a nostrum vended under the denomination of "*lapis antifebrilis.*" He found that it was composed of *arsenious acid* and oxide of lead.—*Knop's Central-Blatt,* Marz 1853.

H. W.

## SULPHATE OF QUINIDINE.

There has been recently distributed among commercial men a circular without date or signature, and with no indication of its origin, announcing a large adulteration of the sulphate of quinine by a product little known, the *sulphate of quinidine*. It has excited much interest among dealers of quinine, and many methods have been suggested for detecting the presence of quinidine in sulphate of quinine.

This new organic base has been studied successively by MM. Henri and Delondre, Winckler, Howard, Zimmer, and Leers. MM. Henri and Delondre, its discoverers, considered it a hydrate of quinine. MM. Winckler and Leers examined a product made by M. Zimmer, of Frankfort, and did not derive their quinidine from the incriminated quinquinas; moreover, they give no processes for obtaining the substance. M. Howard has announced that the base is abundantly contained in the *Quinquina cordiforlia* of New Granada, Bolivia, and Peru.

These chemists are not agreed in the composition and properties of the quinidine, and no one of them states the proportions between the quinine and quinidine contained in the suspected barks.

The most striking characteristics of the quinidine appear to be its constant crystallisation, its very slight solubility in ether, the greater solubility of its sulphate in water, compared with that of the sulphate of quinine.

MM. Bouquet and Schäuffelé have examined a new Granada quinquina imported largely into Europe; it comes from near Fusagasuya, and is known under the name of *Quinquina caqueta*. Twelve kilogrammes of bark have afforded as pure quinine as that extracted from the *Q. calysaya;* the sulphate has all the characters of the sulphate of quinine, and shows no trace of quinidine.

In the black bittern which affords ordinarily the quinidine, MM. Bouquet and Schäuffelé have found some grammes of crystallised products, resembling quinidine in some of their characters, but too different to be confounded with it. The total quantity of this crystallised product corresponded to 3 p. c. by weight of the sulphate of quinine obtained in the treatment of the quinquina essayed. It is easily understood that the works of a large manufacturer might produce these crystallised matters in small specimens, but not for adulterating the sulphate of quinine.

These authors conclude that the properties of the quinidine are so uncertain that it is prudent to wait for more investigation before admitting it among ascertained chemical bases.—*American Journal of Science and Arts*, March, 1853.

---

## SULPHOCYANOHYDRIC ACID IN COMMERCIAL AMMONIA.

Mazade has found syphocyanohydric acid in the ammonia derived from gas-works. It exists, of course, in the form of sulphocyanide of ammonium. Moreau has previously observed the presence of sulphocyanide of ammonium among the products of the distillation of bituminous coal. The reddish tinge presented by some specimens of ammonia—alum made from such ammonia is due to the action of the sulphocyanogen upon traces of iron present.—(*Comptes Rendus*, XXXV., 803.)

# EDITORIAL.

## AMERICAN PHARMACEUTICAL ASSOCIATION.

On the 24th of August the American Pharmaceutical Association is to hold its annual meeting in Boston. We hope that the attendance will be full, and that every section of the country may be represented, otherwise the proceedings will lose much of their influence and value. And, in this connection, would it not be well to consult, in regard both to the time and place of future meetings, mainly the convenience and interest of the majority of the delegates or of those who are eligible to become delegates? An annual change of the place of meeting has undoubtedly some advantages. It is pleasant for the pharmaceutists of New York, or Philadelphia, or Boston, or Baltimore, in their turn, to receive their friends in their respective cities, and to return the kindnesses and hospitalities they have received. Each centre, too, collects a larger representation from its own neighborhood, and thus, *perhaps*, new vigor may be infused into the association. But where is the migration to stop? Are we to follow the example of the American Medical Association, and wander from Boston to St. Louis, from Charleston to New York? Is this the plan that will best promote the interests of the Association? If so, let it be adopted; but if not, let one or two places be selected where trade interests will collect the largest number of members, and at which they can attend the meetings of the Association with the least possible sacrifice of time; and let, too, the time of meeting be appointed so as best to suit the convenience of members at a distance.

---

Statistical Circular.—We give below the circular issued by the New York College of Pharmacy for the purpose of obtaining statistical information in regard to various matters of interest to the profession. Similar circulars have been issued by other institutions. It would have been well that some previous consultation had been held, so that the points of enquiry would have been more uniform in the different States. The questions of the Philadelphia College, for instance, differ widely from the New York circular. We could wish that some distinct enquiries had been addressed to our German brethren. In New York, and in many other cities of the Union, the German apothecaries constitute a large, an educated and a meritorious class. They have here a distinct society, which holds stated meetings, and subscribes for numerous European journals. Many of them would be valuable collaborators of the association, and much useful statistical information could readily be obtained regarding a variety of points which will readily suggest themselves:

CIRCULAR FROM THE COLLEGE OF PHARMACY OF THE CITY OF NEW YORK.

*Dear Sir*,—At a meeting of the National Pharmaceutical Convention, held at Philadelphia, October 6th, 1853, (a copy of its proceedings is herewith presented,) the following resolution (see page 21) was adopted:

"*Resolved*—That the Executive Committee be requested to obtain, through the several Colleges of Pharmacy and Pharmaceutical Associations, previous to our next annual meeting, answers to the following questions, as far as expedient."

The undersigned, having been appointed a Committee by the College of Pharmacy of the City of New York, respectfully request your co-operation with them in obtaining the required information at as early a date as possible, that it may be properly arranged to present at the meeting of the American Pharmaceutical Association, to be held on the 24th of August next, at Boston.

For convenience of arrangement, the Committee propose to send a circular to a prominent druggist of each town, so far as can be ascertained, in this State, soliciting him to fill up the answers to the annexed questions, and to furnish any other useful information that his judgment may suggest.

The statistics of pharmacy in the surrounding country would be very useful, and add much value to the report.

The advantages that will accrue to our profession in the organization of the American Pharmaceutical Association, and the amount of valuable information thus accumulated, induce the Committee to hope that you will not decline a helping hand.

If so disposed to favor us, will you please state, in addition to your answers, what city, town or district, is embraced in your report, including statement of population. The leaf containing questions may be detached, filled up, and addressed to Geo. D. Coggeshall, (Chairman of Committee,) No. 809 Broadway, New York.

Should circumstances, however, deprive us of your aid, you will confer a favor by apprising us to that effect without delay.

Yours very respectfully,

GEO. D. COGGESHALL,<br>
JAMES S. ASPINWALL,<br>
JOHN MEAKIM.<br>
} Committee of College of Pharmacy of the City of New York.

June, 1853.

*Questions proposed by the College of Pharmacy of the City of New York, to obtain Statistics for the National Pharmaceutical Association, to be held at Boston, 24th of August,* 1853.

1. How many Apothecaries and Druggists are there in your city, town, or district?

2. What Pharmaceutical organizations exist—what is the number of their members as compared with the number of Druggists and Apothecaries in the locality?

3. How far is the business of dispensing medicines separated from the office of prescribing?

4. Have you any information in regard to the practice of our art, and the professional character of its practitioners, in your own or other localities, likely to be of advantage to the Association in promoting the objects it has in view?

5. Are there any State Laws for the protection of the interests of the profession of Pharmacy, for the suppression of Empiricism, or in reference to the sale of poisons? (This question the Committee can probably answer pretty correctly in regard to the State of New York. Any information you may possess of such regulations existing in other States will be duly appreciated.)

NEW YORK

# JOURNAL OF PHARMACY.

SEPTEMBER, 1853.

## ON THE MANUFACTURE OF AMMONIA AND AMMONIACAL SALTS.

During the last twenty-five years, the manufacture of liquid ammonia and of ammoniacal salts (more especially the sulphate of ammonia) has received considerable development, inasmuch that in nearly all the principal towns of the kingdom manufactories of these articles are now to be met with. The development of this manufacture has arisen from the immense increase in the production of the raw ammonia furnished by the continued extension of gas-lighting, the low prices at which it is obtainable from this source rendering the application of liquid ammonia, and of ammoniacal salts, accessible to various useful purposes in the arts, manufactures, and agriculture, to which previously the cost of these articles formed an impediment. Liquid ammonia is usually obtained in the commercial scale by submitting a mixture of sulphate or muriate of ammonia and lime to the action of heat, in a closed iron pan or still; the ammonia passes off in the state of vapor, and is condensed by passing through water contained in a series of Woulfe's bottles, formed of lead or earthenware, whence the solutions of ammonia may be drawn off, of any required strength or density. The residuum in the still is either sulphate or muriate of lime, according to the salt employed.

Carbonate of ammonia is obtained by exposing a mixture of sulphate or muriate of ammonia and carbonate of lime to the action of heat enclosed in a retort. Carbonate of ammonia and sulphate or muriate of lime are thus obtained; the former passes off into large leaden chambers, called balloons, where it is condensed in solid masses, whilst the latter remains as a residuum in the retort. The impure carbonate of ammonia thus obtained is then placed in iron pots, and heated, by which means the pure salt is volatilized and collected in suitable receiving or subliming vessels.

The sulphate and muriate of ammonia may be obtained by the action of sulphuric or muriatic acid on certain sulphates and muriates in the carbonate of ammonia contained in the ammoniacal waters of the gas-works or other sources, the sulphuretted hydrogen contained in these waters being got rid of by the assistance of the metallic oxides, &c. The solutions of these salts are then evaporated and crystallized. The sublimed muriate of ammonia (sal ammoniac) is obtained either by heating the crystallized muriate or a mixture of sulphate of ammonia and common salt, or sulphate of ammonia and muriate of lime, in iron pots, and collecting the sublimed salt in suitable receivers, attached by means of luting to the subliming pots.

As the mode of manufacturing these articles varies according to particular circumstances, we shall proceed to mention the chief sources whence ammonia and its salts are obtainable, and describe some of the numerous processes which have of late years been devised for obtaining them in the commercial scale.

*Ammonia from Soot.*—The soot arising from burning the dung of camels and other animals appears to have been the original source of ammonia. Egypt formerly supplied large quantities of muriate of ammonia obtained from this source. Twenty-six pounds of soot are said to yield six pounds of sal ammoniac. From coal soot, also, a considerable quantity of ammonia, in the state of carbonate and sulphate, may be obtained either by sublimation or lixiviation with water. It is chiefly on account of the ammonia contained in soot that this substance forms so valuable a manure.

*Ammonia from Bones, &c.*—The destructive distillation of bones for the purpose of obtaining animal charcoal, used as a decolorizing agent in the refining of sugar and various chemical salts, is a source of ammonia. For this purpose the bones are carbonized in suitable sized retorts, or pots, the products of distillation being water, carbonate of ammonia, the oil called Dippel's oil, and some incondensable gases. The following are the particulars relative to the products as manufactnred, (in France,) on the large scale, of animal charcoal and ammoniacal salts:—Bones, of various kinds, 46,754 tons; silk waste and old leather, 30 tons; sulphuric acid, 11½ tons; common salt, 80 tons; and plaster of Paris, 2¾ tons, were the raw materials employed. The products obtained therefrom were, 2,400 tons of animal charcoal, 44 tons of sal ammoniac, 100 tons of sulphate of soda, 4 tons of liquor ammonia, and 25 tons of sulphate of ammonia. The ammoniacal salts are obtained in this manufactory as follows:

*Sulphate of Ammonia.*—The condensed liquors from the carbonization of the bones are separated into two distinct states, the oily and the aqueous products, the latter of these containing carbonate of ammonia, are treated with sulphate of lime, whence result insoluble carbonate of lime and sulphate of ammonia in solution, which is evaporated and crystallized.

*Muriate of Ammonia.*—This salt is obtained by either of the three following methods:—1. By decomposing sulphate of ammonia by means of common salt. 2. By treating the crude carbonate of ammonia liquors obtained from the distillation of bones with muriatic acid. 3. By decomposing the crude carbonate of ammonia liquors with muriate of manganese, the residuum obtained in the manufacture of chlorine. In either case, the solution of the salts obtained is evaporated and crystallized, and afterwards, if desired, sublimed. 204 lbs. of bones, being carbonized, yield a sufficient quantity of carbonate of ammonia to furnish from 102 to 122 lbs. of sublimed sal ammoniac.

*Carbonate of Ammonia.*—This salt is obtained by submitting a mixture of 65¼ lbs. of sulphate of ammonia, and 99 lbs. of carbonate of lime to distillation, whence is obtained about 41 lbs. of crude carbonate of ammonia, which is afterwards refined.

*Liquid Ammonia.*—This is obtained by heating together in a suitable retort or vessel, 61¼ lbs. of calcined sulphate of ammonia, and 61¼ lbs. of slaked lime. The disengaged gas is collected by absorption in water contained in a series of Woulfe's apparatus, through which it is made to pass.

M. Leblanc, to whom we owe the process of obtaining soda from common salt, originated the following method of manufacturing muriate of ammonia. He employed two tight brick kilns for this purpose, one of which he charged with sulphuric acid and common salt and the other with animal matters. The muriatic acid gas evolved from the one kiln, and the ammonia evolved from the other he caused to pass separately into a chamber lined with lead, containing a stratum of water on its bottom. The two gases here combined with the formation of sal ammoniac.

*Ammonia from Guano.*—Mr. Young took out a patent, November, 1841, in which he describes his method of obtaining ammonia from guano. He fills a retort, placed vertically, with a mixture of two parts by weight of guano, and one part by weight of hydrate of lime or other caustic alkali. These substances are thoroughly mixed by giving a rotary or reciprocating motion to the agitator placed in the retort, a moderate degree of heat is then applied, which is gradually increased until the bottom of the retort becomes red hot. By this means the ammonia is set free, and the uric acid contained in the guano, being decomposed, yields ammonia also. The ammoniacal gas thus given off is absorbed by water in a condenser, whilst other gases, which are given off at the same time, being insoluble in water, pass off. Solutions of carbonate, bicarbonate, and sesquicarbonate of ammonia are produced by filling the condenser with a solution of ammonia and passing carbonic acid through it. A solution of sulphate or muriate of ammonia is obtained by filling the condenser with diluted sulphuric or muriatic acid and passing the ammonia through it as it issues from the retort.

Dr. Wilton Turner took out a patent, March 11, 1844, for obtaining salts of ammonia from guano. The following is his method of obtaining muriate of ammonia in conjunction with cyanogen compounds:—The guano is subjected to destructive distillation in close vessels, at a low red heat during the greater part of the operation, but this temperature is increased towards the end. The products of distillation are collected in a series of Woulfe's bottles, by means of which the gases evolved during the operation may be made to pass two or three times through water before escaping into the air. These products consist of carbonate of ammonia, hydrocyanic acid, and carburetted hydrogen, the first two of which are rapidly absorbed by the water, with the formation of a strong solution of hydrocyanate and carbonate of ammonia. After the ammoniacal solution has been removed from the Woulfe's apparatus, a solution of protomuriate of iron is added to it in such quantities as will yield sufficient iron to convert the latter into Prussian blue, which is formed on the addition of muriatic acid in sufficient quantity to neutralize the free ammonia; the precipitate thus formed is now allowed to subside, and is carefully separated from the solution, and by being boiled with a solution of potash or soda, will yield the ferrocyanate of the alkali, which is obtained by crystallizing in the usual way. The solution (after the removal of the precipitate) should be freed from any excess of iron it may contain, by the careful addition of a fresh portion of the ammoniacal liquor, by which means the oxide of iron will be precipitated, and a neutral solution of ammonia obtained. When the precipitated oxide and cyanide of iron have subsided, the solution of muriate of ammonia is drawn off by a syphon, and the sal ammoniac obtained from it by the usual processes; the oxide of iron is added to the ammoniacal solution next operated upon.

If sulphate of iron and sulphuric acid are used, sulphate of ammonia is the ammoniacal salt produced, the chemical changes and operations being similar to the above. In Doctor Wilton Turner's patent of December 24, 1846, he directs that the urate of ammonia contained in guano be converted into allantoin, oxalic acid and urea. The allantoin is capable of being decomposed into oxalic acid and ammonia by being boiled with a solution of any caustic alkali or alkaline earth. The oxalic acid unites with the alkali used, whilst the ammonia passes over, and may be collected as liquor ammoniæ. Ammonia may also be obtained from the urea above mentioned by boiling it in a still with milk of lime, when it is decomposed into carbonic acid, which unites with the lime, and ammonia which passes into the receiver.

In the specification of his patent of August 11, 1846, Mr. Hills describes his mode of obtaining sesquicarbonate of ammonia from guano. To effect this, the guano is first mixed with charcoal, or powdered coke, the mixture is then heated, and the sesquicarbonate of ammonia obtained by sublimation.

*Ammonia from Urine.*—Stale urine is also a source of ammonia. The urea of the urine undergoes decomposition, with the formation of ammonia. By the addition of sulphuric or muriatic acid, sulphate or muriate of ammonia may be obtained. It is on account of the ammonia contained in stale urine that this substance is employed in the scouring of wool and woollen cloth.

*Ammonia from Peat.*—Mr. Hills, in his patent of August 11th, 1846, specified the following method of obtaining ammonia from peat. The peat is placed in an upright furnace, and ignited; the air passes through the bars as usual, and the ammonia is collected by passing the products of combustion through a suitable arrangement of apparatus to effect its condensation. This plan of obtaining ammonia from peat appears to be precisely similar to that patented by Mr. Rees Reece, (January 23d, 1849,) and made to form an important feature in the operations of the British and Irish Peat Company. The first part of Mr. Reece's patent is for an invention for causing peat to be burned in a furnace by the aid of a blast, so as to obtain inflammable gases and tarry and other products from peat. For this purpose, a blast furnace, with suitable condensing apparatus, is used. The gases, on their exit from the condensing apparatus, may be collected for use as fuel or otherwise; and the tarry and other products pass into a suitable receiver. The tarry products may be employed to obtain paraffine and oils for lubricating machinery, &c., and the other products may be made available for evolving ammonia, wood spirit, and other matters by any of the existing processes. On the 27th of July, 1849, a statement was made in the House of Commons to the effect that 100 tons of peat would produce 2,602 lbs. of carbonate of ammonia, of the value of £32 10s. 2d., and other products of the value of £59 6s. 6d.; the peat costing £8, and the labor of converting it into these valuable products £8 more. An amended statement afterwards appeared in the company's prospectus, from which it appeared that 36,500 tons of peat were capable of yielding sufficient ammonia to furnish, with the aid of the requisite quantity of sulphuric acid, 365 tons of sulphate of ammonia. Dr. Hodges, of Belfast, states that in his experiments he obtained nearly 22¾ lbs. of sulphate of ammonia from a ton of peat. Sir Robert Kane, who was employed by Government to institute a series of experimental researches on the products obtainable from peat, states that he obtained sulphate of ammonia at the rate of 24 8-10 lb. per ton of peat. Messrs. Drew and Stocken patented, in 1846, the obtaining ammonia from peat by distillation in close vessels, as practised in the carbonization of wood. It will thus be seen that peat is a source of ammonia, but that this source is a profitable or economical one, in a commercial point of view, we believe has yet to be determined.

*Ammonia fram Schist.*—Another source of ammonia is bituminous schist, which, when submitted to destructive distillation, gives off an ammoniacal liquor, which may be employed in the manufacture of ammoniacal salts by any of the usual processes. The obtaining ammonia from schist forms part of a patent granted to Count de Hompesch, September 4, 1841.—*Pharmaceutical Journal*, July 1853.

(To be continued,)

---

## ON WHITE OR IMPERIAL RHUBARB.

BY DR. G. WALPERS.

In all works on Pharmacology there occurs a somewhat vague account of a very superior kind of rhubarb, said to be collected for the sole and particular use of the Imperial Court of St. Petersburgh, and distinguished by the name of *White* or *Imperial Rhubarb* (*Radix Rhei alba seu imperialis*). It is described as a rhubarb root in which the white portion so far predominates that only a few red streaks are perceptible upon the surface of a transverse section. No one, however, is from personal knowledge acquainted with this species of rhubarb. In order to put an end to these doubts, I sometime since addressed a letter to Mr. Büchner, Chief Apothecary to the Imperial Court, begging him for a small specimen of this "*Imperial Rhubarb*" for my pharmacological collection, or should the communication of this precious drug be inadmissible, that I might at least have an authentic description of it. Mr. Büchner replied to this request with the utmost promptitude, informing me that, after having instituted the most careful inquiries, it appeared that no such species of rhubarb had at any time been imported for the Imperial family; that it had never occurred in commerce; and, finally, that in neither any public or private collection in St. Petersburgh was there to be found a specimen of this (consequently mythical) root.—*Bonplandia*, for March 15, 1853.

[It was the Russian traveller, Pallas, who first drew attention to the so-called *White Rhubarb*. We extract from his works the passage relating to it: "J'ai vu pendant mon séjour à Kiakta des petits morceaux de rhubarbe blancs comme du lait. Elle est douce au goût, et a les mêmes propriétés que celle de la meilleure qualité. L'apothicaire se proposoit de trier tous ces morceaux, et de les envoyer séparément à Pétersbourg pour la pharmacie de la Cour."—*Voyages de M. P. S. Pallas, en différentes Provinces de l'Empire de Russie, et dans l'Asie Septentrionale, traduits de l'Allemand.* Paris, 4to, 1793, tome iv., p. 219.—Ed. *Ph. Journ.*]

---

## LINIMENTUM ACONITI RADICIS.

BY WILLIAM PROCTOR, JR.

Take of Aconite Root in powder.....four ounces.
Glycerin..................two fluid drachms.
Alcohol, a sufficient quantity.

Macerate the aconite with half-a-pint of alcohol for twenty-four hours, then pack it in a small displacer, and add alcohol gradually until a pint of tincture has passed. Distil off twelve fluid ounces, and evaporate the residue until it measures twelve fluid drachms. To this add two fluid drachms of alcohol and the glycerin, and mix them.

*Remarks.*—This preparation is intended as a substitute for aconitia as an external anæsthetic application. It is used in the following manner: Cut a piece of lint or muslin of the size and form of the part to be treated, lay it on a plate or waiter, and by means of a camel's hair brush saturate it with the *liniment.* Thus prepared it should be applied to the surface, a piece of oiled silk laid over, and kept in place by an adhesive edge or by a bandage. The object of the glycerin is to retard evaporation after application to the skin, and the oiled silk is also used with this view. This preparation is twice the strength of the root, and is exceedingly active. It should not be applied to an abraded surface, and in its use the patient should be cautioned in relation to its poisonous nature, and avoid bringing it in contact with the eyes, nostrils, or lips.—*American Journal of Phnrmacy, July,* 1853.

---

## ON THE MANUFACTURE OF GLYCERIN.

BY CAMPBELL MORFIT, M. D.

Glycerin is generally made, on the large scale, either by directly saponifying oil with oxide of lead or from "the waste" or spent leys of the soap-makers. The first mode of obtaining it is complex and expensive, while in the latter the difficulty of wholly separating the saline matters of the "waste," renders it impossible to obtain a perfectly pure product. In view of these obstacles, and the increasing demand for the article, both in medicine and perfumery, I submit a new process, which has been found, by actual practice, to combine the great and desirable advantages of economy of time, labor, and money.

Take 100 pounds of oil, tallow, lard or "stearin," (pressed lard,) place it in a clean iron bound barrel, and melt it by the direct application of a current of steam. While still fluid and hot, add 15 pounds of lime, previously slaked and made into a milk with 2½ gallons of water, then cover the vessel, and continue the steaming for several hours, or until the completion of the saponification. This is known when a sample of the resulting and cooled soap gives a smooth and lustrous surface on being scraped with the finger nail, and breaks with a cracking noise. By this treatment, the fat is decomposed, its acids unite with the lime to form insoluble lime soap, while the eliminated glycerin remains in solution in the water along with the excess of lime. After it has been sufficiently boiled, it is allowed to cool and settle, and is then to be strained through a crash cloth.

The soap is reserved for sale to stearic candle makers, or else may be reconverted into saleable fat by the process given at pp. 432, 445 Morfit's "*Applied Chemistry.*"

The strained liquid contains only the glycerin and excess of lime. It must be carefully concentrated by steam heat. During evaporation, a portion of the lime is deposited on account of its lesser solubility in hot than in cold water. The remainder is removed by treating the evaporated liquid with a current of carbonic acid gas, boiling by steam heat, to convert any soluble *bi*-carbonate of lime that may have been formed, into insoluble neutral carbonate, allowing repose, decanting or straining off the clear supernatent liquid from the precipitated carbonate of lime, and further evaporating, as before, if necessary, to drive off any excess of water.

As nothing fixed or injurious is employed in the process, the glycerin thus prepared will be absolutely pure.—*Silliman's Journal.*

Baltimore, Md., March, 1853.

## TABLE OF THE QUANTITIES OF ESSENTIAL OILS YIELDED BY NUMEROUS VEGETABLE SUBSTANCES.

We have compiled from the last edition of the Hamburg Pharmacopœia the following table, believing it to be very correct, and likely to be useful to the pharmaceutical body:

| | Yields | of Oil. |
|---|---|---|
| Herba Absinthii, dry | 20 lbs. | 1 to 1½ oz. |
| " " fresh | 100 " | 1 to 1½ " |
| Baccæ Juniperi | 25 " | 3 to 4 " |
| Baccæ Luari | 25 " | 1 to 1½ " |
| Radix Arnicæ, dry | 16 " | about 1 " |
| Cortex Aurantii | 10 " | about 1 " |
| Flores Tanaceti, fresh | 50 " | 2 to 1½ " |
| Herba Majoranæ, dry | 20 " | about 3 " |
| " " fresh | 100 " | about 3 " |
| Herba Menthæ Crispæ, dry | 25 " | 3 to 4 " |
| " " " fresh | 100 " | 3 to 4 " |
| Herba Menthæ Piperitæ, dry | 25 " | 3 to 4 " |
| " " " fresh | 100 " | 3 to 4 " |
| Herba Origani, dry | 25 " | 2 to 3 " |
| " " fresh | 100 " | 2 to 3 " |
| Herba Rutæ, dry | 25 " | about 1 " |
| Herba Sabinæ, fresh | 20 " | 4 to 6 " |
| Herba Salviæ, dry | 25 " | about 3 " |
| " " fresh | 100 " | about 3 " |
| Herba Serphylli, fresh | 100 " | about 1 " |
| Herba Thymi, dry | 20 " | 1 to 1½ " |
| Radix Calami, dry | 25 " | 3 to 4 " |
| Radix Valerianæ, dry | 50 " | about 8 " |
| Semen Anisi | 25 " | 9 to 12 " |
| Semen Carui | 25 " | about 16 " |
| Semen Cumini | 10 " | " 3 " |
| Semen Fœniculi | 25 " | " 16 " |
| Semen Petroselini | 25 " | " 4 " |

| | | | | |
|---|---|---|---|---|
| Caryophilli.................... | 1 | " | " 2½ | " |
| Cortex Cinnamomi............. | 25 | " | " 3 | " |
| Cortex Cassiæ................... | 25 | " | " 3 | " |
| Fructus Cubebarum............ | 4 | " | 4 to 8 | " |
| Macis ........................... | 2 | " | about 3 | " |
| Myristicæ ...................... | 2 | " | 3 to 4 | " |
| Flores Anthemidis, dry......... | 60 | " | about ½ | " |
| Herba Melissæ, fresh........... | 60 | " | 1 to 1½ | " |

---

## PERMANGANATE OF POTASH.

In consequence of the successful use of permanganate of potash in diabetes, under Mr. Sampson, the results of which have been lately published in the *Lancet*, and as it is probable that it will come into more general use, we think a short notice of it will be found useful to our readers.

This salt is formed by the mixture of peroxide of manganese with hydrate of potash; the resulting salt is, however, more abundant if chlorate of potash be used in addition.

There are several modifications of the process: that of Chevillot and Edwards is to ignite one part of peroxide of manganese with one part of hydrate of potash, dissolve the resulting mass in water, decant the red solution and evaporate, rapidly at first, till small needles appear, then cautiously, that crystallization may go on regularly. Wöhler's (*Pogg.* xxvii., 626) process is as follows: Chlorate of potash being kept in a state of fusion over a spirit lamp, hydrate of potash is first added to it, and then an excess of finely divided peroxide of manganese, which immediately dissolves, forming a splendid green solution. The mixture is then heated till the whole of the chlorate of potash is decomposed, and the mass when cold is boiled with a small quantity of water, whereupon the green color of the solution changes to red; finally, the liquid is decanted from the peroxide of manganese while still hot, and set aside to crystallize by cooling. It crystallizes in all proportions with perchlorate of potash, with which it is isomorphous; the latter salt crystallizes in splendid red crystals when a small quantity of permanganate of potash is added to its solution. With equal parts of the two salts, the crystals are nearly black.

Gregory's (*J. Pharm.*, xxi., 312; also *Ann. Pharm.*, xv., 237) consists in adding to a finely divided mixture of eight parts of peroxide of manganese and seven parts of chlorate of potash, a solution of ten parts of hydrate of potash in a very small quantity of water, evaporating to dryness; igniting the finely-pounded mass in a platinum crucible over a spirit lamp till the whole of the chlorate of potash is decomposed, (for which a low red heat is sufficient,) and proceeding as described above. It is readily decomposed by organic matter, so that if it is required to filter the solution previous to crystallization, the neck of the funnel should be filled with asbestos.

The composition of permanganate of potash, according to Mitscherlich, is

| | By calculation. | | By experiment. |
|---|---|---|---|
| $KO$ | 47.2 | 29.65 | 30.385 |
| $Mn_2O_7$ | 112.0 | 70.35 | 69.580 |
| $KOMn_2O_7$ | 159.2 | 100.00 | 99.965 |

The crystals are soluble in sixteen parts of water at 60°.

The dose generally found to agree best with the stomach is about three grains, given in three or four tablespoonfuls of water, three times a day, a little before meals; much larger doses, (as much as ten or twelve grains,) however, have been given, but the dose should be gradually increased.—*Pharmaceutical Journal*, July, 1853.

## ANHYDROUS VALERIANIC ACID.

Chiozza has obtained anhydrous valerianic acid by the method which Gerhardt has applied to the isolation of acetic and butyric acids. When oxychlorid of phosphorous, $P\ Cl^{3}\ O^{2}$, is brought into contact with valerianate of potash, a violent reaction takes place and the odor of the oxychlorid disappears. By treating the mass with a weak solution of carbonate of potash, and then with ether, and evaporating the ethereal solution, the anhydrous acid is obtained as a limpid, highly mobile liquid, lighter than water, and possessing a feeble odor of apples. The liquid boils at 215°, and distils over perfectly colorless: its vapor irritates the eyes and provokes coughing. The reaction by which the anhydrous valerianic acid is obtained is represented by the equations,

$$P\ Cl^{3}\ O^{2} + 3\ (C^{10}\ H^{9}\ O^{3},\ KO) = PO^{5}\ 3\ KO + 3\ (C^{10}\ H^{9}\ O^{2}\ Cl)$$

$$3\ (C^{10}\ H^{9}\ O^{3},\ KO) + 3\ (C^{10}\ H^{9}\ O^{2}\ Cl) = 3\ KCl + 3\ (C^{10}\ H^{9}\ O^{3})$$

the oxychlorid of valeryl, $C^{10}\ H^{9}\ O^{2}\ Cl$, is here first set free, and then reacts on another portion of valerianate of potash.

By the action of oxychlorid of benzoyl on valerianatè of potash, the author has also obtained a compound of anhydrous valerianic with anhydrous benzoic acid represented by $C^{10}\ H^{9}\ O^{3} + C^{14}\ H^{5}\ O^{3}$. It is an oily liquid, heavier than water, and leaving an odor like that of anhydrous valerianic acid. By distillation it is separated into anhydrous benzoic and anhydrous valerianic acids. Alkaline solutions transform it into valerianates and benzoates.

By the action of aniline upon anhydrous valerianic acid, Chiozza has prepared valeranilide crystallizing in magnificent rectangular tables fusing at 115° C. Its formula is $N\ C^{12}\ H^{6},\ C^{10}\ H^{9}\ O^{2}$.—*American Journal of Science and Arts*, March, 1853, from *Comptes Rendus*, xxxv., 568.

# ON ERGOT OF RYE.

BY H. L. WINCKLER.

The author at the beginning of the harvest of last year collected ergot of rye, which he has dried at 139° Fahr., pulverized, and extracted, first with ether and then with water.

The watery extract was treated with strong alcohol, and separated from albuminous matter by filtration. The spirit was distilled off, and the residue brought to dryness. During this operation a small quantity of a brown powder (the ergotine of Wiggers) was precipitated, and again dissolved in the concentrated liquid.

The ethereal extract contained the fatty oil, which was equal to 34 per cent. of the ergot of rye. The residue of the watery extract treated with alcohol (Winckler's extractive ergotine) dissolves readily in alcohol and water under the precipitation of a light brown powder (the ergotine of Wiggers). It has a bitterish cooling taste, and afforded, when distilled with quick lime, a distillate with the odor of herrings, containing propylamine or trymethyline, but no ammonia. The residue consisted of a compound of secaline (that is, the before-mentioned volatile base) with ergotine (Wiggers). The latter body Winckler regards as an acid.

By treatment of ergot of rye with alcohol acidified with sulphuric acid, the author extracted a red ferruginous coloring matter, which has a great resemblance to bluthämatin.

The chemical constituents of ergot of rye are, according to the author, secaline in combination with ergotine, the red ferruginous coloring matter with a base yet to be eliminated, albumen soluble in water and in a coagulated condition, a large quantity of fatty oil, which in the normal grain appears to be replaced by amylon, fungus sugar, (Wiggers,) which disposes the watery extract of ergot of rye so strongly to fermentation, formiates and phosphates. These are the most important constituents. The specific action of the ergot of rye can only be ascribed to the secaline compound or the coloring matter, or to both of these compounds together, as, according to all experience, it does not belong to the fatty oil.

The powdered ergot of rye intended for medical purposes should be dried at a temperature not exceeding 139° Fahr., and preserved completely dry in a vessel impermeable to the atmosphere. The powder preserved in this manner appears almost odorless, of a light grey blue color, but evolves the peculiar odor of ergot of rye directly it is moistened with water. The watery extract, particularly that prepared with finely-powdered ergot, in the cold, or treated with cold water and then evaporated in a water bath, possesses the peculiar odor of ergot of rye, affords by distillation with caustic lime a considerable quantity of secaline and ammonia, and contains without doubt the greatest portion of the active constituents of the ergot of rye, but it cannot be kept. The spirituous tincture, prepared with alcohol of 40 per cent., by several days' digestion, at an ordinary temperature, from finely pulverized ergot, appears of a dark brown color, contains all the active constituents of the ergot of rye, and very little fatty oil, which separates in a crystalline form at very low temperatures.

The spirituous extract is best kept and most effective when it is prepared by twice extracting the fine powder with an equal quantity of cold distilled water, clarifying the concentrated extract, and treating it with alcohol of 80 per cent. as long as a precipitate results on the addition of a fresh portion. The spirituous fluid is, after 24 hours, separated from the precipitate by filtration; the filtrate subjected to distillation in a water bath, and the residue evaporated to the consistence of an extract. The extractive ergotine prepared in this way is a little hygroscopic, possesses a light brown color, a slight narcotic odor, dissolves under the separation of a little ergotine (Wiggers) in water, and evolves when treated with a solution of caustic potash, in a high degree, the penetrating odor of secaline. By distillation of the concentrated watery extract with caustic lime a very concentrated solution of secaline is also obtained.

Winckler recommends for further investigations on the activity of the ergot of rye the pure muriate of secaline, the neutral compound of secaline with ergotine, the red coloring matter, and the neutral compound of ergotine with ammonia. Winckler has found the compound of ergotine with secaline (ergotinate of secaline) in the black sporous mass of *Lycoperdon cervinum.*—*Central-Blatt.*

---

## NEW METHOD OF ESTIMATING THE VALUE OF CHLORINATED LIME.

Dr. Penot has so far altered the method of Gay-Lussac for the estimation of chlorinated lime, that he employs an alkaline solution of arsenious acid; and instead of a solution of indigo, a colorless iodized paper, which becomes blue by the smallest quantity of free acid.

This test paper is prepared in the following manner:—1 gramme of iodine, 7 grammes of crystallized carbonate of soda, 3 grammes of potato starch, and ¼ of a litre of water, are heated until perfect solution and decoloration ensue; after which, so much water is added to the solution that the whole measures ½ a litre. White paper is soaked therein, and then dried. This is the iodized paper.

For the preparation of the test liquid, 4,44 grammes of arsenious acid, with 13 grammes of crystallized carbonate of soda, are dissolved by heat in ¾ of a litre of water, and the mixture diluted with water to form 1 litre. 10 grammes of the chlorinated lime, to be estimated, are dissolved in the usual way, in 1 litre of water, an alkalimeter of which is poured into a glass. The alkalimeter then is filled with the test liquid, and from this so much poured, by degrees, into the solution of chlorinated lime, until a drop of the latter, when placed on the iodized paper, ceases to color it. The degrees employed give direct the degree of chlorinated lime, or the number of litres of chlorine gas contained in 1 kilogramme of the chlorinated lime tested. For the estimation of the correctness of the results obtained, the process may be reversed, that is, the solution of chlorinated lime poured into an alkalimeter of the test liquid until a drop of the mixture colors the iodized paper blue. Thus, when the chlorinated lime contains, in the kilogramme, 90 litres of gas, or when 90 degrees are obtained in the first process, 111 degrees must be found by the second one.

When very weak chlorinated lime is tested, 10 degrees of test liquid, with 90 degrees of water, are used in the alkalimeter. The quantity sought is, then, the tenth of that found.—*Bullet. d. Mulhouse and Annals of Pharmacy.*

---

## SAFE METHOD OF DETERMINING THE QUANTITY OF WATER IN IODINE.

Bolley weighs 1 gramme of iodine in a small evaporating dish, adds to it 6 or 8 times its weight of mercury, rubs the mixture carefully, and heats the dish in a water bath until it ceases to lose weight. The loss is water. The greater part of the mercury may be separated again by pressure.—*Polyt. Central-Blatt.*

## THE PRODUCTION OF IODINE IN FRANCE.

According to Payen, the manufacture of iodine in France affords 300,000 kilogrammes of sulphate of potash, 340,000 kilogrammes of chloride of sodium, 3,450 kilogrammes of iodine, or an equivalent quantity of iodide of potassium, 250 kilogrammes of bromine or bromide of potassium, and 2,000,000 kilogrammes of dry lixivated residue. The consumption of iodine in the last year has risen so high that the quantity produced in France is not sufficient for French commerce, and on that account foreign iodine must be introduced. —*Annals of Pharmacy, July,* 1853.

---

## THE ANÆSTHETIC PROPERTIES OF THE LYCOPERDON PROTEUS—COMMON PUFF BALL.

BY MR. W. B. RICHARDSON.

The author's attention had been directed to the fact, that the smoke of the common puff ball was used in the country for stupefying bees, and the idea struck him that it would be worth while to ascertain if the same agent would produce narcotism in higher classes of animals. Several weeks since, he commenced a series of experiments with the fumes of the fungus, and had continued them to the present time. He found it possible to produce the most perfect anæsthesia with the fumes. His experiments had been made on dogs, cats and rabbits, and had been witnessed by Drs. Willis, Crisp, Cormack, Snow, and several others. He had administered the narcotic fumes in the impure state, and in a clarified state obtained by passing them through a solution of caustic potass. When an animal was exposed to a large quantity of the narcotic vapor, the narcotism came on very speedily, and the insensibility was most decided, but recovery soon took place. Dr. Willis and Mr. Richardson had removed a large tumor from the abdomen of a dog that had been placed under the influence of the narcotic. No sign of pain was shown during the operation, and the animal did well afterwards. The fumes were obtained by burning the fungus. When a moderate quantity was inhaled slowly, the narcotism came on and passed off slowly, the animal exhibiting all the symptoms of intoxication, with convulsions, and sometimes vomiting. Several animals had been intentionally destroyed by the narcotic. It destroyed life slowly; a dog would often inhale the fumes for twenty minutes or half an hour after being completely narcotised, previous to expiring. The heart's beat, in all cases, survived the respirations. The lungs, after death, were pale; there was no sign of congestion in any organ; the blood retained its red color, but did not coagulate quickly; cadaveric rigidity set in in two or three hours. During recovery from a protracted nacotism, an animal would sometimes be quite conscious, but insensible to pain. Mr. Richardson had himself inhaled the clarified fumes of the fungus; they produced in him symptoms of intoxication and drowsiness, but he did not breathe them long enough to become completely narcotised. Mr. Richardson was able to afford but little information as to the nature of the narcotic agent contained in the fumes. Many of the fungi possessed narcotic properties, and had been supposed to possess an alkaloid resembling morphia; but the subject had never been thoroughly investigated. He should only say, concerning the narcotic principle contained in the puff-ball—1st. That it was of a most volatile nature; 2ndly. That it was not absorbed by alcohol, water, or strong alkaline solution; 3rdly. That if the fungus was burned in oxygen gas, the narcotic principle still remained in the fumes, and produced its effect, if free oxygen was breathed with it. The fungus had been given to two animals without effect. In Italy, it was fried and eaten as food. In conclusion, Mr. Richardson said, that he had been anxious only to show that a volatile narcotic principle, capable of causing anæsthesia by inhalation, did exist in one of the fungi; it remained to be seen whether other fungi possessed a similar principle, and whether from a fungus an anæsthetic could be obtained that might be used in practice, with as little trouble to the operator and with less danger to the patient than ether or chloroform.

The President (Dr. Forbes Winslow) asked, if Dr. Snow had any remarks to make.

Dr. Snow corroborated Mr. Richardson's observations, having witnessed several of his experiments. There could be no doubt that the fungus did possess a very volatile narcotic principle, capable of causing insensibility to pain. As yet, however, the narcotic was not so practicable as chloroform. The subject deserved and required further research.—Medical Society of London, from the *Medical Times and Gazette*, June 11, 1853.

---

## ON THE PREPARATION OF LIQUID PERCHLORIDE OF IRON AS A HÆMOSTATIC AGENT.

BY M. BURIN DU BUISSON, OF LYONS.

It is known that a great many substances have the property of precipitating albumen from its solutions.

Almost all the acids precipitate it white; acetic acid converts concentrated solutions of albumen into jellies.

Strontia, baryta and lime form with albumen precipitates which are insoluble in water.

Almost all the metallic salts are precipitated by albumen, and the white precipitate insoluble in water, which this substance forms with bichloride of mercury, is well known. To the other metallic salts which possess this property, sulphate of copper, but more especially perchloride of iron, must be added.

Perchloride of iron possesses, indeed, in the highest degree, the property of combining instantaneously with albumen, and of forming with it a precipitate under the form of a consistent and insoluble magma, as Dr. Pravaz has just proved, and every one now knows the importance of the application which this skilful practitioner has recently made of the aqueous solution of this salt for instantaneously coagulating the blood in the arteries, as regards its special employment for the cure of aneurisms in man.

Perchloride of iron unites, indeed, all the qualities desirable (and even exclusive) for fulfilling the object to which Dr. Pravaz has so happily applied it—great hæmostatic power, perfect harmlessness, and solubility in water: it remained, therefore, only to find a mode of preparation which would enable us to obtain this salt always very pure, and its aqueous solution at a maximum density, which might be always and everywhere identical, indispensable conditions for attaining the object proposed by Dr. Pravaz, who has been kind enough to entrust this task to us. The following are the results we have arrived at:

LIQUID PERCHLORIDE OF IRON, OF DR. PRAVAZ.

| Take, | Grammes. |
|---|---|
| Commercial sulphate of iron | 1,000 |
| Water | 3,000 |
| Pure iron filings | 100 |
| Sulphuric acid | 15 |

The whole is introduced into a matrass, or, better still, into an enamelled cast iron vessel, and allowed to digest on a sand bath until the disengagement of gas entirely ceases; it is filtered, and 500 grammes of liquid hydrosulphuric acid are added to the liquor, and the whole is left to repose for twelve hours; at the end of this time, the solution is boiled for half an hour and filtered.

200 grammes of pure concentrated sulphuric acid are added to the filtrated liquor; the mixture is placed in a porcelain capsule, or an enamelled cast iron vessel, which must not be more than half filled, and boiled, and pure nitric acid is added in small portions until the last addition causes no disengagement of red vapors; it is then removed from the fire, the liquor is diluted with from 25 to 30 times its weight of cold water, and all the iron is precipitated in the state of peroxide with a slight excess of liquid ammonia: the precipitate is washed by decantation with pure water a great number of times, and it is dried in the air by spreading it in thin layers on a cloth.

The dry and pulverized oxide is afterwards calcined at a red heat in a shallow wrought iron vessel, so as not to raise the temperature too high; the astringent saffron of Mars, of the shops, is thus obtained, which is no other than pure peroxide of iron, when it is thus prepared.

The perchloride of iron is afterwards obtained in the following manner:

| | Grammes. |
|---|---|
| Peroxide of iron as above prepared...... | 200 |
| White and pure hydrychloric acid....... | 1,000 |

It is allowed to act without heat for five or six hours, and then the vessel is placed in a boiling water bath and heated until the oxide is almost entirely dissolved; this operation must be performed in a porcelain capsule of known weight; the liquid is decanted in order to separate the undissolved oxide, and it is carefully evaporated on the sand bath, stirring continually to the consistence of a thick syrup, the weight of which is then determined: a quantity of distilled water equal to half this weight is then added; the heat is then continued for a short time, and the whole is poured into a filter; the capsule and filter are washed with a fresh quantity of water, equal to the first, and sufficient of this liquid is then added to the first liquid to obtain a homogeneous mixture having the constant density of 43·5 to 44°.

By operating thus, we obtain a very limpid liquid, having only a slight acid reaction, but perfectly pure, at the maximum of saturation, and always identical, which may be preserved without any deposition of salt, provided that it be kept in a well corked bottle; it is of a deep brown color by reflected, and of a greenish golden yellow by transmitted light, or in a thin layer.

Five or six drops of this liquid, mixed with the white of an egg suspended in 20 grammes of water, are sufficient for causing the whole to assume, in less than a quarter of a minute, the form of a mass which, on reversing the vessel which contains it, remains adhering to the bottom of the vessel, and it detaches itself only after a very long time, when the water begins to separate partially, in the same manner as the serum of coagulated blood.

This preparation, therefore, combines all the conditions required for realising all the anticipations to which the observations of Dr. Pravaz have justly given rise.—*Journal de Chimie Medicale*, June, 1853.

# ON THE PREPARATION OF LACTATE OF PROTOXIDE OF IRON.

BY M. C. J. THIRAULT.

In the preparation of lactate of iron by the processes described in chemical works, difficulties are frequently encountered, especially in the concentration of the liquor for the purpose of obtaining the salt in crystals. Even should a first crystallization be obtained without difficulty, on concentrating the mother-liquors in order to obtain a second crystallization, the liquid acquires a reddish tint, owing to the peroxidation of the salt, which now refuses to crystallize. Another difficulty presents itself in drying the lactate of iron when obtained. If certain precautions be not taken the salt, instead of being of a yellowish-white with a tinge of green, acquires a reddish-yellow color, in which case it is in great measure peroxidized.

All these difficulties, which I have expertenced in making the salt for the first time, in addition to the facility with which lactic acid combined with lime may be artificially prepared, induce me to publish the processes which I have always found successful.

There are two processes for obtaining solution of lactate of protoxide of iron, either of which may be employed with equal success. The one consists in the direct action of lactate acid on iron filings, and the other in the double decomposition of protosulphate of iron and lactate of lime. But to whichever of these the preference is given, it is essential in carrying out the process according to my mode of operating, to have a small quantity of lactic acid in reserve.

The following is the mode of operating if the former of the two processes indicated above be adopted:

After having prepared lactate of lime in the usual way, by artificial means, it is necessary to test the degree of purity of the salt, as it is difficult to get it always in the same state, for not only does it frequently contain carbonate of lime, but the amount of water present is always variable. It should be ascertained, therefore, what quantity of sulphuric acid of a definite strength is required for the complete decomposition of a given quantity of the lactate.

For the preparation of lactate of iron a certain quantity of the lactate of lime is mixed with the required quantity of sulphuric acid for its decomposition, the latter being mixed with ten or twelve times its weight in water, and allowed to stand in contact with it, without heat, for forty-eight hours, the mixture being stirred from time to time. It may then be filtered through a cloth, to separate the sulphate of lime, when a solution of lactic acid, sufficiently pure for the purpose intended, will be obtained.

If it be desired to get the lactic acid in a greater state of purity, the decomposition of the lactate of lime may be effected with oxalic acid instead of sulphuric acid, but for the purpose referred to this is unnecessary, as the small quantity of sulphate of lime which it would retain when sulphuric acid is used would be deposited during the concentration of the solution.

Two-thirds of the lactic acid, obtained in the manner indicated, is to be added to iron filings in an iron vessel, and the action promoted by the application of heat. When the iron ceases to be acted upon the liquor is to be filtered, and if the directions above given have been followed it will be in a condition favorable to crystallization. The solution, as it filters, should be received in a vessel immersed in warm water, and this should be subsequently covered. After five or six days the sides of the vessel will be found to be covered with a crystalline coat of lactate of iron. It only remains to dry the salt, which is very easily effected by first washing it with a mixture of one part of lactic acid and eight parts of spirit, and afterwards exposing it to a temperature of from 60° to 70° Fahr., on filtering paper or on a chalk-stone.

In order to effect the crystallization of the mother-liquor, some of the free lactic acid, which was kept in reserve, is to be added to it, together with some iron filings, and the mixture rapidly evaporated, while the hydrogen gas, resulting from the action of the acid on the iron, is being evolved. The lactate is thus preserved from undergoing peroxidation, and the whole of the liquor may be exhausted of its salt.

An equally satisfactory result with that above described may be obtained by double decomposition, but as it is necessary in this case to use very weak solutions of sulphate of iron and lactate of lime, and subsequently to concentrate the liquor in order to effect crystallization, the peroxidation of the salt must be prevented by keeping up the disengagement of hydrogen in the manner already described.—*Journal de Pharmacie and Chemist.*

---

# EDITORIAL.

## VARIA.

### AMERICAN PHARMACEUTICAL ASSOCIATION.

*Second Day—Afternoon Session.*

[AMERICAN PHARMACEUTICAL CONVENTION.—From the *Boston Traveller* we learn that the Convention was organized on the morning of Thursday, the 25th, by the appointment nf William A. Brewer, of Mass., as President; G. D. Coggeshall, of N. Y., Alex. Duval, of Richmond, Va., and C. B. Guthrie, M. D., of Memphis, Tenn., as Vice-Presidents; Edward Parrish, of Philadelphia, Recording Secy.; Wm. B. Chapman, Cincinnati, Corresponding Secy.; Alfred B. Taylor, Philadelphia, Treasurer; and Wm. Proctor, Jr., T. B. Merrick, N. Y., and Joseph Laidley, Va., Executive Committee. We subjoin from the *Traveller* a synopsis of the debate on the Drug Inspection Law.]

The Drug Law was then taken up, and Mr. Fish offered the following:

*Resolved*, That in the opinion of this Association all varieties of drugs that are good of their kind should be admitted by the special examiner.

On this resolution an animated discussion arose, in which several gentlemen took part.

Mr. Merrick, of New York, made an able and effective speech in support of the resolution. He first asked the question is the law for the special examination of drugs a good one? and in answer to this urged the following objections to it: It is in conflict with the liberty we all ought to enjoy in business. The difference in the success of different druggists depends mainly upon the reputation, good or bad, which they acquire by their knowledge, skill and probity in the selection and sale of medicines, or by the inferiority in their stocks of drugs, which results from a want of these qualities. The direct aim of this law is in good measure to deprive druggists of the advantages resulting from this competition. He looked upon all laws of the kind as checks to human progress. He further objected to the drug law on the ground that after a trial of three or four years it has not been found to work well. The office of special examiner is placed in the hands of persons unfitted by education and previous pursuits to execute so important a trust. He urged that physicians were less qualified than practical druggists for the station. He reviewed the late instructions of the department to the special examiners, and pointed out its defects. He would rather trust his eyesight to tell the quality of many articles, such especially as aloes, senna, rhubarb, &c., than any estimate founded on the standards given. The specific gravity of the essential oils is no criterion of their strength in a majority of cases. The idea that the value of Peruvian barks could be ascertained by the amount of alkaloids they contain was combated, and the doctrine maintained that all barks have their particular uses, and all should be allowed to enter our ports if *good of their kind.*

The next speaker was Mr. Colcord, of Boston. He was pleased with many points in the report of the committee, but not prepared to adopt it as a whole, nor to vote for this resolution. He likes mackerel No. 1 and good of its kind, but would as soon eat No. 3 mackerel as to vote for this resolution.

Mr. Fish said he also liked No. 1 mackerel, but had eaten No. 3, and was willing to allow any one that privilege, even though it might not be considered good of its kind. In reference to the cinchona bark, he wished to say that during an experience of 26 years in the drug trade, he had found Maracaibo bark to meet the wants of a great majority of the people in his section of the country. During the prevalence of spotted fever, as an epidemic, in the valley of the Connecticut, in the years 1803, '4, '12 and '13, the medical profession relied entirely upon that bark, and fought successfully that dire disease with it; and it was not until a later period that any of the officinal barks came into use, which were, of course, found preferable. That bark still holds its place, and forms nine-tenths of the consumption of the people, and is, in a vast majorify of cases, preferred. He regarded the strict construction placed upon that section of the law as an actual prohibition of many valuable remedies. Under it, nit. potassa was inadmissible, as well as any bark nonofficinal. He coincided with Mr. Merrick in his views regarding the law, and now desired to pursue such a course as to render its operation less objectionable.

He believed the intent of the law was simply to exclude *adulterated* or *deteriorated* drugs, but was not applicable to any article in its natural state that possessed remedial powers. He conceived that the examiners had assumed judicial powers and undertaken to decide upon what should or should not be admitted, with regard to quality, upon grounds wholly inapplicable, as has been illustrated recently in Philadelphia. He did not believe that a bark, to possess remedial powers, should, of necessity contain quinine. The false Angostura (Strychnos-pseudo Quina) was the most valuable anti-periodic known, but contained not a particle of quinine. He regarded the present operation of the law as a step backward rather than in advance, and earnestly hoped that a more liberal spirit would finally prevail.

Dr. Guthrie replied to the arguments urged for the adoption of this clause of the report; reviewing the causes which led to the enactment of the law of 1848; giving a history of the state of the drug trade in the West and South before such law, and the present condition of the trade. Dr. Guthrie urged the necessity of a high and consistent stand being taken by this association; urged the importance of our action as to its future usefulness and bearings upon the profession of Pharmacy in the United States; its effect upon the medical profession; its importance to the community at large.

The American Pharmaceutical Association stands as the representative of the profession, and the profession stands as the curators and conservators of the public health; community looks to them not only that every article dispensed by them be "good of its kind," but that the kind be good, and not only good but the best.

The exhibition of articles sold by our profession are at the best hard to take, and we can do no less than to offer such as will require the smallest amount to produce the same effect.

Dr. Guthrie argued that instructions of the Secretary of the Treasury were on this subject sufficient, and that notwithstanding the execution of the law from its being made a political appointment, a matter of great regret, and calculated to eventually destroy the whole force and effect of the law, from the frequent changes in an office, the execution of which requires great experience and an extensive and minute acquaintance with drugs in general--and urged that the association should protest against such changes, unless called for by prominent and experienced dealers in such articles.

Dr. Guthrie gave to the association many instances that had fallen under his observation while collecting information as to the practical effects of this law under the instructions of the late Secretary of the Treasury, going to show the beneficial effects of the law, and gave it as his opinion that great good had resulted therefrom, not only in its immediate effects, in keeping out of market inferior drugs, but in begetting an inquiry and increased demand for good drugs. He also urged the subject of home adulteration as having been greatly checked by the action of the law, and closed by an earnest and warm appeal to his brethren of the profession to stand firm, unfalteringly, on the clear ground of right, regardless of any outside pressure, come that pressure from what source it may.

Mr. Coggeshall would be glad to have a decision upon this vexed and tedious question, a decision now by this body that so far as its influence extends, it may be settled at once and for ever. This is the third time that this question has come before meetings of this kind, the Conventions of 1851 and '52, and now the National Pharmaceutical Association—it has twice been earnestly debated at much length, its claims each time fully and fairly considered, and it has twice been rejected by an emphatic vote. Is there consistency in bringing up this matter year by year in the very same words? In regard to the standards he was very well satisfied with those contained in the instructions lately issued by the Secretary of the Treasury as far as they go, and it is remarkable how well the ground is covered by them. He considered the present barks, or the great bulk of them, imported under the names of Carthagena and Maracaibo, as altogether different from and inferior to those of 25 and 30 years ago, when they were subjected to the examination reported in the foot notes of the U. S. Dispensatory. And that European rhubarb was not a legitimate article of medicine, but is used as an adulteration of Russian and Chinese, or as a substitute in whole or in part for them—the true article of Russian rhubarb being literally unknown out of the principal cities.

The question on the adoption of the resolution was then taken and lost; after which, an adjournment to nine o'clock in the morning was carried.

---

Cowhage Ointment.—M. Blatin recommends an ointment formed by rubbing up about seven grains and a half of mucuna pruriens with an ounce of lard as a mild counterirritant. Of this ointment seven or eight grains is to be rubbed upon the surface for from ten to twenty minutes. It produces an eruption similar to that caused by the sting of nettles, and attended with a slight burning stinging pain, which soon diminishes and passes off in half an hour.

---

Mucilage of Tannin.—Tannic acid has been used with much advantage in case of opthalmia arising from granular lids; but however finely the tannin may be powdered, the roughness and hardness of the minute particles still cause a good deal of pain and irritation. To obviate this, M. Hairion proposes the following formula for a mucilage, which he has used with much success:

Pure tannin.................................. 5 grammes.
Distilled water..............................20 grammes.

Dissolve in a mortar, and add—

Gum arabic.................................10 grammes.

Mix intimately, and strain through linen.

The mucilage thus formed is smooth, homogeneous, and of the consistence of syrup.

LANTH'S MIXTURE.--A nostrum under the title of Lanth's mixture has obtained considerable repute in the treatment of cutaneous diseases. It is composed of:

Chloride of Barium..............................gr iii Ss.
Whytt's stomachic tincture........................ ℥ i.
Distilled water.................................... ℥ iij.

Whytt's stomachic tincture consists of:

Yellow bark.......................................℥ iij.
Gentian.........................................
Orange peel......................................*aa* ℥ i.
Proof spirit......................................oi Ss.
Cinnamon water.................................. ℥ viij.

---

PULVIS ANTIMONIALIS.—A late number of the *London Medical Times* contains an analysis of twenty specimens of antimonial powder obtained from as many reputable druggists in London. In two instances, sesqui-oxyde of antimony, which is commonly esteemed the active ingredient of the medicine, had been substituted for antimonial powder, the specimens consisting solely of that substance. The other eighteen specimens contained antimonious acid, sesqui-oxyde of antimony, and phosphate of lime; the proportion of these ingredients however varies considerably, more or less sesqui-oxyde however being contained in all of them. The antimonious acid varied from 30.4 to 52.40 per cent.; the sesqui-oxyde of antimony from 0.34 or 3.97 per cent.; and the phosphate of lime from 45.03 to 68.57.

---

FERRUGINOUS COLLODION.—M. Aran recommends a mixture of equal parts of Bestucheff's tincture and ordinary collodion as an external application in erysipelas. According to M. Aran the mixture forms a thinner pellicle, but one more supple, elastic, and less liable to crack than the *ordinary* collodion.

---

TULLY'S MATERIA MEDICA AND THERAPEUTICS.—We have received the seventh number of Dr. Tully's work, and are rejoiced to see its publication is regularly continued. When Dr. T. reaches the individual articles of the materia medica we hope to enrich our columns with some of the results of his long experience and close observation.

NEW YORK

JOURNAL OF PHARMACY.

OCTOBER, 1853.

## ON CREASOTE.

BY EDWARD N. KENT.

Those who have had occasion to notice the article which has recently been sold under the name of Creasote, have doubtless observed a remarkable difference between it and that formerly sold under the same name. It is well known that creasote was formerly prepared exclusively from wood-tar, and was generally imported from England. The new article is obtained from Germany; and in a recent examination of it, I have found it to be carbolic acid, or hydrated oxide of phenyle, and is consequently prepared from coal-tar. A slip of pine wood, dipped first into this, and then into hydrochloric acid, becomes blue, which is not the case with creasote prepared from wood-tar. In all other qualities it is so similar to creasote as to be scarcely distinguishable from it, except by its less disagreeable odor, which has doubtless caused it to come so generally into use. It is applicable to all uses to which creasote is applied, and, though described by chemists under a different name, I am disposed fully to concur with those who consider carbolic acid to be creasote in a purer form than that obtained from wood-tar.

It is well known that carbolic acid may be easily contained by agitating the oil produced by the distillation of coal-tar, with a strong solution of caustic alkali, and the subsequent decomposition of the alkaline solution by an acid. But the article thus obtained cannot be purified by any of the processes described in chemical works, so as to remain colorless or compare in purity with that prepared by the German manufacturing chemists. To obtain this desirable result I have devoted much labor; and, as the process has not, to my knowledge, been previously published, will proceed to describe the method of manufacture and purification which has proved successful, with the hope that it may be interesting and profitable to some of our manufacturing chemists, who may be induced to engage in its manufacture.

When coal-tar is subjected to distillation, a small quantity of light oil and water first pass over, but the principal product is a heavy oil, amounting generally to a little more than twenty-five per cent. of the measure of the tar. The residue is pitch. Carbolic acid, in an impure state, is obtained from the above heavy oil, by agitating it with strong caustic lye; but, as the crude coal oil contains generally a large per centage of napthaline and other impurities, I prefer to rectify it and collect the product in two separate portions, the first of which should be used for the preparation of creasote. In this rectification, it is convenient to use twelve parts of the crude heavy oil, distil off eight parts of "rectified oil," change the receiver, and continue the distillation nearly to dryness. The second portion of the distilled product contains an abundance of napthaline, which is most easily removed by continually using this portion over again in subsequent rectifications, by adding it to more crude oil, sufficient to make twelve parts for another operation. By continually using this crude portion over again, in the above manner, the napthaline and other impurities are removed, by drawing off the residue remaining in the still at the end of each rectification.

By exhausting the rectified oil with a strong solution of

caustic soda, about twenty-five per cent. of carbolic acid is obtained from it. The caustic soda should be as strong and as free from carbonic acid as possible, and for this purpose it cannot be well prepared by the cold process of leeching, which is used by soap manufacturers. I have succeeded best by boiling one pound soda ash with one gallon of water, and then adding to the boiling solution one pound hydrate of lime, in small portions at a time, and, after boiling about fifteen minutes, covering the vessel, and letting it settle till cold. The supernatant lye, decanted off *clear*, is ready for use. A very strong solution of perfectly caustic lye is thus obtained, but if less lime or more water be used, it will not answer well. It is almost impossible to filter the strong lye through the lime residue, but, if it is left till cold, the residue becomes hard and firm, and the lye may then be easily decanted. The lime residue may then be washed with another gallon of water, left to settle, decanted, and this dilute solution used instead of water for making the strong lye in a subsequent operation. The hydrate of lime for the above purpose is best prepared by slaking it with one-third its weight of water, in a vessel loosely covered, and leaving the mixture till the aqueous vapor has combined with a small portion of lime, which would otherwise remain anhydrous.

The best plan for obtaining the creasote is to mix the rectified oil with an equal measure of the strong caustic lye, stir it occasionally for half a day, draw off the alkaline solution, and again treat the oil in the same manner with half the measure of caustic soda first used. This removes all the creasote contained in the oil, if the lye is good, and in this case a sample of the oil, agitated with a little fresh lye, no longer gives to the latter a dark color. It is best not to heat this mixture, as by so doing the oil becomes rapidly oxidised, and confers a dark color on the alkaline solution, which renders it difficult to be separated. After the first treatment with caustic lye, a large portion of the alkaline compound remains dissolved in the supernatant oil, which renders it necessary to use a second portion of caustic soda to remove it, in the manner above described.

The alkaline solution of creasote (or carbolic acid) may be decomposed with almost any acid, but strong sulphuric acid is the most convenient and economical, and this produces a hot solution of sulphate of soda, which becomes a crystalline mass on cooling, while the creasote separates readily to the top, and may easily be removed either before or after the crystallization of the sulphate of soda.

The crude creasote thus obtained is of a light brown color, but soon becomes very dark, and holds water, resin, sulphate of soda, and the substance which becomes brown by oxidation. Of these substances the three first can be removed by distillation, and the last by oxidation and subsequent distillation, but for this purpose a powerful agent must be resorted to. Chromic acid is reduced by it to oxide of chromium, but it is not effectual in perfectly oxidising all of the brown impurity. Nitric acid converts the creasote into carbozotic acid, and consequently cannot be used. Concentrated sulphuric acid answers the purpose admirably, and, in short, this is the only agent which has proved effectual in the purification. For this purpose the acid must be in the most concentrated state, and consequently the crude creasote must first be rectified, to remove water from it, before adding the strong acid, otherwise the latter will become diluted, and less active.

In the rectification of the crude creasote, the first portion which passes over contains water, and should be set aside, to be again separated. When no more water passes over, the rectified product should be collected by itself, in a dry vessel, and the distillation continued nearly to dryness. The residue should be removed from the still while hot, as it consists of resin and sulphate of soda, which solidifies on cooling. Strong sulphuric acid, in the proportion of one pound to a gallon, is now to be added to the rectified creasote, stirred well, and left till next day. The acid dissolves in the oil, and causes it to become of an orange color; but, if the oil contains water, the acid becomes diluted, and separates from the oil: hence the necessity of the above precaution in separating the water. Oxidation commences slowly in the cold, and the oil becomes charged with sulphurous acid, but heat is requisite to complete the oxidation of the impurities, although this also decomposes a portion of the creasote. The mixture is therefore to be distilled gently, nearly to dryness; and the residue of resinous matters drawn off while hot. The product is of a yellow color, which is due to its being saturated with sulphurous acid, but by exposure to the air for some time, this is mostly removed, and the creasote becomes of a pale yellow color. In this state it would probably answer for many purposes; but if it is required to be colorless, it is only necessary to wash it with an excess of solution of carbonate of soda, and again rectify it in a glass retort.

*New York, September 19th*, 1853.

---

# MEMORANDA OF SOME OF THE ARTICLES IN THE PHARMACEUTICAL DEPARTMENT OF THE NEW YORK EXHIBITION OF THE INDUSTRY OF ALL NATIONS.

BY BENJAMIN CANAVAN.

CRYSTALLIZATIONS.—Some very handsome specimens of, from Howards and Kent, England.

EMERY STONE.—Two specimens, one marked "Turkey;" the other, "Naxos." They do not differ in appearance from ordinary stone, and would not be likely to be considered of any value, if accidentally met with. From England.

BOTANICAL SPECIMENS.—A number of very well-culled samples, consisting not alone of the leaves, but also the flowers, and some of the other characteristic parts, giving a pretty good idea of the whole plant as it grows. A specimen of Sem. colchici in this collection is so remarkably plump, that, if met with in the market it would be supposed to have been wetted. From J. H, Kent, *surgeon*, England.

MAGNESIA—Calcined, and Carbonate of, and strong solution of: Subject to examination, it was said, but none appeared open for that purpose. From Jennings, Cork, Ireland.

CAFEINE AND ALOINE.—The specimen of Cafeine is passing beautiful, resembling on its surface the very finest white fur that can be *imagined.* The specimens of Aloine, compressed as they are under glass, have a good deal the appearance of arnica flowers, without their yellow corollas. From J. H. Smith Edinburgh.

MUSTARD.—A show-case containing specimens of white and black mustard seeds, in different degrees of preparation, from whole to finished. Those marked "finished" were indeed so, having entirely moulded and shrunk to nothing. From New-castle-on-Tyne . . . A specimen from Harrison, Eaton, and Co., Cincinnati, is of fine color, pungent taste, and good flavor.

CRYSTALS OF SALTPETRE.—Some mammoth specimens from Croton Laboratory.

OIL OF PEPPERMENT, HOTCHKISS'S.—Some specimens of this well-known article, which took a premium at the London Exhibition.

DOUBLE SULPHATE OF ZINC AND AMMONIA.—A dirty-looking salt, having the following inscription:

$$Zn\ O,\ S,\ O,^3 + N.\ H.^4\ O,\ SO^3 + 7HO$$

ISAIAH DILKE, *fecit.*

MEAT-BISCUIT.—A specimen now three years old, apparently in good keeping, which had been in the search for Sir John Franklin, on board the Arctic Expedition.

BLACK LEAD CRUCIBLES.—From a manufactory in New Jersey. Said to be from seven to ten times better than the imported article.

CHEMICALS U. S.—A large assortment of the manufacture of Powers and Wightman, amongst the curious of which is a large vat of crystallized alum, capable of holding several persons; for the rest, they bear a favorable comparison with any others in the Exhibition, judging from appearance, which is all that can be done in those circumstances. Their gallic acid is very much improved, being in beautiful silken crystals. A specimen of crystallized sulphur should be noted.

PHARMACEUTICAL PREPARATIONS.—A very extensive assortment from Gehe and Co., Dresden, among which are Rad. Sarsa Lissabon, resembling our Vera Cruz more than any other variety. Rad. Sumbul.: this is in circular pieces, flat, about an inch thick, and three to six in diameter, very light-colored and peeled. Rad. Salep.; Rad. Rhei Austri., similar to English rhubarb. Rad. Irid. Flor., smoothed into suitable pieces for the use of children when teething. Sem. Fœnicul. Cretic., much larger than the usual variety. Sem. Cydoniæ Russic et Germ., the former of which are large, dark, and appear to be formed by the agglutination of several seeds together; the latter resemble our own. Semen Lycopodii: this appears to be ordinary Lycopodium, and is, therefore, a *pollen*, not a semen. Bezetta Rubra; this is a bundle of red, thin, gauze-like cloth, which I do not recognize: for the rest, it is remarkable for great elaboration and Gothic style. Alkaloids, &c., from E. Merck, Darmstadt. From O. Herman, Acid Phosphoric Glacial; most beautifully transparent. Alum of iron, and a deep garnet-colored salt, intituled, "Kali Zooticum Rubrum Gmelim. Specimens of sulphur cast into heads, &c.

PHARMACEUTICAL PREPARATIONS FROM FRANCE—Among which are Extr. Glycyrrhizæ, prepared in vacuo, of a light yellow color, similar to that of the root, and a specimen of very fine Pulv. Glycyrrhiza. There are also castor-oil beans, honey, pretty white, very dark yellow, and pretty fair white wax, with three barks.

Ecorce de Bois de Piment,
" " " Rose,
" " " Dentelle,

whether medicinal or not, does not appear, from Hayti.

Matanzas sends sulphate of quinine, of very fair appearance, and a few other chemicals; and from British Guiana we have an unique specimen of isinglass, in large thick pieces. Annatto seeds, somewhat like seed-lac in appearance, and distinguished by an eye in one end, black in the centre, surrounded by a yellowish areola. Cassava, Laurel-oil, and India-rubber milk, or the article in the fresh and fluid state. A variety of Barks, among which I observe Simarouba and Cusparia, and a sample sulphate of Bebeerin, made from the *Nectandria Rhodiœi;* and lastly, though not the least, Castor-oil, *without taste or smell*, from Ponce, Porto Rico. There is a quibble in this: good castor-oil has always been free from taste or smell, but, nevertheless, very nauseous from its oiliness, a quality which is discoverable by taste and one of which it is physically impossible to deprive it. Many suppose that it is this disagreeable quality from which it is freed, but are already, or soon will be, undeceived. This, reflection tells me, as I have never had the curiosity to try the article.

---

## CHEMICAL AND PHARMACOLOGICAL EXAMINATION OF KINO.

The author first satisfied himself by a comparison of the most trustworthy statements, that the officinal kino known among druggists as the East Indian, should more correctly be called African, because it is for the most part the air-dried juice which exudes from incisions made in the stems of several species of Pterocarpus: P. erinaceus, and P. senegalensis growing in the forests of Senegambia, and P. indicus and P. marsupium, growing upon the coast of Malabar, and other parts of the East Indies.

These so-called oriental varieties of kino all present the following physical characters: color, garnet-red; fracture, conchoidal. When chewed, they color the saliva red by transmitted, and violet by reflected light. The taste is purely astringent. The fragments of kino treated with distilled water, dissolve partially, communicating a yellowish-red color to the water, which, when allowed to stand, and even when excluded from the air, deposits a fine orange-colored powder, forming a deposit of sometimes three layers. This is again almost entirely dissolved by hot water or alcohol. But neither boiling water or alcohol dissolve kino completely, a more or less swollen skeleton of each individual fragment always remaining. The addition of distilled water to the tincture causes a faint cloudiness, which disappears again spontaneously. Ether produces a precipitate in both aqueous and alcoholic extracts, but both become clear on standing. When the tincture containing ether is evaporated, it becomes turbid at the boiling point, from the separation of cinnamon-colored flocks, which subsequently re-dissolve with violent agitation of the liquid. Ether does not take up anything, even from finely-powdered kino.

Tincture of kino reddens litmus somewhat more distinctly than the aqueous infusion. The former is precipitated by alkalies; the latter only by carbonate of ammonia; neither give any precipitate with lime-water or tartrate of potash and antimony. Protochloride of iron gives with the aqueous infusion a deep green color, and green flocks separate after some time. Perchloride of iron gives a greyish or yellowish-green bulky precipitate; lead salts give various precipitates, according as the infusion is prepared with hot water or cold, when air has access or the contrary.

African kino burnt in a porcelain crucible leaves about two per cent. of ash, consisting of phosphate of soda, carbonate of lime, phosphate of magnesia, traces of sulphate of lime, and silicate of iron. When submitted to dry distillation, it gives off an odor resembling vanilla, acid water then passes over (perhaps formic acid) and some empyreumatic substances not examined; pyrogallic acid could not be detected. Heated upon platinum foil it swells up, evolving first agreeable and then acid vapors.

As the author could not succeed in effecting a simple separation of the astringent principle of kino, the behavior of various reagents with aqueous and alcoholic infusions was more carefully examined. The separation of the tannic acid by means of a solution of gelatine, recommended by Gerding, is imperfect; but if, on the other hand, a prepared animal skin is employed, only a little gallic acid is left in the liquid, inasmuch as the red coloring matter enters into combination, together with the tannic acid, forming a red leather. The contact of oxygen with Gerding's coccotannic acid gave a different result; a stream of oxygen passed through the aqueous infusion of kino does not cause any perceptible alteration of the tannin, even after long warming, the coloring matter alone appearing to be oxidized. The opinion that the red coloring matter is a product of the alteration of the tannic acid, is rendered improbable by the action of sulphurous acid, which gives to the aqueous infusion a yellow color, although the red substance is not converted into anything resembling tannic acid, but is partially precipitated in the form of orange-colored flocks, which re-dissolve in alkalies with a red color; the tannic acid gave the same reactions as before, and in the evaporated liquid crystals of the sulphate of the alkali used were formed. Moist chlorine behaved in a similar manner, with the exception that the yellow precipitate floated in a colorless liquid, and the tannic acid itself appeared to be altered.

The products obtained by the action of caustic potash upon raw kino, and those obtained by treating the powdered gum with hydrochloric acid for the purpose of separating the earthy bases, were submitted to analyses, and found to correspond closely with the substance called kino red by Gerding.

Strong nitric acid decomposes all the constituents of kino, especially when heat is applied; nitric oxide and hydrocyanic acid are evolved, and the liquid contains nitropikric acid and oxalic acid.

Hennig attempted to separate the tannic acid of kino by taking advantage of the fact that ordinary tannic acid is dissolved by acetic acid, and remains in solution even on the addition of water, while the red substance of kino is at first completely precipitated, on diluting the solution in acetic acid with water. Raw kino in fine powder was digested for some days with concentrated acetic acid, the liquid evaporated, and the residue digested with very cold water, until it began to acquire color. The product obtained in this way was, however, too small.

The fractional precipitation of the solution of kino by means of metallic salts, especially acetate of lead, yielded larger quantities of tolerably pure tannic acid. This salt first combines, apparently in substance, with the "kino red;" subsequent precipitates always contain larger percentages of oxide of lead and larger quantities of tannic acid, but the acetic acid set free somewhat disturbs the result. For this reason the aqueous infusion of kino was treated with successive portions of hydrated oxide of lead, but still the tannic acid obtained, though large in quantity, was impure. Finally, Hennig found that the most advantageous process was to precipitate the concentrated alcoholic decoction of kino with subacetate of lead, added drop by drop, until only a few drops of pure water filtered out of the brownish-red jelly which was formed; the mass was then digested in very cold distilled water, until it began to communicate a color to it, when it was poured off, and filtered rapidly. This liquid contained the greater part of the tannic acid. This process may be supposed to consist either in a combination of the acetate of lead with the red coloring matter of the kino only, and that the tannic acid is mechanically retained until the alcoholic jelly is saturated with water, or that both substances form lead salts, and that the contact with water causes a decomposition, in consequence of which tannic acid is set free. It is advisable to use a slight excess of subacetate of lead, rather than not, for the quantity of tannate of lead dissolved in that case is insignificant compared with the freedom of the tannic acid from coloring matter.

After the addition of a sufficient quantity of moist hydrated oxide of lead, the slightly reddish-colored tannate of lead was separated and introduced into a retort, when it was dried in a stream of hydrogen gas. Hennig obtained from two analyses the following results, corresponding with Berzelius's formula for tannic acid of oak:

| | | | |
|---|---|---|---|
| C | 14 | 53.16 | 52.7 |
| H | 10 | 3.71 | 3.9 |
| O | 8 | 43.13 | 43.5 |

The analysis of the lead salt gave:

| | | | | |
|---|---|---|---|---|
| C | 18 | 34.02 | 33.00 | 34.55 |
| H | 18 | 5.67 | 5.93 | 5.92 |
| O | 10 | 25.19 | 26.67 | 25.23 |
| PbO | 1 | 35.12 | 34.40 | 34.30 |

The elements are here nearly in the same proportions as in Rochleder's catechuic acid, and the difference may be owing to an admixture of acetic acid.

Hennig is of opinion that the red coloring matter so intimately combined with the tannic acid, may be obtained best by treating the aqueous infusion from which the above-mentioned yellow deposit has separated, with finely-powdered hydrated oxide of lead, until the liquid is nearly decolorized. The substance obtained from the lead compound in the ordinary manner, gave on analysis:

| | | | |
|---|---|---|---|
| C | 11 | 43.65 | 43.71 |
| H | 5 | 3.31 | 3.31 |
| O | 10 | 53.04 | 52.98 |

Basic acetate of lead is better suited to the separation of this red coloring matter than neutral acetate; however, the lead compound prepared with the former is not one with an excess of base, but shows that the above empirical formula must be multiplied by 5:

| | | |
|---|---|---|
| C | 55 | 38.08 |
| H | 25 | 2.88 |
| O | 50 | 46.16 |
| PbO | 1 | 12.88 |

Hennig calls this substance kinoic acid.

The third substance contained in African kino is very difficult to obtain colorless, and free from the above acid. Hennig endeavored to prepare it by digesting the already-mentioned spontaneous deposit from the aqueous infusion with successive quantities of water, until it was no longer colored upon standing, and gave no reaction with perchloride of iron, then extracting it with strong alcohol, saturating the tincture with neutral acetate of lead, and drying the precipitate, collected on a filter under the air-pump. Analysis gave 25.29 per cent. oxide of lead and

| | | | |
|---|---|---|---|
| C | 29 | 41.74 | 41.74 |
| H | 22 | 4.99 | 4.73 |
| O | 25 | 53.27 | 53.53 |

corresponding closely with the formula of Jahn's pectic acid. This substance appears to be more prone to alteration by external influences than the former, and passes finally into ulmic acid, which partly constitutes the residue left on the extraction of kino by water or alcohol.

The quantitative relations of the several constituents of kino may be represented in the following order:

Kinoic acid
Tannic acid and a trace of gallic acid
Pectin
Ulmic acid
Inorganic salts with a trace of earthy bases.

Bischoff and Mohr have already put forth the opinion that the astringent substance in kino is identical with ordinary tannic acid, at least in reference to the characteristic precipitation with persalts of iron, and the possibility of obtaining this reaction with various kinds of kino, tormentilla, and other plants, induced Hennig not only to give up the opinion that coccotannic acid is a definite substance, but likewise to regard the different kinds of tannic acid, which precipitate persalts of iron green or grey, and are admitted by chemists to be in almost every case distinct substances, as intimate mixtures of tannic acid, which give a blue precipitate with persalts of iron, and some modifying substance, such as a yellow or red coloring matter. He found, however, that the tannic acid from kino differed from that of the oak in two particulars, viz., the solubility in ether and the reaction with potasso-tartrate of antimony; but he considers that the minute and probably inappreciable quantity of kinoic acid mixed with the tannic acid might be sufficient to account for these discrepancies.

The red substance which Hennig calls kinoic acid corresponds with the coloring matters associated with tannic acid in elm-bark, catechu, cinchona-bark, coffee, &c., and cannot, in kino at least, be regarded as a product of the oxidation of tannic acid, but is probably the derivative of a colorless substance, for, according to Pereira, the fresh juice of the kino-tree has but a faint reddish tint.

This red substance is more readily soluble in alcohol than in cold water, and to it the alcoholic solution owes not only its intense red color but likewise its acid reaction, It gives a yellowish-brown precipitate with perchloride of iron, and a brownish-red one with acetate of lead. It partly separates from the hot aqueous solution on cooling. From these characters many who have previously examined this substance inferred that it was a resin, an opinion which Mohr opposes. A. W. Buchner states that he has detected catechin in kino, and ascribes to it the production of a green precipitate with persalts of iron. Hennig, however, expresses his conviction that catechin is not present in true kino, and is only a constituent of those drugs which are varieties of catechu, although frequently confounded with kino, viz., Uncaria or Nauclea Gambir, the product of Erythina monosperma.

The behavior of this red coloring matter towards the tannic acid is remarkable, for it not only adheres to it with obstinacy, perhaps holding it, together with the pectin, for some time in solution, but likewise gives reactions with acids, bases, and salts, in a manner resembling the conjugate acids. Hennig considers that the red coloring matter of kino originally existed in a colorless state, combined with the tannic acid, and that during its subsequent alteration by the air, in consequence of the absorption of oxygen, the state of combination is not destroyed, but continues, perhaps, even until the formation of ulmin has taken place.

The presence of pectin in kino has been conjectured by Pereira. He considers "that kino consists principally of a peculiar substance (eucalyptin) analogous somewhat to pectin and tannic acid," and he infers this especially from its behavior with alkalies and the precipitate formed with lime-water. Still this precipitate could not be prepared with African kino, which is not the produce of Eucalyptus resinifera. The vegetable gelatine is the cause of the kino swelling in water and alcohol, and gives rise to the formation of the substance deposited from solutions of kino, even when air is excluded, and gradually becoming more insoluble on further treatment with indifferent menstrua. It is this circumstance which has led to the opinion that kino is a gum, although no one has ever obtained from it a substance soluble in water, and precipitible in alcohol. But the pectin, in its combinations with earthy bases, or with tannic acid, must behave in a very variable manner with reagents, unless, indeed, we must ascribe to the difficultly-removable kinoic acid (Vauquelin obtained only a *red* gum) at least such an influence upon the pectin, that it separates so quickly from cold water, but is then dissolved by alcohol as well as by hot water.—*Archiv. der Pharmacie*, February, 1853.

# ON THE MANUFACTURE OF AMMONIA AND AMMONIACAL SALTS.

Continued from p. 264.

*Ammonia from the Ammoniacal Waters of Coal Gas-works.*—The chief source whence ammonia is now obtained, is the ammoniacal waters produced by the distillation of coal, as performed at gas-works. A great number of processes have been devised for the purpose of obtaining ammonia and ammoniacal salts from these waters in the most convenient and economical way, the principal of which we now proceed to notice. As most of these processes have for their object the obtaining of more than one of these salts, we have found it preferable to describe them in the order of priority of invention rather than under the head of each particular salt. Mr. Ledsom took out a patent, March 2, 1827, for improvements in the manufacture of muriate of ammonia. In this process a quantity of the ammoniacal liquor obtained from the distillation of coal is converted into muriate of ammonia by saturating it with muriatic acid. When this has been done, the liquor is to be evaporated and the salt reduced to a crystalline state. The crystals are then to be dissolved in water, and lime added to the liquor in the proportion of fifty pounds of lime to 100 pounds of muriate of ammonia. The gas passed off from the retort in the process of distillation, having been conducted through water for the purpose of cooling it and separating the tar, is now to be passed through this liquor, when the sulphuretted hydrogen which it contains, uniting with the ammonia, for which it has a great affinity, becomes soluble in the water, and remains principally in the purifier. But if any portion of the sulphuretted hydrogen happens to pass over, it is arrested by another vessel of water containing the mixture above described. When the muriate of ammonia in the liquor has become spent, the liquor is to be drawn off from the purifier, and a fresh supply introduced, and the spent liquors may be restored by another quantity of muriatic acid. Messrs. Midgley and Kyan patented, November 4, 1837, the following process for obtaining ammoniacal salts, and at the same time preventing the usual nuisance arising from the vapors evolved from manufactories when the ammonia is extracted from ammoniacal liquor, according to the modes of manufacture previously in use. For this purpose, the patentees submit the ammoniacal liquor to the action of lime, in the following manner:—To 500 gallons of the liquor they add 250 lbs. of quick lime, slaked with a sufficient quantity of water. This is poured on to a grating which is employed for the purpose of preventing large pieces from passing through, and is kept well agitated. It is then placed in a still, in which it is heated to from 170° to 200° Fahr. The ammonia thus becomes evolved, and is then passed into acid in which salts are formed, which are obtained in solution. When the ammonia is worked off, the residuum is cleared out, and a fresh charge put in. Mr. William Watson took out a patent, November 8, 1838, for improvements in the manufacture of liquid ammonia, applicable to the purposes of dyeing, scouring, and other manufacturing processes. "In this process," states the patentee, "which I have invented, I manufacture the liquid ammonia from gas-water, and I dispense entirely with the use of sulphuric or muriatic acid, and of course with the evaporation and crystallization. I make it in the following manner:—The gas-liquor, or gas-water, I put into a retort or any other suitable vessel, along with fresh-slaked lime, the quantity of which is to be determined by the quality of the water; by the application of heat, a tolerably pure liquid ammonia is disengaged, which, getting passed into water, forms a solution of ammonia. When this distillation has been carried so far that a considerable portion of the steam or the vapor of water proceeds from the retort along with the ammonia, the ammoniacal solution already formed, is to be removed—this I call the first portion; and what is collected afterward by a continuation of the process, I call the second portion; and, being very impure, it is put back into the retort.

with the mixed charge of gas-water. The first portion must be again submitted to distillation, with or without a small quantity of lime, and the same precaution must be observed as before: that is, so long as the principal portion of what proceeds from the retort or boilers is ammoniacal gas, it must be passed into water; and when this ceases to be the case, as, by continuing the heat, the water, as well as the ammonia will evaporate, the solution of ammonia already formed must be removed. This may be called the first portion of the second distillation. The process may be continued then until all or nearly all of the ammonia is distilled; this second portion is to be returned, as before, to the retort. The first portion of this second distillation is a solution of ammonia sufficiently pure for common purposes; but it may be still further purified by distilling it a third time in the same manner as before, preserving that portion only which is made by the absorption of the ammoniacal gas in water, and returning to the retort the latter products of the process, which consist of ammonia and water mixed with impurities." Mr. Croll's process (patented July 29, 1840) for obtaining the salts of ammonia is of two kinds: in one of these dilute sulphuric or muriatic acid is employed to abstract the ammonia from the gas, and in the other the chloride and sulphate of manganese and muriate of iron are employed for the same purpose. In the latter case a vessel used in the manufacture of gas for holding wet lime for the purposes of gas purifying, is filled with a solution, composed of 1 cwt. of chloride of manganese to forty gallons of water, and the gas is forced through this solution in the usual way by the pressure of the retorts, by which means the ammonia is absorbed. As soon as this solution is saturated with ammonia, it is drawn off, and the vessel fresh charged. Sulphate of manganese and muriate of iron may also be employed in the same way to absorb the ammonia produced in the manufacture of coal-gas.

In the case of using sulphuric acid, a vessel more commonly employed for washing gas is filled with a solution composed of 100 gallons of water to two pounds and a half of sulphuric acid, spec. grav. 1.845, and the gas is passed through it as usual, until it has attained the spec. grav. of 1.70, and is saturated with ammonia. It is then drawn off, and the vessel charged anew.

When muriatic acid is used, it is applied in the same manner as regards proportion, the acid being of spec. grav. 1.65 before it is mixed with the water: the solution of muriate of ammonia is to be drawn off when it has acquired a density of 1.176. In order to obtain the ammoniacal salts (when a salt has been used for purification), the insoluble part of the mixture is allowed to settle, and the clear liquor, which contains muriate of ammonia and sulphate of soda is drawn off. These must be separated from each other, either by crystallizing salts of ammonia from that of soda, or by evaporating both to dryness, and subliming the ammoniacal solution. The salts formed by the use of the chloride of manganese and salts of zinc may be obtained by the same means.

Mr. Croll thus describes the peculiar mode of manufacturing or reproducing the salts by the double decomposition of salt, and the residuum and precipitates of chloride of manganese:— To twelve ounces of the dry precipitate, add one pound of common salt, mix them intimately together, and submit them, in a suitable furnace, to a heat scarcely perceptible in the dark, for two or three hours; then to 140 pounds of this mixture add forty gallons of water. It is then fit to be used for purifying gas from ammonia, and the residuum which the gas leaves in passing through it is to be heated in like manner. The insoluble part of the solution before mentioned may be brought to its original state by dissolving it in the acid forming one of its constituents, or dissolving it in sulphuric or muriatic acid, by which means a sulphate or muriate of soda is obtained. In Mr. Waterton's patent, dated August 27, 1840, for the manufacture of ammonia, two methods of effecting the proposed object are there described. The first consists in making a saturated solution of common salt in water, and mixing it with a quantity of finely pulverized carbonate of ammonia, about equal in weight to the salt contained in the solution. The mixture is agitated in a close vessel for six or eight hours, and as much carbonic acid gas is passed therein as it will absorb (but the introduction of this gas is not absolutely necessary, although the patentee prefers it), the liquid is then separated from the solid matter by filtration and pressure. The solid matter is chiefly bicarbonate of soda, and the liquid holds in solution muriate and carbonate of ammonia, and common salt, and sometimes a small portion of the bicarbonate of soda.

The liquid is now placed in a distilling vessel, and the carbonate of ammonia being distilled over into a suitable receiver, a solution of muriate of ammonia and common salt remains in the still. This solution is evaporated to such a consistency as will cause the separation of the common salt by crystallization, and the salt thus crystallized is separated from the liquid by any convenient method. The liquid is then evaporated until it attains the proper specific gravity for crystallizing, and it is transferred into suitable vessels for that purpose. The crystals produced by these means are nearly pure muriate of ammonia, and when pressed and dried, may be brought into the market without further purification, or they may be sublimed into sal ammoniac.

The other mode of manufacturing sal ammoniac consists in taking a quantity of liquid containing ammonia, either in the caustic state, or combined with carbonic, hydrosulphuric, and hydrocyanic acids (as in the case of the ammoniacal liquor of the gas-works), and rectifying it by distillation until the distilled portion contains from twenty to twenty-five per cent. of carbonate of ammonia. If the liquid contain any other acids than those above mentioned, a sufficient quantity of lime is used in the distillation to decompose the ammoniacal salt. The distilled liquid being now mixed with as large a quantity of powdered common salt as it will dissolve, is agitated for several hours, and as much carbonic acid gas is passed into it as it will absorb. The remainder of the operation is the same as before described in the first method of manufacturing muriate of ammonia.

In 1841, Mr. Laming took out a patent for manufacturing carbonate of ammonia, by mixing together its separate acid and alkaline constituents instead of by the decomposition of an ammoniacal salt. One of the processes used is to cause ammonia and carbonic acid gas obtained separately from any convenient sources, to traverse a succession of leaden chambers, maintained at as cool a temperature as was conveniently practicable, and so contrived as to favor the admixture of the dissimilar gases. In this process it is not essential that the two gases be present in their combining proportions; it is preferable that the carbonic acid be in greater abundance than will combine with the ammonia which is present. Sometimes a stratum of water, or of water impregnated with ammonia, is placed in one or more of the leaden chambers, and carbonic acid and ammonia in the form of gas are introduced; in which case, it is stated, a larger proportion of carbonic acid gas is found in the resulting salt or saline solution than when only the hygrometic moisture of the aëriform fluids is present. In Mr. Astley's process of manufacturing muriate of ammonia, the bittern or muriate of magnesia, obtained from the sea-salt works, was employed as the source of muriatic acid, and the parings of skins, horns, and other animal matters, furnished the ammonia. The animal matters were saturated with the bittern in stone-rooms heated by brick flues, and being afterwards subjected to a red heat in a close kiln, muriate of ammonia was obtained.

A valuable improvement in the mode of obtaining ammonia from ammoniacal solutions was patented in the name of Mr. W. E. Newton, patent-agent, November 9, 1841. The real patentee, we believe, was Mr. Laming, of Clichy Chemical Works, near Paris. This improvement consisted in the application of the well-known still invented by Mr. Coffey for the distillation of spirit, to the production of ammonia, either pure or more or less impure, according to the purpose for which it is required, from any liquid from which by the agency of steam it may be eliminated, either alone or in conjunction with vapor, carbonic acid, or other volatile matters, the presence of which do not prevent the application of ammonia to one or more useful purposes.

This apparatus, or ammonia-still, is an upright vessel, divided by horizontal diaphragms or partitions into a number of chambers. It is proposed to construct the vessel of wood, lined with tin, and the diaphragms of sheet iron. Each diaphragm is perforated with many small holes, so regulated both with regard to number and size, as to afford, under some pressure, passage for the elastic vapors which ascend during the use of the apparatus, to make their exit by a pipe opening from the upper chamber. Fitted to each diaphragm are several small valves, so weighted as to rise whenever elastic vapors accumulate under them in such quantity as to exert more than a certain amount of pressure on the diaphragm. A pipe also is attached to each diaphragm, passing from about an inch above its upper surface to near a cup or small reservoir, fixed to the upper surface of the diaphragms next underneath. This pipe is sufficiently large to transmit freely downwards the whole of the liquor which enters for distillation at the upper part of the upright vessel, and the cup or resrvoir, into which the pipe dips, forms, when full of liquid, a trap, by which the upward passage of elastic vapors, by the pipe, is prevented. The vessel may rest on a close cistern, contrived to receive the descending liquid, as it leaves the lowest chamber, and from this cistern it may be run off by a valve or cock, whenever expedient. The cistern, or in its absence the lowest chamber, contains the orifice of a pipe which supplies steam for working the apparatus. The exact number of chambers into which the upright vessel is divided is not of essential importance; but the quantity of liquid and the surface of each diaphragm being given the distillation within certain limits will be more complete, the greater the number of chambers used in the process. The liquid undergoing distillation in this apparatus necessarily covers the upper surface of each diaphragm to the depth of about an inch, being prevented from passing downward through the small perforations, bp the upward pressure of the rising steam and other elastic vapors; and, on the other hand, the steam being prevented by the traps from passing upwards, by the pipes is forced to ascend by the perforations in the diphragms; so that the liquor lying on them becomes heated, and, in consequence, gives off its volatile matters. When the ammoniacal liquid accumulates on one of the diaphragms, to the depth of an inch, it flows over one of the short pipes into the trap below, whence it overflows into the next diaphragm, and so on.

The management of the apparatus varies in some measure with the form in which it is desirable to obtain the ammonia. When the ammonia is required to leave the upper chamber, in the form of gas, either pure or impure, it is necessary that the steam which ascends, and the current of ammoniacal liquor which descends be in such relative proportions that the latter remain at or near the atmospheric temperature during its passage through some of the upper chambers, becoming progressively hotter as it descends, until it reaches the boiling temperature; in which state it passes through the lower chambers, either to make its escape, or to enter a cistern provided to receive it, and in which it may for some time be maintained at a boiling heat. On the contrary, if the ammonia, either pure or impure, be required to leave the upper chamber, in combination with the vapor of water, the supply of steam entering below must bear such proportion to that of the ammoniacal liquid supplied above, that the latter may be at a boiling temperature in the upper part of the apparatus.

Solutions of ammoniacal salts, which have had their respective acids abstracted by any of the usual means, afford, by being thus treated, ammoniacal gas, either alone or in combination with water of considerable purity; but the apparatus is equally serviceable in obtaining similar results, more or less impure, from the ammoniacal waters obtained by the distillation of coals, or of bones or other animal matters, as well as from stale urine. Acids and certain other matters contained in these impure liquids, may first be partly removed by lime and other well-known means; and some of them will be further removed during the passage of the ammonia through the apparatus, care being taken to use them so dilute that the vapor which escapes with them shall be sufficient in quantity to prevent the solidification of the ammonia by the carbonic acid which rises with it, and the consequent obstruction of the passages. Instead of being furnished with perforations, valves, and pipes, the diaphragms may have plain surfaces, and each be bent upwards at one of its sides, so as not entirely to separate the contiguous chambers. The diaphragms should be bent upwards at opposite sides alternately, thereby permitting the descending fluid to fall as a cascade from the right-hand side of one diaphragm on to the next below; and then from the left-hand side of that one to the next in succession, and so on until the whole of the diaphragms are occupied with liquid. In this case the liquid will be heated by the contact of the ascending steam sweeping over its extensive surface; and also by the steam acting on the under sides of the diaphragms on which the liquid rests.

Mr. Philippi's process for obtaining ammoniacal salts, as patented by him, July 21, 1842, is that of decomposing the ammoniacal waters of the gas-works by means of sulphate or chloride of manganese, the gas being passed through the solutions contained in suitable cisterns or apparatus. Mr. Philippi also describes an arrangement or apparatus suitable for obtaining ammonia and ammoniacal salts from gas-liquor. For this purpose gas-liquor is acted upon by lime in a common distilling apparatus, heated by steam or otherwise, by means of a worm or injection; the ammonia set at liberty by the heat escapes into a second boiler similar to the first one through a connecting-pipe—the condensing of the ammoniacal vapors heats the second boiler, in which there are lime and ammoniacal waters. A third boiler is employed with the same effect, after which there is a leaden worm, in which the vapors circulate. This worm is surrounded by cold ammoniacal water, and descends into a leaden vessel, in which is deposited a solution of alkali, which at first is very strong, but becomes weaker as the distillation goes on. The alkali is withdrawn before it descends below 220°, but as a part of the ammonia is in a gaseous state, there are two other vessels prepared after the first one, the whole forming a Woulfe's apparatus. The solution of lime of the second vessel, which is not saturated after one distillation, is put into the second boiler, that the lime and ammonia which are dissolved in the liquid may be used. If muriate, sulphate, or carbonate of ammonia be required, the vapors may be condensed in suitable vessels containing muriatic, sulphuric, or carbonic acids.

For the purpose of obtaining ammonia sufficiently pure for many purposes in the arts from gas-water, Mr. Laming patented, July 13, 1843, the substitution of a solution of muriate of lime for the mineral acids usually employed, This process is as follows: he first mixes with gas-water a sufficient quantity of muriate of lime in solution to convert the carbonate of ammonia which is present into muriate of ammonia, and, after having separated the carbonate of lime which forms, the remaining solution is exposed for an hour to a boiling temperature. This solution, after having been cooled, is first agitated with enough hydrated oxide of iron to combine with all its sulphuretted hydrogen; secondly, with lime enough to saturate the muriatic acid which is present; and, finally, it is distilled. The ammonia will be found in the water that comes over, in a tolerably pure state.

In Watson's patent of January 16, 1844, the following description of apparatus for manufacturing sulphate of ammonia is given. An iron boiler capable of holding a charge of about 260 gallons of ammoniacal gas-liquor is provided, furnished with a bent pipe or tube, connecting the boiler with a leaden vessel open at the top. Into the boiler a quantity of slaked lime may be placed with the ammoniacal liquor, which has the effect of hastening the operation, and producing a salt of a purer quality. The leaden vessel is partly filled with sulphuric acid (if sulphate of ammonia be required) in the proportion of about one pound weight of sulphuric acid, sp. g. 1.700 to every gallon of water. This acid must be diluted with three to four times its weight of water. When heat is applied to the boiler the ammonia is driven off, and on coming into contact with the acid in the leaden vessel combines with it with the formation of solution of sulphate of ammonia, which is afterwards drawn off, and crystallized. By the use of muriatic acid on muriate of lime, a solution of muriate of ammmonia may be obtained.

Johnson's process (patented 1845) for obtaining sulphate of ammonia, is to put the ammoniacal liquor of the gas-works into a boiler similar to a steam-engine boiler, having a pipe passing from the top into a vessel containing a solution of alkali, lime, or of sulphate of iron or manganese, into which the pipe dips; another pipe passes from the top of this vessel to the bottom of a second, containing dilute sulphuric acid. The liquor being put into the boiler, heat is applied, and the hydrosulphate of ammonia being the most volatile of the salts contained in the liquor, passes over; first its hydrosulphuric acid is absorbed by the contents of the first vessel, and the ammonia by the acid contained in the second vessel with the formation of sulphate of ammonia. After the hydrosulphate of ammonia has all passed over, the liquid remaining in the boiler may be drawn off and neutralized in the usual way with sulphuric acid, and thus muriate of ammonia may be obtained.

Mr. Johnson patented, August 11, 1845, a method of obtaining ammoniacal salts, by passing coal-gas on its way from the retorts to the gasometer, through vessels containing certain metallic salts, such as sulphate of iron as the cheapest, previously pounded very fine, and moistened with just enough water to bring the pulverized iron to a pasty consistency. Sulphate of ammonia is thus obtained.

Mr. Hills patented, August 11, 1846, the following process relative to the manufacture of ammoniacal salts. To obtain muriate of ammonia he employs muriate of magnesia, which he either mixes in the state of powder with the coal in the manufacture of gas, or he puts it in a small iron vessel placed within the same retort, or when several retorts are used at the same time, one retort may be used to contain the muriate of magnesia alone; in either case, the muriatic acid liberated from the decomposition of the muriate of magnesia by means of heat combines with the ammonia to form muriate of ammonia, which is collected in the ammoniacal liquor.

In the same patent Mr. Hills describes his improved apparatus for obtaining ammonia from ammoniacal liquors. This apparatus is similar in construction to a condenser which is in common use for the distillation of alcohol, and which in form is a four-sided vessel, furnished with shallow pans fixed to the alternate sides. The ammoniacal liquor flows through pipes placed under the upper shelves or pans, thus keeping them cool, whilst itself receives an accession of heat, and then flows into the top pan of the lower series. When this top pan is full, the liquor flows over into the next of the series, and so on to the bottom. The pans in the lower series are kept hot by pipes which pass under them in a zig-zag form, through which pipes hot water, steam, or hot air circulates. The liquor in passing through this apparatus, has its ammonia sublimed into the upper part, the water running out by a pipe at the bottom.

*Pharmaceutical Journal, August.*

To be continued.

---

## NOTE ON CUCUMBER OINTMENT.

BY WILLIAM PROCTER, JR.

Several years ago (April, 1847) I published in this Journal a note on the preparation of Cucumber Ointment, since when it has gradually come more into use as an emollient application to irritated parts of the skin. It may not be improper to again call attention to the preparation and the mode of preparing it:

Take of Green Cucumbers (suitable for table use) 7 pounds *av.*
" Lard (the purest and whitest) - - 24 ounces "
" Veal suet (selected) - - - - 15 ounces "

The unpared cucumbers, after being washed, are reduced to a pulp by grating, and the juice expressed and strained. The suet is cut in small pieces, and heated over a salt water bath until the fat is fused out from the membranes; the lard is then added, and when liquefied is strained through muslin into a wide-mouthed earthen vessel capable of holding a gallon, and stirred until it commences to thicken, when one-third of the cucumber juice is added, and beaten with the ointment by means of a wooden spatula until its odor has been almost wholly extracted. The part that separates by standing is decanted, and the other two-thirds consecutively incorporated and decanted in the same manner. The jar is then closely covered and placed in a water-bath until the fatty matter entirely separates from the exhausted juice. The green albuminous coagulum which floats on the surface is then skimmed off, and the jar put aside in a cool place that the ointment may solidify. The crude ointment is then separated from the watery liquid on which it floats, melted, and strained; a part into a jar, and closely sealed for keeping, the remainder into a mortar, and triturated with a little rose-water until it is very white and creamy, for present use. It is usual to keep this ointment in glass jars covered with rose-water, to prevent access of the air.—*American Journal of Pharmacy.*

---

## FLUID EXTRACT OF HYOSCYAMUS.

The following formula was communicated by Mr. Charles Augustus Smith, of Cincinnati, who states that the preparation it affords has been much used and liked in that city. When made from carefully dried and good hyoscyamus, it must be a fair representative of the plant.

Take of Hyoscyamus leaves (garbled) eight ounces (Troy.)
" Diluted alcohol - - - a sufficient quantity.
" Sugar - - - - eight ounces (Troy.)

Reduce the hyoscyamus to a uniform coarse powder; pour over it a pint of diluted alcohol; allow it to macerate for twenty-four hours; put it into a suitable percolator, and, when carefully packed, pour gradually on it diluted alcohol, until three pints of tincture has passed. The flow should be very slow, that thorough exhaustion of the leaves shall take place. The tincture is then evaporated to ten fluid ounces—the sugar dissolved in it while hot, and when cold, two fluid ounces of alcohol (835 sp. gr., or as much as is sufficient to make the whole measure a pint) is added, and the fluid extract passed through a fine muslin strainer.

This preparation affords an admirable means of prescribing henbane in fluid preparations. The alcohol of the tincture is avoided, and the trouble of incorporating the solid extract superseded. It is of the same proportional strength as the fluid extract of valerian, and the dose varies from 15 drops to half a teaspoonful, the latter dose being equivalent to two or three grains of extract.

When the apothecary has in possession solid extract of hyoscyamus of *ascertained* good quality, a fluid extract of similar strength may be obtained by triturating half an ounce of the extract with ten fluid ounces of water till dissolved;—eight oz. of sugar dissolved in it, and finally sufficient alcohol to make it measure a pint, and strain. Practically, henbane yields but five per cent. of extract; the above recipe assumes it to be 6¼ per cent., a difference altogether proper in view of the possible injury to the juices in preparing the extract originally.—*American Journal of Pharmacy*, September, 1853.

## CHEAP METHOD OF PREPARING CHROME RED.

BY PROFESSOR RUNGE.

This process consists in the decomposition of chloride of lead by bichromate of potash: 448 lbs. of litharge, 60 lbs. of chloride of sodium, and 500 lbs. of water are intimately mixed. As soon as the mass becomes white and swells up considerably, more water is added to prevent its becoming too hard. After about four days the mass consists of a compound of chloride and hydrated oxide of lead. Without separating the mother-liquor which contains undecomposed chloride of sodium and soda, 150 lbs. of powdered bichromate of potash is added, the whole well stirred together, and finally washed.—*Polytechn. Notizblatt.* No. 1.

---

# EDITORIAL.

## OUR INDUSTRIAL EXHIBITION.

The chemists and pharmaceutists of our own country have not contributed so liberally as might have been desired to the Exhibition of Reservoir Square. We miss the ample collection of raw material, of crude drugs, which formed a marked feature in the London Exhibition. There is no attempt even at a collection of the medical plants of our own country. From the size of the building and the mode of arrangement necessarily, perhaps, adopted, it is difficult to find the various articles; and the catalogue, made up in haste, and before many of the articles had been received, is no reliable guide. Still there is much to interest the pharmaceutists; and the beauty of the products exhibited by some of our own manufacturing chemists makes us regret that the number sent is so limited. Place has been already given in another part of the present number to some notes made by Mr. Canavan, after a cursory visit, and without making any pretensions to a complete list, we will here add somewhat to the survey. On another occasion, and particularly on the publication of the Annotated Catalogue we will recur to the subject.

A marked feature in the Exhibition is the collection of Gehe and Co., of Dresden agents, Khrœl and Co., 161 Pearl Street). It forms, indeed, an extensive cabinet of the materia medica, amounting to no less than 1,080 different specimens, admirably put up for exhibition; besides these, there is an extensive assortment of homœopathic medicines, and of the various apparatus used by apothecaries and chemists. Many of the articles are not used in this country, being specimens of trivial herbs, &c., employed in Germany and on the continent of Europe. Others, as patchouli (Herba plectanthri graveolentis) are used only in perfumery, but many are rare and curious. The whole collection, we believe, is for sale, and would prove a valuable acquisition to one of our colleges. As evidence of the completeness of the collection, there are found among the alkaloids and peculiar principles obtained from plants

Meconine, in needle-formed colorless crystals.

Menispermine, from menispermum cocculus, in colorless pearly scales.

Narcotine, amorphous, instead of crystalline.

Ononine, white and apparently amorphous. The ononis spinosa is a thorny shrub, whose roots are sometimes employed in Europe to make a diuretic infusion.

Papaverine, a crystalline powder not quite colorless.

Peucedanine, from peucedanum officinale, not used. Passes for stimulant and diaphoretic.

Picrotoxine, the active principle of cocculus indicus (from menispermum cocculus), amorphous; should be in colorless crystals.

Rhabarberin, a dark, extract-like mass.

Rhein, a bright yellow amorphous powder. The Rhabarberin of Brandes?

Solanine, from solanum dulcamara.

Theobromine, white and amorphous.

Elaterine, colorless crystals.

Quassine, quassite, from quassia amara, dark, extract-like mass, not at all like the principle described by Wiggers.

Sanguinarine, red and amorphous, impure.

Berberine, from berberis vulgaris, the common barberry, a lemon-yellow powder.

Bebeerine, from nectandria rodiæi, a light-brown amorphous powders.

Sulph. Bebeerine, in transparent brown scales. The specimen is less highly-colored than that of the same substance sent by Merck.

Atropine, from atropa belladonna, a white crystalline powder.

Asparagine, hard transparent crystals, larger than peas.

Asaron?

Æsculin, from æsculus hippocastaneum, a yellowish powder.

Aconitine, amorphous, and not freed from coloring matter.

Meconic Acid, in beautiful pearly scales, the only specimen in the Exhibition.

Veratrine; the specimens of Merck and those of Rosengart and Denis are both whiter than the one in Gehe's collection.

Caffeine.

Anemonine, from anemone nemorosa, colorless crystals.

Anemonic Acid, amorphous.

Hippuric Acid, white, tolerably good crystals.

Chinic Acid.

Gentisin Cristallizatum, marked in the English catalogue as Gentianin; in fine lemon silky crystals. Gentisic Acid of Lecomte?

Filicin, from aspidium filix mas. Filicic Acid? Cream-colored and amorphous.

Glycirrhizin, a brownish amorphous mass of an intensely-sweet taste.

Hæmatoxylin, the coloring principle of hæmatoxylon campeachianum, brownish crystals; probably colored from exposure to light.

Jalapin, amorphous and colorless.

Inulin, small grains, slightly colored.

Phlorizin, from the root of the pear and apple-tree, colorless and amorphous.

Conin, coneiine, conicin, coneia, the liquid alkaloid from conium maculatum.

Nicotin, a yellowish oily fluid, marked in the catalogue as the poison of Bocarmé.

Bruceuon Purum, bruceine, amorphous, almost colorless, masses.

Bruceum Sulphuricum, sulphate of bruceine, in large and almost colorless crystals, resembling a good deal commercial oxalic acid.

Cantharidin, in small, white, prismatic crystals.

Cetrarin, the bitter principle of cetrarin islandaic, white, amorphous.

Chelidonin, from chelidonium majus, in colorless crystals.

Chinidum Purum Cristillizatum, pure quinidine in crystalline masses, not intensely bitter.

Codein Purum, well-defined, colorless large, prismatic crystals; the specimen from Merck's laboratory is, however, much finer.

Colocynthin, an amorphous, light-yellow powder.

Columbin Crystallizatum, minute nearly colorless crystals.

Cubebin, minute colorless crystals.

Daturin, minute colorless crystals.

Delphinin Purum from Delphinia Staphysagrium, amorphous powder.

Digitalin, a very dark, soft extract.

Digitalin Purum, yellowish-gray, and apparently amorphous.

Piperin, in very fine yellow crystals.

Salicin, in minute crystals, not so white as the specimen furnished by Merck.

Santonin, the active principle of the flowers of the Artemisia Judaica, and A. contra, in very beautiful crystalline plates; the finest specimen, however, of santonin is furnished by Powers and Weightman, of Philadelphia; it is superior even to that of Merck.

We have not gone over all of the peculiar principles found in this beautiful collection. Of quinine alone there are specimens of the acetate, arseniate, citrate, hydrochlorate, sulphate, neutral sulphate, and valerianate. We shall recur to the Exhibition in our next number.

NEW YORK

# JOURNAL OF PHARMACY.

NOVEMBER, 1853.

## ADMISSION OF DRUGS INTO THE U. STATES.

### Report of the Committee appointed by the Pharmaceutical Association.

New York, October 7, 1853.

Mr. Alfred B. Taylor,

*Philadelphia.*

Dear Sir:—Will you do me the favor to furnish a copy of the Report of the Committee appointed by the Pharmaceutical Association, of which you were Chairman, on the subject of "Admission of Drugs into the United States." The object of this request is, that the report may be published in the *New York Journal of Pharmacy.*

In my opinion, the gentlemen comprising that Committee, and those advocating its adoption in Convention, were treated with great discourtesy in the report being refused a place in the published report of the Proceedings of the Convention. I think it due to them, as well as to the public generally, that it should be brought before the community.

You are no doubt aware of my views on the question involved, they agree in the main with those of the Committee. It is fortunate that the framing of this report has fallen into such able hands as the document for itself shows.

Your early attention to the above will be acknowledged by

Yours very respectfully,

T. B. MERRICK.

---

PHILADELPHIA, October 9, 1853.

MR. T. B. MERRICK,

Dear Sir:—I herewith transmit you a copy of my Report, as requested; you are at liberty to make what use of it you please.

I must say that I learned with some regret that it was excluded from the published proceedings of the Association, not that I, by any means, insist on the views there expressed being infallibly right, and those of others opposed, wrong; but I am in favor of the fullest freedom of thought and speech. As Paul says, "Let every man be fully persuaded in his own mind." I am convinced that the opinions there set forth are correct, but if not, I am open to conviction, only, however, by argument. I should have much liked to have seen published in the "proceedings" both the report and also the arguments against it. I think it would have been not only interesting, but also useful in arriving at the truth; for it is only by hearing the arguments on both sides of any question that we can hope to arrive at a just conclusion.

Hoping that the opinions advanced in the report may coincide with the "sober, second thought" of druggists and pharmaceutists throughout the country, I trust that next year we may read, in the "published proceedings" of the Association, at least the following resolution: "*Resolved*, That in the opinion of this Association, all varieties of drugs that are good of their kind should be admitted by the Special Examiner of Drugs and Medicines."

Believe me, yours very respectfully,

A. B. Taylor.

---

August, 24, 1853.

## TO THE AMERICAN PHARMACEUTICAL ASSOCIATION.

The Committee to whom was referred the subject of the inspection of drugs, for the purpose of "endeavoring to arrive at some practicable means of fixing standards for imported drugs," respectfully report—

That they have devoted considerable time and attention to the subject, and have become pretty fully aware both of the importance and the difficulty of devising a plan whereby the standards for imported drugs may be rendered uniform at the different ports of entry.

Since our last Convention, the subject has in a measure been taken out of our hands by the Hon. Secretary of the Treasury, who has issued a circular of instructions, (for the guidance of the various Examiners,) containing a list of specified standards for a number of drugs. This list, though as yet very incomplete, and, in the opinion of the Committee, in a number of points faulty, has been considered as affording a sort of sample of what is wanted.

The Committee, in attempting to continue the list, so as to comprise the leading articles of the Materia Medica, have found a great deal of difficulty; and, in consequence, have determined rather to offer their suggestions as to the most practicable means of fixing standards for imported drugs, than to offer a series of standards, which was their first intention.

To decide between articles of so high a standard as to be just below passable, and others of so low a standard as to be barely admissible, or, in other words, between the best rejected and the worst admitted drugs, is a task requiring the exercise of sound judgment and the nicest discrimination. In the case of chemical preparations, many of the gums, gum resins, some of the roots, woods, barks, &c., it will perhaps be no very difficult matter to assign satisfactory standards; that while they will exclude adulterated and deteriorated articles, will not interfere with the business arrangements of the honest importer; whereas, in the case of herbs, leaves, flowers, extracts, many of the essential oils, &c., it will be very troublesome, if not utterly impossible, to devise means whereby they may be uniformly judged of.

After a careful consideration of the subject, the Committee believe that the opinion advanced by one of its members (Dr. Stewart) at our last Convention, that "all varieties of drugs that are good of their kind should be admitted by the Special Examiners," is correct, and that it forms the only safe and just basis on which to found a rule whereby the Examiner should be governed. If an article is to be condemned on the ground that it will or may be used for adulterating purposes after it is imported, it is difficult to see where will be the limit to these stoppages. Copaiba is adulterated with Castor Oil; Essential Oils with Turpentine; Bromide is substituted for Iodide of Potassium; must we on this account exclude all these articles, and say there shall be imported no more Castor Oil, or Oil of Turpentine, or Bromide of Potassium? and so on to the exclusion of perhaps one half of the articles now imported. This *would* be stopping adulteration with a vengeance!

The question naturally arises, what constitutes "good of their kind," a question much more readily asked than answered. To define precisely what drugs are so, involves a thorough knowledge of the Materia Medica, of the properties and appearances of the articles composing it, of their deterioration by age, moisture, and other causes, together with the adulterations they are liable to, and the means of detecting them.

The Committee have thought that this can be the most readily and effectually settled by the method they are now about to propose. We have prepared and herewith present two lists, embracing all the articles recognized by the United States Pharmacopœia, as constituting the Materia Medica, together with the preparations that are officinal in that work. The first list comprises chemical preparations, and such other articles as we think it practicable to devise standards for; while the second list is composed of herbs, roots, flowers, &c., which cannot so well be judged of by their chemical constituents as by their physical and apparent properties. It will be seen that we have also included in this second list the essential oils, tinctures, extracts, &c., articles that unfortunately are often adulterated or deteriorated, but many of which, we must confess, we are at a loss how to test, even when we suspect them to be so.

We propose that these lists be considered by the Association, article by article, so that we may have the opinion of the Association as to what articles they may consider it practicable to adopt standards for. If there appear on the first list any articles for which the Association deem it impossible or useless to adopt standards, let such names be stricken from the list; while, on the other hand, if there are any on the second list for which standards are thought practicable, let them be transferred to the other list. When the list is arranged, let it be apportioned off amongst the different Pharmaceutical Associations present, whose duty it shall be, carefully to examine the articles assigned to them, especially as regards their deterioration and adulteration, and to devise tests for the detection of such adulterations, and at the same time to arrange standards of purity, whereby they may be judged, not only by the drug examiners, but also by druggists and physicians. The whole to be reported to this Association at its next annual session. We are of opinion that in this way a large amount of very valuable information may be collected, and that the fixing of standards is a task of too great magnitude to be arrived at with satisfactory results in any other way.

In the late Circular of Instructions, issued by the Treasury Department, bearing date June 4th, 1853, there are several points to which this Committee would except. The first section reads as follows: "To avoid the recurrence of a difference of opinion between the officers of the Customs as to what particular articles of commerce should be considered drugs and medicines, and as such subject to special examination by the Special Examiner of Drugs and Medicines, it is thought proper to state that, in conformity with the evident spirit and intent of the law, it is required that all articles of merchandize, used wholly or in part as medicines, and found described as such in the standard works specially referred to in the Act, must be considered drugs and medicines; and that all invoices, therefore, of such articles, in whole or in part, must be submitted to the examination of the Special Examiner of Drugs and Medicines, before they can be permitted to pass the Custom-house." We think this is unjust, and *evidently not* in conformity with the spirit and intent of the law, since it includes such articles as White Lead, Arsenic, Litharge, Lapis Calaminaris, Musk, Mastic, and a variety of other articles, (which are generally, if not always, far from being pure,) extensively used in the arts, and to a very limited extent in medicine, and which must hereafter be entirely excluded from our markets if they are to be judged of by their medicinal fitness.

In the article of galls, of which we suppose there are used in the arts a thousand pounds to every one that is used in medicine, what does the importer, or consumer who uses them for dyeing purposes, care whether they are of the standard strength that is proper to be used in medicine? Is it just that he should be made to pay the high price of such an article, when he could get an article half as good, that is, one of which he would have to use twice as much, for perhaps one fourth the price of the other.

Again, "Saccharum" (sugar) is an article of the Materia Medica, and is extensively used in medicinal preparations, and is "found described as such in the standard works specially referred to in the Act." For all this, we do not believe that it is "in conformity with the evident spirit and intent of the law" that this article must be considered as a drug or medicine, and therefore submitted to the examination of the Drug Examiner.

We think there should be a wide and liberal discrimination made between articles used for manufacturing purposes, and those not so used; that the manufacturer, on giving sufficient security that it should be used only in manufacturing, should be allowed to import and use any material that might best suit his views and purposes.

We think that European Rhubarb should be admitted.

We think that some of the standards are too high for practical purposes. The standard named for Opium is 9 per cent. of pure Morphia: this corresponds to 11.89 per cent. of crystallized sulphate of morphia, an average which we believe is seldom obtained from the best commercial article of Opium. We think that in this and in all similar cases the particular process by which the result is arrived at should be given. A simple statement of 9 per cent. of pure morphia is not (though it might seem so at first sight) sufficiently definite. Crystallized morphia is considered quite as pure as morphia precipitated from its solution by means of ammonia; while in the one case it has two equivalents of water of crystallization,* whereas in the other it has none, thus making a considerable difference in the product, 9 per cent. of anhydrous morphia containing in reality as much morphia as 9.55 per cent. of the crystallized variety; or a lot of Opium that would yield 9 per

* Fowne's Chemistry, page 389.

cent. of pure crystallized morphia, would afford only 8.47 per cent. of anhydrous morphia.

The standard of Elaterium, as containing 30 per cent. of Elaterin, we consider too high.

In the case of Rhubarb, particularly in powder, or of Senna, we do not consider the amount of soluble matter as any fair criterion of their strength or quality. The 40 per cent. of soluble matter required in Rhubarb might be obtained from sugar, sawdust, or indeed from any other adulteration, while a great part of the 28 per cent. of the soluble matter requisite in Senna might be obtained from cynanchum oleœfolium, or any other leaves that might be mixed with it as an impurity or adulteration.

In regard to secret or patent medicines, we believe the law gives the Examiner no right to exclude them, unless they fall under its condemnation. The only part of the law which can possibly apply to them, reads as follows:

Section 3rd.—"And be it further enacted, That if, on examination, any drugs, medicines, medicinal preparations, whether chemical or otherwise, including medicinal essential oils, are found, in the opinion of the Examiner, to be so far adulterated or in any manner deteriorated, as to render them inferior in strength and purity to the standard established by the United States, Edinburgh, London, French, and German Pharmacopœias and Dispensatories, and thereby improper, unsafe, or dangerous to be used for medicinal purposes, a return to that effect shall be made upon the invoice, and the articles so noted shall not pass the Custom-house," &c., &c.

Now we contend that there is no standard given for these medicines in any of these Pharmacopœias; therefore, they cannot, by adulteration, deterioration, or any other process, be rendered inferior to standards which do not exist.

We have not heard it urged that these articles are either adulterated or deteriorated, but simply their composition is not known, and however praiseworthy or desirable it may be to exclude them, we do not consider that, under the law as at present existing, this is a valid objection. If an importer wishes to import a mixture of Salicine and Quinine, and has it put up in bottles, labelled "equal parts of Salicine and Quinine," the Examiner, on finding that it is just what it purports to be, is as certainly bound to pass it, as if it were pure quinine, simply labelled as such; whereas, if such a mixture were to be examined by the proper standard for quinine (which it does not pretend to be) it would, as a matter of course, be condemned as not coming up to that standard. The same principle undoubtedly holds true with regard to patent or secret medicines. For example: if a purgative pill, (the composition of which is unknown, further than it is Mr. A. B. C.'s Purgative Pill, and that the purgative dose is four pills,) is presented at one of our ports for entry, it would most certainly be unjust to say, that because it does not correspond with the "Compound Cathartic Pill" of the United States Pharmacopœia, and is inferior in strength to that, the dose of which is only three pills, (a correspondence that was never intended,) it must be rejected. We believe that if on examination these pills are found to be not adulterated, not deteriorated, but just what they purport to be, under the law as at present framed, the Examiner of Drugs is bound to admit them.

We would wish to have it understood, most distinctly, that it is not against the exclusion of secret medicines we are arguing, but against their illegal exclusion. We have a law, let us stand by it; if it does not suit us, let us alter it. We would most heartily say *Amen*, not only to a law prohibiting the importation of medicines whose composition was not correctly and exactly known, but would also recommend that the State Legislatures should pass such laws as would prevent the sale of any medicinal preparation whatever, the composition of which was not entirely public.

We learn that a lot of pills are now at the Philadelphia Custom-house, having been rejected under the recent instructions of the Hon. Secretary of the Treasury, and that gentleman has determined that, if possible, they shall be analysed. Supposing an analytic chemist could be found of sufficient skill to return the following as their composition: "Ext. Colocynth. Comp. gr. ij; Pulv. Rhei gr. i; Pulv. Jalapæ gr. i; Ext. Gentianæ gr. i" in each pill, a form which, (though simple, and just such as occurs daily with an apothecary engaged in compounding prescriptions,) would defy the skill of any chemist to give a correct proximate analysis. What then? Is it the province of the Examiner to say that they contain too much Extract of Colocynth, or that they don't contain enough Rhubarb? Is it his province to sit in judgment, and say to one importer, "these pills are not safe for you to take because they don't suit your case;" and to another, "you can have them because your physician has given you a prescription for just such pills?"

We think that the construction recently put by the Hon. Secretary of the treasury upon the 4th Section of the Law, as passed by Congress, 26th June, 1848, is erroneous and illegal. That section reads as follows:

"And be it further enacted, That the owner or consignee shall, at all times, when dissatisfied with the Examiner's return, have the privilege of calling, at his own expense, for a re-examination, and on depositing with the Collector such sum as the latter may deem sufficient to defray such expense, it shall be the duty of that officer to procure some competent analytical chemist, possessing the confidence of the medical profession, as well as of the colleges of medicine and pharmacy, if any such institutions exist in the State in which the Collection District is situated, who shall make a careful analysis of the articles included in said return, and a report upon the same under oath; and in case the report, *which shall be final*, shall declare the return of the Examiner to be erroneous," &c, &c., making the report of the analytical examiner *final.*

The recent clause in reference thereto, reads as follows:

"The appeal from the report of the Special Examiner of Drugs and Medicines, provided for in the Act, must be made by the owner or consignee within ten days after the said report; and in case of such appeal, the analysis made by the analytical chemist is expected to be full and in detail, setting forth clearly and accurately the name, quantity, and quality of the several component parts of the article in question, to be reported to the Collector under oath or affirmation.

"On such report being made, a copy of the same will be immediately furnished by the Collector to the Special Examiner of Drugs and Medicines, who, if the report be in conflict with his return made to the Collector, and he have cause to believe that the appeal and analytical examination have not been conducted in strict conformity with the law, may enter his protest in writing against the reception and adoption by the Collector of such report and analysis, until a reasonable time be allowed him for the preparation of his views in the case, and their submission to this department for its consideration."

This, it will be seen, makes that report *not final*, and, we think, in the hands of an examiner disposed to be captious, will cause a great deal of unnecessary expense and delay.

There has recently been a considerable amount of opposition raised to the law, in consequence of the obstructions thrown in the way of legitimate business, not because spurious or adulterated drugs have been rejected, but because, through either ignorance or misapprehension of the spirit of the law, a great deal of vexation and expense has been caused by the delay that has not unfrequently occurred in the admission of drugs, about the quality of which there could be no reasonable doubt.

As an illustration, we would state that there are now at the Philadelphia Custom-house, under sentence of condemnation, three importations of quinine, comprising in all 750 ounces, part of which was imported 7th of May last, (and which it is believed is of very excellent quality,) since which time the owners have been trying in vain to get it "passed."

We *know* that in Philadelphia importers have *often* ordered their drugs through other ports. because they could get them with less trouble and delay than by having them entered at Philadelphia.

We believe that while the Drug Law has been beneficial in its action on the character of the drugs imported into this country, it has, in many instances, subjected honestly disposed importers to serious losses and delays.

The best devised system of standards and tests will be of no avail, unless the officers to whom is entrusted the execution of the law have the requisite qualifications of judgment and ability, or, in other words, are honest and competent; and, we think, that such officers, acting under a few general instructions, relying on a correct knowledge and sound judgment, with a determination not to admit adulterated or deteriorated drugs, will find much less trouble in carrying out the law satisfactorily than they would under more complicated instructions.

We would condemn the stringent application of the law that would unnecessarily oppress the honest importer, and would recommend that, in reference to articles used for manufacturing or mechanical purposes, as liberal a construction as is consistent with safety should be manifested, and thus remove a very plausible objection of those who wish the law abolished on the alleged ground that more harm than good results therefrom.

(Signed,) ALFRED B. TAYLOR, } *Committee.*
JOHN MEAKIM, }

[The other Members of the Committee did not sign or see the report. They were, JAMES BURNETT, of Boston, and Dr. D. STEWART, of Baltimore.]

# MEMOIR ON SQUILL.

BY M. TILLOY.

## First Analysis.

Two hundred and fifty grammes of squill, dried and coarsely powdered, put into a displacement vessel, were treated with ether, until it passed through tasteless. This ether, distilled, left as a residue, an odorous fatty matter, of yellow color, of the consistence of lard, pitchy, like resin mixed with a little oil, and of an acrid and very bitter taste. It dissolved entirely in the alcohol and the alkalies; the acid separated it from the latter, under its own form and with its own properties. Put into boiling water, it communicated to it an acid and bitter taste, aided by a very minute portion of the saccharine matter which was dissolved in it, and which we detected after the evaporation of the water. Heated in a capsule, it liquified and was ultimately decomposed, leaving a not very bulky charcoal. It inflamed on contact with an ignited body better than the fat oils, and less easily than the essential oils. By means of repeated washings in boiling water, the acrid and bitter taste is entirely removed from the fatty matter.

These same 250 grammes of squill were washed, in the same apparatus, with alcohol of 90° until it passed through tasteless. This liquid was very *acrid* and still *bitter;* distilled, it gave a residue of yellowish color still containing fatty matter which had escaped the action of the ether, and which may be entirely removed by a new washing with the latter.

The saccharine matters carried away by the alcohol were separated with distilled water; there then remained a resiniform substance, of a light amber color, which was the *acrid* principle.

This substance possesses some of the characters of the resins; it softens in hot water, dissolves in the alkalies and alcohol, but not in ether, when placed on incandesent coals, it fuses, swells up, gives out much smoke, and exhales the odor of urea. The dilute acids have no action on it.

It gives to alcohol all its acrid taste, producing on the tongue the effect of arum-root. Its action on animals is most energetic; a very small dose kills a rabbit. In the dose of 5 centigr., it kills a dog.

These same 250 grammes of squill were afterwards made to undergo washing with distilled water. The water contracted a slightly saccharine and bitter taste. Evaporated to the consistence of a soft extract, the mucous portion separated by means of alcohol at 90°. Then a bitter and slightly saccharine extract was the residue of the distillation of the alcohol. By re-dissolving this extract in water, and filtering through animal charcoal, the liquid was deprived of all its bitterness, and remained saccharine without any other taste. I did not think it necessary to ascertain whether or not this sugar was crystallizable.

## SECOND ANALYSIS.

We repeated the process of our former analysis, with the following modification, namely: decoloring the alcoholic tincture of squill with tribasic acetate of lead, and precipitating, after filtration, the lead from the acetate remaining in the liquor, with a few drops of sulphuric acid. By this means we obtained the results announced, and the same as by the first analysis. We find this mode more economical and more prompt.

## THIRD ANALYSIS.

Fresh squill was rasped and treated with boiling water; the settled liquid was divided into two equal parts.

The first part was treated in the same way as for extracting digitaline, by means of subacetate of lead, tannin, protoxide of lead, &c., &c. The tannin having precipitated only partially the acrid and bitter principles which the water still retained, these not very satisfactory results showed us that this plan could not be applied with advantage to the extraction of the active principles of the squill.

The second part of this same aqueous solution was filtered cold through animal charcoal, to which it abandoned all its bitterness and acridness. There only remained an insipid and sweet taste. After having washed this charcoal with water, and having dried it, it was treated hot with alcohol, which removed the acrid and bitter principles retained by the charcoal. Distilled, it gave as a residue the same substances as in the first two analyses, which led me to think that this last mode might be usefully employed in the extraction of quinine and strychnine; but having been able to free the charcoal from it only by means of alcohol, and not by means of sulphuric acid, this process does not present any real advantage.

The volatile principle of M. Vogel, decomposable by boiling water, remains to be spoken of. Notwithstanding my researches, made with all precautions, into the products of volatilisation, I was able to discover nothing, and I am convinced that it does not exist. But I have found a *pungent* matter, alterable by boiling water, as indicated by M. Vogel, which, however, is neither *fugaceous* nor *volatile;* it is a multitude of small crystals interposed in the parenchyma of the bulb, in needles of silky appearance, without taste, insoluble in water, alcohol, and ether.

Isolated and suspended in a very small quantity, these crystals occasion, when we rub ourselves with them, a smarting and, after a moment, a redness and very distinct small blisters; it is a similar effect to that of stinging-nettles. Treated with boiling water, these crystals are disaggregated, and lose their form and action. The dilute acids dissolve them, and they are precipitated as a white powder by saturation with ammonia or any other alkali.

Their composition is that of nitrate of lime, which we recognised in all its properties. To extract these crystals from fresh or dried squill, it is cut into small pieces, which are agitated in water, in which it is allowed to macerate for not longer than a quarter of an hour, it is decanted, being kept stirred all the while. The crystals obtained are washed after having been allowed to deposit. It was to these crystals that the stinging action was due, for it was in vain that we rubbed ourselves with the liquid which held them in suspension, when they had settled to the bottom of the vessel.

From the foregoing, it is proved that the acrid principle is the most active substance of squill. As regards the bitter principle which is obtained by the repeated washings of the fatty body in boiling water, and which may be entirely isolated from the acrid principle, I have not been able to study its therapeutical effects without exposing myself to the penalties which the law inflicts on those who, not being physicians, practise as such. I gave some to a dog, which appeared to me to be rendered slightly unwell by it. Squill contains therefore—

1. A very acrid and poisonous substance, soluble in alcohol, but not in ether.

2. A very bitter principle, yellow, soluble in water and alcohol.

3. A fatty matter, tasteless, soluble in ether, and not in alcohol, when it is perfectly free from the acrid and bitter principles.

4. Citrate of lime, the stinging action of which is purely mechanical.

5. Finally a mucous matter and sugar.—Extract of a letter from M. Tilloy to M. Soubeiran; *Journal de Pharmacie*, June, 1853, and *Pharmaceutical Journal.*

# ON THE MANUFACTURE OF AMMONIA AND AMMONIACAL SALTS.

Concluded from p. 304.

A great variety of processes have been patented within the last few years by Mr. Laming and Mr. Hills, having for their object the purification of coal-gas and the obtaining of ammonia and ammoniacal salts. In his patent of November 4, 1847, Mr. Laming claims the use of the undermentioned salts for the above-named purposes, the solution of which is absorbed into sawdust, or other porous material, and placed in the purifying vessel of the gas-works, viz., chloride of calcium, the muriates and sulphates of manganese, iron, and zinc; the carbonates of manganese, iron, zinc, and lead. The oxides of manganese, iron, zinc, or lead, may also be added to any of the above materials. The ammonia or ammoniacal salts contained in the spent purifying materials may be removed by heat or washing.

The specification of the same patent contains an account of certain modes of treating the ammoniacal liquor of gas-works, so as to obtain from it and sulphate of lead, a solution of sulphate of ammonia. and either an oxide or carbonate of lead, of sufficient purity to serve as, or be converted into, white lead.

Mr. Laming converts the hydrosulphate of ammonia contained in gas-liquors into carbonate of ammonia by the following process: A mixture of deutoxide of copper and charcoal, or other form of carbon in fine powder, in the proportion of twelve parts by weight of the former to one of the latter, is introduced into a retort made red hot, and furnished with an eduction-pipe, which passes through cold water, and finally enters into the gas-liquor. The formation of carbonic acid gas soon takes place, by the union of the carbon with the oxygen of the metal, and this gas combining with the base of the hydrosulphate of ammonia contained in the gas-liquor, converts it into carbonate, with liberation of hydrosulphuric acid. When the carbonic acid gas ceases to come away, nearly all the carbon will have disappeared from the retort, and the copper which it contains become reduced to the metallic state. The charge is then drawn and left to cool, while a second charge of similar materials is being worked off, during which time the copper re-absorbs oxygen from the air, and becomes again deutoxide of copper, which may then be used anew with fresh carbon.

Mr. Hills, in the patent of November 28, 1849, claims the use of his sub-sulphates, the oxychlorides, and the hydrated or precipitated oxides of iron, (which he prefers to use in a rather damp state,) either by themselves or mixed with sulphate of lime, or sulphate or muriate of magnesia, baryta, strontia, potash, or soda; and he causes them to be absorbed into or mixed with sawdust or peat charcoal in coarse powder, or breeze, or other porous or absorbent material, so as to make a very porous substance easily permeable by the gas. This material is to be put into a purifier, (a dry lime purifier will answer the purpose,) and the gas is to be passed through it; by this means, the ammonia and other products are absorbed. By the admission of air and application of heat to the material so saturated with ammonia, this substance is driven off and collected by passing it through a condenser, or the ammonia may be fixed by an acid, and converted directly into sulphate or muriate of ammonia. If sulphate of lime or sulphate of magnesia be present in the purifying material, these salts will be decomposed with the formation of sulphate of ammonia, which may then be washed out of the purifying material, concentrated by evaporation, and crystallized.

Mr. Laming, in his patent of April 23, 1850, claims the use of muriate of iron, of muriate of iron decomposed by lime into chloride of calcium and oxide of iron, of sulphate of iron decomposed by its equivalent quantity of chloride of sodium, adding to the solution of muriate of iron thus produced, enough hydrate of lime to decompose it into chloride of calcium and precipitated oxide of iron. In these, and in various modified forms of the same process, muriate of ammonia may be obtained from the purifying material when it has served its purpose, and has been removed from the purifying vessel. Mr. Laming also claims the use of a mixture of sulphate of lime and sulphate of iron, of a mixture of hydrated or precipitated oxide of iron with carbonate of lime, magnesia, carbonate of magnesia, or magnesian limestone, of chloride of magnesium or sulphate of magnesia and water, phosphate of lime dissolved in hydrochloric acid, and, lastly, of a mixture containing sulphate of magnesia or chloride of magnesium or calcium, or one or more of them in combination with oxide of copper, and mixed or not with lime or magnesia, or both or either, or both of the carbonates of those earths. In all these cases, the salts employed are mixed with sawdust or some other porous substances, and the material so compounded is placed in the purifying vessels of the gas-works. The gas, in its passage through the purifiers, gives up its ammonia, which is afterwards obtained as sulphate or muriate of ammonia, by washing the material when it has become fully saturated with ammonia.

Messrs. Crane and Jullien, in their patent of January 18, 1848, describe a method of manufacturing ammonia in the state of carbonate, hydrocyanate, or free ammonia, by passing any of the oxygen compounds of nitrogen, together with any compound of hydrogen and carbon, or any mixture of hydrogen with a compound of carbon or even free hydrogen, through a tube or pipe containing any catalytic or contact substance, as follows: Oxides of nitrogen, (such for instance as the gases liberated in the manufacture of oxalic acid,) however procured, are to be mixed in such proportion with any compound of carbon and hydrogen, or such mixture of hydrogen and carbonic oxide or acid as results from the contact of the vapor of water with ignited carbonaceous matters, and the hydrogen compound or mixture containing hydrogen, may be in slight excess, so as to ensure the conversion of the whole of the nitrogen contained in the oxide so employed, into either ammonia or hydrocyanic acid, which may be known by the absence of the characteristic red fumes on allowing some of the gaseous matter to come in contact with atmospheric air. The catalytic or contact substance which Messrs. Crane and Jullien prefer, is platinum, which may be either in the state of sponge, or asbestos coated or covered with platinum. This catalytic substance is to be placed in a tube, and heated to about 600° Fahr., so as to reduce the temperature of the product, and at the same time prevent the deposition of carbonate of ammonia, which passes onwards into a vessel of the description well known and employed for the purpose of condensing carbonate of ammonia. The condenser, for this purpose, must be furnished with a safety-pipe to allow of the escape of uncondensed matter, and made to dip into a solution of any substance capable of combining with hydrocyanic acid or ammonia where they would be condensed. A solution of salt of iron is preferable for this purpose.

Mr. Hills took out a patent, October 19, 1848, for improvements in treating certain salts and gases or vapors, in which he describes a method of distilling the volatile solution of ammonia for the purpose of producing ammonia of a more highly concentrated character. For this purpose he employs a tower, circular by preference, which should be about ten diameters in height; this is to be furnished with gratings, placed from 3 to 4 feet apart throughout the whole height of the tower; the spaces between each being filled with coke, pieces of earthenware, or other substances, to form greatly divided media. The volatile solution to be distilled, whether pure or combined with other matters is to be introduced at the top of the tower, and allowed to percolate through the coke, while, at the same time, a jet of steam or heated air is introduced at the bottom, which, in its ascent, meets the ammonia distributed over a great amount of surface, by which means the more volatile parts of the ammonia become vaporized and carried off by the steam; this being collected at the top and conveyed to a refrigerator and condensed, while the waste liquor escapes at the bottom of the tower. As an auxiliary to this apparatus, another tower is placed on the top of that already described. This the patentee calls a concentrator: it is filled with the same materials as the other, and furnished with a coil of pipe, through which the solution of ammonia is to be passed when introduced to the lower tower; the vapors arising from this partially vaporize the ammonia in the pipe, while, at the same time, the more aqueous parts of the vapors are condensed before passing off to the condensor.

Dr. Richardson's process, patented January 26, 1850, for manufacturing sulphate of ammonia, consists in subliming the double salt of sulphate of magnesia and ammonia obtained by the following method: The ammoniacal liquor of the gas-works is added to a solution of sulphate of magnesia, with application of heat, until the solution is rendered nearly neutral; the precipitate is then allowed to subside, and the clear liquor drawn off, concentrated by boiling to from 50° to 60° Twaddle, (spec. grav. 1,250 to 1,300,) and crystallized. If preferred, the gas-water may be neutralized by sulphuric acid before it is added to the solution of sulphate of magnesia. The double salt of sulphate of magnesia and ammonia may also be obtained by subjecting the sulphate of magnesia, either in solution or in a damp state, to a current of ammoniacal gas, obtained by the distillation of gas-water, guano, or any other matter from which ammonia can be procured by destructive distillation with quick-lime; the ammoniacal gas being purified before using by passing it through water.

Michiel's mode of obtaining sulphate of ammonia, patented April 30, 1850, is as follows: The ammonical liquors of the gas-works are combined with sulphate and oxide of lead, which is obtained and prepared in the following way: Sulphuret of lead, in its natural state, is taken and reduced to small fragments by any convenient crushing apparatus. It is then submitted to a roasting process, in a suitably arranged reverberatory furnace of the following construction: The furnace is formed of two shelves, or rather the bottom of the furnace and one shelf, and there is a communication from the lower to the upper. The galena or sulphuret of lead, previously ground, is then spread over the surface of the upper shelf, to the thickness of about 2 or 2½ inches, and there it is submitted to the heat of the furnace. It remains thus for about two hours, at which time it is drawn off the upper shelf and spread over the lower shelf or bottom of the furnace, where it is exposed to a greater heat for a certain time, during which it is well stirred, for the purpose of exposing all the parts equally to the action of the heat, and at the same time the fusion of any portion of it is prevented. By this process the sulphuret of lead becomes converted, partly into sulphate and partly into oxide of lead. This product of sulphate and oxide of lead is to be crushed by any ordinary means, and reduced to about the same degree of fineness as coarse sand. It is now to be combined with the ammoniacal liquors, when sulphate of ammonia and sulphuret and carbonate of lead will be produced.

In order to obtain sulphate and muriate of ammonia with the greatest possible economy, Mr. Spence patented, November 12, 1850, the following process: A series of two or more, say, for instance, four cylindrical boilers are placed at such a distance, one above the other, that the contents of the upper boiler may be drawn off into the one next below it. Each boiler is furnished with a cock to allow of the passage of the contents of the boiler from one to the other throughout the series. Each of these vessels contains gas liquor, from a reservoir of which a pipe passes to the upper boiler, which is also furnished with an exit-pipe. Into the lower boiler high-pressure steam is passed, which soon causes the gas-liquor to boil, and the vapor of ammonia and water passes off through an exit-pipe into the boiler placed next above it in the series, the liquor in which is thus also brought to boil, the vapor of ammonia and water passing off from it in the same way to the boiler next above it, and so on throughout the series. By the time the vapor of ammonia passes off from the uppermost boiler it has become so concentrated, that on passing it into sulphuric or muriatic acid, a concentrated solution of either of those salts is obtained, of sufficient specific gravity to crystallize without evaporation, and thus a considerable saving in fuel and time is effected, and the ammoniacal gas-liquor is most thoroughly exhausted. Fresh supplies of ammoniacal liquor are constantly furnished to the uppermost boiler from the reservoir; whilst the partially exhausted liquors are run from the higher to the lower vessels in succession, and the exhausted liquors run off to waste from the lowermost vessel of the series. As the gas-liquors often contain some fixed ammoniacal salts, Mr. Spence recommends the addition of lime to the contents of the boilers, in order to render free the ammonia contained in such salts.

Mr. Wilson patented, December 7th, 1850, the following process of obtaining sulphate of ammonia from the waste products of coke-ovens and other furnaces. For this purpose, he employs the following apparatus: An iron column lined with lead, or a brick column well lined with fire-bricks and well-burnt clay, is filled with coke or round pebbles; this column has an area or cross section five or six times that of the chimney connected with the coke ovens, and is from 12 to 15 feet in height; at the bottom of this column, which can be supported on cross bars, is a space of 3 feet left clear, in which is placed a cistern, constructed of the same materials as the column, and another similar cistern is placed at the top of the column, its bottom being pierced full of holes. The lower cistern is then filled with sulphuric acid so diluted, that when saturated with ammonia it shall not form a solution of sufficient density to cause, on evaporation by the heat of the column, an incrustation of sulphate of ammonia. The gaseous products of combustion are then made to pass through the lower cistern up the column of coke, and as the acid liquor of the lower cistern is continually forced by suitable means into the upper perforated cistern, the ammonia, in its passage upwards, comes into contact with the acid trickling down through the column, and is thus prevented from passing off with the other products of combustion, which are conveyed by an exit-pipe into the chimney. When the acid liquor has become neutralized by the ammonia, it is drawn off, filtered, evaporated, and crystallized, a fresh supply of acid being placed in the lower cistern.

Mr. Laming patented, August 12, 1852, the following method of manufacturing sulphate of ammonia from the ammoniacal liquor of gas-works. The ammonia is first separated in its simple form, or as carbonate of ammonia, by any known means, after which it is converted into sulphite of ammonia, by causing streams of sulphurous acid to be brought into contact with it, and the sulphite of ammonia is finally converted into sulphate by exposing it to the combined influences of atmospheric air and water.

Dr. Ure, in his *Dictionary of Arts and Manufactures*, states that 7,200 gallons of ammoniacal gas-liquor treated with 4,500 lbs. of sulpuric acid, sp. grav. 1,625, produces 2,400 gallons of solution of sulphate of ammonia, of sp. gr. 1,150. As a gallon of solution of ordinary sulphate of ammonia, of the above strength, contains three pounds of crystallized sulphate, it follows that in the above case the product is at the rate of one pound per gallon of gas-liquor, which is almost double the quantity ordinarily obtained.

The quantity of ammoniacal liquor obtained at one of the London gas-works, during one year, from the distillation of 51,100 tons of coal, was 224,800 gallons.

*Ammonia Meter.*—In order to determine the strength of any given solution of ammonia, Mr. J. J. Griffin, of Baker Street, has constructed a useful instrument termed an ammonia meter. This instrument is founded on the following facts:

That mixtures of liquid ammonia with water possess a specific gravity, which is the mean of the specific gravities of their components; that in all solutions of ammonia a quantity of anhydrous ammonia, weighing 212½ grains, which he calls a *test-atom*, displaces 300 grains of water, and reduces the specific gravity of the solution to the extent of .00125; and, finally, that the strongest solution of ammonia, which it is possible to prepare at the temperature of 62° Fahr., contains in an imperial gallon of solution one hundred test-atoms of ammonia.

The ammonia meter is accompanied by a table, containing six columns of numbers. The first column shows the *specific gravity* of the solutions; the second column the *weight* of an imperial gallon in pounds and ounces; the third column the *per-centage* of ammonia by weight; the fourth column the *degree* of the solution, as indicated by the instrument, corresponding with the number of *test-atoms* of ammonia present in a gallon of the liquor; the fifth column shows the number of *grains* of ammonia contained in a gallon; and the sixth column the *atomic volume* of the solution, or that *measure* of it which contains one test-atom of ammonia. For instance, one gallon of liquid ammonia, sp. grav. 880 weighs 8 lbs. 12-8 oz. avoirdupois, its per-centage of ammonia, by weight, is 33.117, it contains 96 test-atoms of ammonia in one gallon, and 20400.0 grains of ammonia in one gallon; and; lastly, 104.16 septems, containing one test-atom of ammonia. Although no hydrometer, however accurately constructed, is at all equal to the centigrade mode of chemical testing, yet the Ammonia Meter, and the table accompanying it, will be found very useful to the manufacturer, enabling him not only to determine the actual strength of any given liquor, but the precise amount of dilution necessary to convert it into a liquor of any other desired strength, whilst the direct quotation of the number of grains of real ammonia contained in a gallon of solution of any specific gravity, will enable him to judge at a glance of the money-value of any given sample of ammonia.—*Pharmaceutical Journal*, September, 1853.

---

# ON THE PURIFICATION OF GLYCERINE, AND ITS EMPLOYMENT IN THE ARTS.

*Report by M. Chevallier on a Paper by M. Bruère-Perrin.*

It is well known that the discovery of Glycerine dates from 1782 or 1783; that it is due to Scheele, who made known the fact that oils and fats contain a saccharine matter which is obtained by treating two parts of oil with one part of litharge, adding some water, and applying heat, and afterwards separating and purifying the saccharine matter which is found in the mother-liquor. Scheele published the results of his investigations on this subject in a communication bearing the title *De Materia Saccharina peculiari Oleorum expressorum et pinguedinum*, which appeared in the *Transactions of the Royal Academy of Sweden*, in 1783. In this publication Scheele gave the name of *sweet principle of oils* to glycerine, from the fact of its having a saccharine character, and of its solution yielding a syrupy product on being evaporated.

The discovery of Scheele was circulated through the scientific journals, and especially Crell's Journal for 1784, and afterwards the Chemical Works of Bergmann, edited by Guyton de Morveau.

By the subsequent extension of scientific investigation it was established that oils are composed of fatty acids and glycerine, and that the latter, which plays the part of a base, is separated in saponification.

Glycerine, although it has been well known to chemists, and although it has been produced in very large quantities since the development of the industrial arts in France, was not employed, being considered a product of the laboratory, curious, but not susceptible of any useful application.

The first use to which glycerine was applied was in medicine; in fact, the sweet principle of oils was first employed as a remedy for diseases of the ear by an English surgeon. This application of it having been made known, the attention of medical men was directed to glycerine, and soon afterwards it was recommended as a valuable application for diseases of the skin. Trials of it were made in Paris by Bazin and Cazenave; in London, by Yearsley, Wakley, and others; and in Russia, by Dr. Dallas, of Odessa, who, without hesitation, pronounced glycerine to be the best of cosmetics. It was established from the experience of these medical men that glycerine, when applied to the skin, penetrates and softens it, and promotes cicatrisation of cracks and fissures.

The memoir of M. Bruère-Perrin relates to the means of purifying glycerine. It is known that as usually obtained it has a disagreeable odor, and that it has been proposed to purify it by passing through it a current of carbonic acid gas to precipitate the lime which it contains. According to M. Bruère-Perrin, this mode of operating only removes the excess of lime present, and not that combined with fatty acids.

M. Bruère-Perrin adopts the following method for effecting the object required: 1st. He determines, by means of oxalic acid, the quantity of lime existing in the liquid to be purified. 2d. The proportion of lime being thus determined, he adds to the liquid a quantity of sulphuric acid sufficient to convert the lime into insoluble sulphate of lime. 3d. He then concentrates the liquor in a tinned copper pan, stirring it briskly during the concentration by an agitator kept in motion by machinery. During the concentration there is a disengagement of vapors, having a disagreeable odor, and a partial decoloration of the liquid takes place at the same time. 4th. When the liquid has acquired a density of 1.075, it is allowed to cool, and then passed through a filter, to separate the sulphate of lime; the excess of acid which has been used in the previous part of the process is now saturated with carbonate of potash, and the liquid again evaporated, with constant agitation, until it has a specific gravity 1.19, when it will deposit a certain quantity of sulphate of potash in a gelatinous mass; it is then allowed to cool, strained, and the deposit washed with a small quantity of water, to which a little spirit has been added. 5th. It is again evaporated, still keeping it agitated, and after bringing it to a specific gravity of 1.24 while hot, it is left to cool, when a further precipitation of sulphate of potash takes place, from which it is filtered.

The product resulting from these operations is of an amber color, free from any marked odor, having a sweetish taste, and being unctuous to the touch. In this state it is treated while cold with animal charcoal, and filtered. It is now free from color or any sensible odor.

Glycerine, like water, mixes with aqueous liquids, with alcohol, and with acetic acid; it moistens bodies without rendering them greasy; like oil, it is unctuous to the touch, and does not evaporate when exposed to the air. It is easily charged with the aroma of volatile oils; it does not become rancid, nor does it ferment.

M. Bruère-Perrin has introduced glycerine into toilet soaps, and has used it in the preparation of cosmetic vinegar, aromatized spirits, and several other articles of perfumery. We are assured that the soap with glycerine retains its original soft consistence, and that the unctuosity of the glycerine is imparted to the skin. We have tried several of these preparations and verified the descriptions given of them.—*Journal de Chimie Médicale.*

---

## COLLEGE OF PHARMACY

### OF THE CITY OF NEW YORK.

The regular Course of Instruction, comprising Lectures on Chemistry, Materia Medica and Pharmacy, will commence on Monday, the 7th of November, next, and be continued on Monday, Wednesday, and Friday evenings of each week, until the 1st of March, at the Chemical Lecture Room, of the

Medical College, in Thirteenth Street, between the Third and Fourth Avenues, which location has been selected to secure the superior accommodations there offered by Prof. Doremus, in the use of his complete Chemical Apparatus, and also the privilege of the students being allowed access, free of charge, to the course of Chemical Lectures delivered before the New York Medical College, thus affording unusual facilities in the study of Organic Chemistry.

*Lectures on Materia Medica and Pharmacy*, from 7 to 8 o'clock, P. M., by Prof. B. W. McCready, M.D., and *Lectures on Chemistry*, from 8 to 9 o'clock P. M., by Prof. R. O. Doremus, M. D.

Tickets for the Course on Materia Medica and Pharmacy, at $7, and on Chemistry, $7, may be procured of James S. Aspinwall, 86 William street; Geo. D. Coggeshall, 809 Broadway; John Meakim, 497 Broadway.—*New York, October*, 1853.

---

# EDITORIAL.

Proceedings of the American Pharmaceutical Association, at the Annual Meeting, held in Boston, August 24th, 25th, and 26th, 1853. Published by direction of the Association. Philadelphia: Merrihew & Thompson, printers, Merchant street, above Fourth.

The Proceedings of the Pharmaceutical Association appear in a neat pamphlet of forty-eight pages. It contains the Minutes of the Proceedings, the Reports of the different Committees appointed by the Association, Reports relating to the Statistics of Pharmacy from the Massachusetts, the Philadelphia, the Cincinnati, and the New York Colleges, with some scattered facts on the same subject from some of the Southern and Western States; the Constitution and Code of Ethics, as passed at the last meeting of the Association, are reprinted, though forming no part of the Proceedings, and the whole is concluded by a list of officers of the Association for the present year, by the Roll of Members, and by the list of Special Committees, who are to report at the meeting to be held at Cincinnati, on July 27th, 1854. The first Report published in detail is that of the Executive Committee, and in it are found several recommendations which we hope may be promptly acted on. One of these is the issue of a cheap and accurate edition of the United States Pharmacopœia. It would appear that but 1,500 copies of the Pharmacopœia are published in its present form, and that this number is sufficient to supply the demand for the ten years which elapses before the appearance of a revised edition. Even in our large cities the place of the Pharmacopœia is to a great extent supplied by the United States Dispensatory and similar works, and confusion and mistakes are undoubtedly occasioned by confounding the formulæ of different colleges. Another recommendation of the Committee is, that the Association should propose Prize Questions for competition. The following are proposed, by way of example, by the Committee:

"*a.* It is conceded that Digitalis of American growth is less active and efficient as an arterial sedative and diuretic than that of English origin. Is this deterioration due to the less abundant formation of *digitalin;* to its modification; or to any other definable cause?

*b.* What are the impediments, if any exist, to the free cultivation of Colchicum Autumnale in the United States, so as to preserve its power unimpaired; and is it true that the recent cormus is more active than the same carefully dried, and if so, why?

*c.* Do Hyoscyamus and Belladonna, grown in the United States, contain the active principles in the same proportions as the European plants?

*d.* Spigelia is admitted to possess positive anthelmintic power. Does this power reside in a distinct, well-defined principle, capable itself of producing the effects of Spigelia; if so, isolate and describe it?

*e.* The best essay on extemporaneous pharmacy, which shall treat of the incompatible combinations most usually prescribed, the best manner of avoiding them, and the most efficient methods of proceeding in effecting the union of substances that are physically incompatible, as emulsions, certain liniments, certain pill ingredients, &c.

*f.* For the best essay on the identification of volatile oils when mixed, their preservation, and the actual effects of light and air on them, under the ordinary circumstances that they are kept in the shop, so as to decide the question whether all of them, or only part, should be kept in the dark, to prevent change?

*g.* For an essay which shall develop the commercial history of all drugs indigenous to the United States, as Senega, Spigelia, Serpentaria, &c., as regards the manner and places of their collection for the supply of commerce, the annual amount collected, and the channels through which they enter general commerce.

*h.* For the best essay on the construction and material of pharmaceutical apparatus, including that for evaporation, distillation, and solution more especially as regards economy, convenience, and effectiveness, with a view to the ordinary wants of a thorough pharmaceutist."

A Committee is recommended on the subject of Home Adulterations, their nature, extent, and *locality*, and on the best means of preventing them.

The Committee on the Sale of Poisons, Mr. Procter, Chairman, presented a long report. After a cursory notice of the Legislation on the subject in France, Germany, and Great Britain, the report reverts to the United States. It appears that in Ohio, New Hampshire, and New York, there exist special Acts upon the subject. The Ohio law enacts—

"Sec 1. That it shall not hereafter be lawful for any apothecary, druggist, or other person in this State, to sell or give away any article belonging to the class of medicines, usually denominated poisons, except in compliance with the restrictions contained in this Act.

Sec. 2. That every apothecary, druggist, or other person, who shall sell or give away, except upon the prescription of a physician, any article or articles of medicine belonging to the class usually known as poisons, shall be required:

1st. To register in a book kept for the purpose, the name, age, sex, and color of the person obtaining such poison.

2d. The quantity sold.

3d. The purpose for which it is required.

4th. The day and date on which it was obtained.

5th. The name and place of abode of the person for whom the article is intended.

6th. To carefully mark the word "poison," upon the label or wrapper of each package.

7th. To neither sell nor give away any article of poison to minors of either sex.

Sec. 3. That no apothecary, druggist, or other person, shall be permitted to sell or give away any quantity of arsenic less than one pound, without first mixing either soot or indigo therewith, in the proportion of one ounce of soot or half an ounce of indigo to the pound of arsenic.

Sec. 4. That any person offending against the provisions of this Act, shall be deemed guilty of a misdemeanor, and, upon conviction thereof, shall be fined in any sum not less than twenty, nor more than two hundred dollars, at the discretion of any court of competent jurisdiction.

Sec. 5. This Act to take effect and be in force from and after its passage."

The New Hampshire law requires that

"Every apothecary, druggist, or *other person*, who shall sell any arsenic, corrosive sublimate, nux vomica, strychnia, or prussic acid, shall make a record of such sale in a book kept for that purpose, specifying the kind and quantity of the article sold, and the time when, and the name of the person to whom such sale is made, which record shall be open to all persons who may wish to examine the same."

The other sections exempt physicians' prescriptions, and provide a penalty of $100 for the violation of the first section. Mr. Edward H. Parker of Concord, N. H., in giving this information states, that the law is almost if not entirely ineffectual, and that not more than *one* in five of the druggists pretend to keep such a record, and some are not even aware of its existence. The effect has been to confine the sale of poisons to the druggist, as "grocers and shopkeepers rarely, if ever, retail arsenic or other poisons specified in this law."

While in New York—

"Every apothecary, druggist, or other person, who shall sell or deliver any arsenic, corrosive sublimate, prussic acid, or any other substance or liquid usually denominated *Poisonous*, without having the word "poison" written or printed npon a label attached to the phial, box, or parcel, in which the same is sold; or who shall sell and deliver any tartar emetic, without having the true name thereof written or printed upon a label attached to the phial, box, or parcel containing the same, shall, upon conviction, be adjudged guilty of a misdemeanor, and shall be punished by a fine not exceeding one hundred dollars."

It would appear from the statements of the Committees that an immense quantity of strychnia is used in this country, though we have never heard that it was used to adulterate beer. Besides the quantity imported, it is stated that between five and six thousand ounces are annually manufactured from about 120,000 lbs. of nux vomica. One manufacturer in Philadelphia alone made 1,840 ounces from 40,000 of the vomica nut, in the year ending June 3rd. According to Mr. G. L. Simmons, of Sacramento, California, large quantities of strychnia are used in that new State, chiefly for the destruction of noxious animals.

The reports of the different colleges on the state of pharmacy in their respective States are contained in an appendix. These reports are necesarily exceedingly imperfect, though they contain much interesting information. We have not space, however, to make any extracts from them.

On the whole, the "Proceedings," largely owing to the energy and industry of Mr. Procter, are valuable, and calculated to exert a beneficial influence. We have to regret the comparatively small number of delegates in attendance, and the partial manner in which the different States were represented. Thirty-eight members were present. Of these, three were from Pennsylvania, all from Philadelphia; four from the City of New York; nineteen from Massachusetts, of whom sixteen were from Boston, and one each from Lowell, Newburyport, and Fitchburg; three from Virginia, all from Richmond; two from Cincinnati, Ohio; two from Vermont; and one each from Connecticut, Tennessee, Maine, Indiana, and New Hampshire. The selection of eminent druggists, residing in different States, as correspondents, made by the Convention, according to a Provision of the Constitution, will go far to remedy this effects, and to extend the influence of the Convention.

NEW YORK

# JOURNAL OF PHARMACY.

DECEMBER, 1853.

## ON THE ALKALOIDS OF THE CINCHONAS.

BY L. PASTEUR.

It is about half a century since *cinchonine*, previously noticed by Dr. Duncan of Edinburgh, was first isolated by Gomès, a physician of Lisbon. To its presence he attributed the action of the cinchona barks; but he misunderstood its alkaline nature, which was not thoroughly appreciated until about 1820 by MM. Pelletier and Caventou; at this period these chemists also discovered *quinine*. About twelve years afterwards, two other French chemists recognized a third alkaloid, to which they gave the name of *quinidine*, in the yellow jesuit's bark. In the year 1829, Sertuerner, who had already become celebrated by his discovery of morphine, pointed out the existence, in the mother-waters, of sulphate of quinine, of an uncrystalizable base, which he called *quinoidine*, and to which he attributed wonderful febrifuge properties.

The general properties of quinine and cinchonine are pretty well known; but with regard to quinidine and quinoidine, the most contradictory opinions prevail. I believe I have got rid of all the difficulties. The results of my labors also exhibit quite new molecular relations between the various alkaloids of these barks. The following are the new facts at which I have arrived.

1. *Cinchonicine.*—When cinchonine in any saline combination is exposed to the action of heat, it is converted into a new base isomeric with, but quite distinct from cinchonine. I call it *cinchonicine.* All the salts of cinchonine may serve for the preparation of cinchonicine; but in order that the conversion may be easily and completely effected, it is necessary to place the salt in certain conditions. In general, when salts of cinchonine are heated, they fuse and become decomposed immediately; and if the fusion of the salt be not effected by some means at a temperature sufficiently distant from the point of decomposition, the cinchonicine will certainly be formed, but destroyed immediately by the further action of the heat. Ordinary sulphate of cinchonine for instance, when heated directly, becomes fused and then immediately destroyed, furnishing a fine red resinous matter, which is the product of the alteration of cinchonicine. But if a little water and sulphuric acid be added to the sulphate before subjecting it to the action of heat, it remains fused even after the expulsion of all the water at a low temperature; and it is sufficient to keep it in this state at a temperature of 248°–266° F. for three or four hours, to convert it entirely into sulphate of cinchonicine. The production of coloring matter is very trifling, nearly inappreciable.

I prove, by facts which will be accepted by all chemists, that if heat plays a great part in this transformation of cinchonine, the vitreous, resinoid state of the product has a certain influence; and the present case of isomerism certainly related to those metamorphoses, of which mineral chemistry offers us several examples, such as soft sulphur, red phosphorus, and vitreous arsenious acid.

2. *Quinicine.*—All that has been stated in the preceding section with regard to cinchonine applies equally to quinine. Any salt of this base, heated in the same manner as the salt of

cinchonine, is also converted into a new base isomeric with quinine. I call this new base *quinicine*. The most convenient mode of preparing it consists in adding a little water and sulphuric acid to the sulphate of quinine of commerce, and exposing it to the heat of an oil-bath of 248°–266 F. for three or four hours; the salt remains fused even after the expulsion of all the water, and becomes completely converted into sulphate of quinicine, with a very minute production of coloring matter.

As regards the general properties of cinchonicine and quinicine, they offer well-marked analogies with the isomeric bases from which they are derived. They especially present the greatest resemblance to one another. Both of them are nearly insoluble in water, but very soluble both in absolute and ordinary alcohol. They both combine readily with carbonic acid, and expel ammonia from its saline combinations in the cold. They are both precipitated from their solutions in the form of fluid resins in the same manner as quinine under certain circumstances. They both deviate the plane of polarization to the right. They are very bitter and febrifuge.

3. *Quinidine.*—The contradictions to be met in the works of chemists with regard to this substance all arise from a fact which has escaped them, namely, that under the name of quinidine two very distinct alkaloids have been confounded; these are nearly constantly associated by mixture in commercial quinidine, if it has not been purified by several successive crystallizations. Thus the quinidine discovered in 1833 by Henry and Delondre is quite a different thing from that which is now called by that name in Germany and France, and the German product is very often mixed in considerable proportion with that discovered by Henry and Delondre. All the details of the properties and composition of these two quinidines will be found in my memoir. I will only add, that one of them, for which I retain the name of *quinidine*, is hydrated, efflorescent, *isomeric with quinine*, deviates the plane of polarization to the right, and possesses, like quinine, the character

of acquiring a green color by the successive addition of chlorine and ammonia; whilst the other, to which I give the name of *cinchonidine*, is anhydrous, *isomeric with cinchonine*, exercises a rotary power to the left, and does not exhibit the green coloration. This is now the most abundant of the two in commercial samples. It is always very easy, by exposing a recent crystallization of cinchonidine to warm air, to ascertain whether it contains any quinidine. All the crystals of the latter base effloresce immediately, retaining their shape, and standing out of a dead white amongst the clear crystals of cinchonidine. We may also recur to the character of the green coloration by chlorine and ammonia.

There are consequently four principal alkalies in the cinchona barks, quinine, quinidine, cinchonine, and cinchonidine.

4. *Action of Heat on Cinchonine and Cinchonidine.*—I have submitted the two new bases quinidine and cinchonidine to the moderate action of heat, as I had done with quinine and cinchonine, and with exactly the same results; that is to say, the two new bases are converted into isomeric bases, weight for weight, with the same facility and under the same conditions as quinine and cinchonine. But, moreover, and this is undoubtedly one of the most important facts in this investigation, the two new bases obtained by the transformation of quinidine and cinchonidine are identical, the first with quinicine and the second with cinchonicine. In this manner we arrive at this remarkable result, that of the four principal bases contained in the cinchona barks, namely, quinine, quinidine, cinchonine and cinchonidine, the first two can be converted, weight for weight, into a new base, quinicine, which proves that they are themselves isomeric, whilst the two others are converted under the same conditions into a second base, cinchonicine, which proves that they are also isomeric.

The molecular relations, to which these results call the attention of chemists, take a new character when we compare the rotary powers of the six preceding alkalies. Quinine deviates to the right, quinidine to the left—both to a considerable extent. Quinicine deviates to the right, but to a very small extent compared with the rotary powers of the two others. The same relations are presented by the three other isomeric bodies, cinchonine, cinchonidine, and cinchonicine. Cinchonine deviates to the right, cinchonidine to the left, both considerably; cinchonicine, on the contrary, produces very slight deviation to the right. The most logical interpretation of these results is the following:—The molecule of quinine is double, formed of two active bodies, one which deviates considerably to the left, and the other very slightly to the right. The latter, which is permanent under the influence of heat, resists isomeric transformation, and remaining without alteration in the quinicine, gives this its feeble deviation to the right. The other group, which on the contrary is very active, becomes inactive when the quinine is heated so as to become converted into quinicine; so that quinicine is nothing but quinine in which one of the active constituent groups has become inactive. Quinicine would also be quinidine in which one of the active constituent groups had become inactive; but in quinidine this very active group would be right instead of left as in quinine, but still united with the same slightly active right group, which being permanent remains in the quinicine, and gives it its weak right deviation. I might repeat all that I have said word for word, applying it to cinchonine, cinchonidine and cinchonicine, which are respectively constituted like their three congeners; they offer exactly the same relations.

5. *Quinoidine.*—I shall not enter into the detail of the experiments which I have undertaken upon quinoidine; but there is one point to which I wish to call the attention of manufacturers of sulphate of quinine and of the companies who collect the barks of cinchonas in America. Quinoidine is always a product of the alteration of the alkalies of the cinchonas. It has two distinct origins. It is produced in the operations for the manufacture of sulphate of quinine, and especially in the forests of the New World, when the wood-cutter, after stripping the bark from the tree, exposes it to the sun to dry it.

Then the salts of quinine, cinchonine, &c. contained in the bark, become converted into resinous and coloring matters, which form the greater part of the quinoïdine of commerce. I have ascertained, in fact, that when a salt of quinine or cinchonine in a dilute or concentrated solution is exposed to the sun even for a few hours, it becomes changed to such an extent that the liquid acquires an extremely dark reddish-brown color. This change, moreover, is of the same nature as that which is effected by the influence of an elevated temperature. I believe, therefore, that considerable loss of quinine, cinchonine, &c. would be avoided, and that the extraction of these bases would be rendered more easy, if the bark was shaded from the light when collected, and dried in the shade. The manufacturer of quinine ought also to avoid the action of a bright light.—*Comptes Rendus*, from *Chem. Gazette*, Sept. 1, 1853.

---

## ON TRUE AND FALSE CREASOTE.

BY GORUP-BESANEZ.

Creasote has been seldom the object of scientific investigation since its discovery. The consequence is, that our knowledge of this interesting body remains very imperfect. Indeed, as great a confusion has prevailed as with phenylic acid, a body whose properties exhibit so great an agreement with those of creasote as to give rise to the belief that they were both identical, and that the difference only depended upon some accidental impurities. This is the view which has been more and more developed amongst chemists, and found an important support in the fact that the substance mostly found at present in commerce under the name of creasote, is nothing else than impure phenylic acid, and is obtained from coal tar, which can be easily proved by the determination of its boiling point, and its behavior to chloride of iron, &c.

The creasote which I examined was obtained from Batka, of Prague, who prepares it extensively from wood tar, particularly from that of the beech wood. Its characteristics and general behavior agree completely with the description given of creasote by Reichenbach, its discoverer. It is an oily, strongly refracting, slightly yellowish fluid, of a penetrating, disagreeable, smoky, peculiar odor, totally distinct from phenylic acid. It tastes burning sharp; produces on the mucous membrane of the tongue a white film. In spirit and ether it is completely soluble; in water little; yet, when shaken with water, it communicates its taste and odor, as well as its reactions. In sulphuret of carbon it is entirely soluble; on the contrary, only partly so in acetic acid. In solution of ammonia it is likewise soluble, and somewhat colors it, but on the water bath all the ammonia is evolved. Muriatic acid produces no change; on the contrary, it mixes with concentrated sulphuric acid completely, and assumes a purple, violet color. A splinter of pine wood moistened with muriatic acid assumes, when immersed, not the slightest trace of a blue or a violet color, and chloride of iron, free from oxygen, produces not the least blue violet coloration, which this reagent does in very dilute solutions of phenylic acid. Nor could I obtain it crystallized, although completely deprived of water, when I repeatedly exposed it to low temperatures. The specific gravity of the crude product ranged between 1,046 and 1,049. By the observation of its behavior in high temperatures, with reference to its boiling point, the following results were obtained: At 194° Fahr. slight ebullition took place. After a deposit had exhibited itself on the neck of the retort, between 140° and 158°, and a milky turbid fluid had began to pass over, consisting of water with a very fetid oil of a lower specific gravity than the water, the boiling proceeded with a continued elevation of the thermometer, and became stronger at 320°, but then almost ceased. The liquid passing over between 248° and 325° was now clear, and possessed a peculiar odor, differing from the crude products. At 390° the boiling was again stronger, and now a body distilling in oily streaks passed over rapidly, while the thermometer rose to 398°, and now remained some time stationary; after which, it rose slowly to 406°, and then until its last portion was distilled over to 421°.

These relations show, what could scarcely have been previously doubted, that the crude product was a mixture of several compounds. The circumstances that the greater portion passed over at a temperature between 397° and 406°, and that the thermometer remained some time stationary at this temperature, which is given in works of chemistry as the boiling point of creasote, show that this portion is the chief constituent of the crude material.

The next object was, therefore, the pure preparation and isolation of the creasote. For this purpose a large quantity of the crude product was distilled, and that passing over between 397° and 406° was intercepted. This was now rectified, and allowed then to stand in a closed vessel for a day over fused chloride of calcium, and, lastly, a third time rectified. Here it was observed that the thermometer remained standing for a time at 397°, but it always rose during the distillation, if even slowly. The product purified in this way was subjected to elementary analysis, with the following per centage results:

| | 1 | 2 | 3 | 4 | 5 | 6 | 7 | 8 |
|---|---|---|---|---|---|---|---|---|
| Carbon.... | 75,32 | 75,72 | 75,54 | 74,76 | 75,82 | 75,02 | 74,78 | 74,68 |
| Hydrogen.. | 7,84 | 7,94 | 7,85 | 7,95 | 7,98 | 7,95 | 7,98 | 7,84 |
| Oxygen.... | 16,84 | 16,34 | 16,61 | 17,29 | 16,30 | 17,03 | 17,24 | 17,48 |
| | 100,00 | 100,00 | 100,00 | 100,00 | 100,00 | 100,00 | 100,00 | 100,00 |

The properties of the creasote purified in the above way, by fractional distillation, were the following: Colorless, oily, not or only a little acid, after a long time becoming dark, strongly refracting light, of a peculiar penetrating smoky odor, and biting, burning taste, of 1,040 specific gravity at 52° Fahr., not crystallizable, and also remaining fluid at very low temperatures, in water little soluble, in spirit and ether, and sulphuret of carbon soluble in all proportions. Only partly dissolved by ordinary acetic acid. Dissolves sulphur, and coagulates albumen. Kills animals, in doses of 5 to 10 drops, in a few minutes' time, with convulsions. Preserves meat and animal substances in general.

From these properties and others, there can be no doubt that the body examined by me is very different from phenylic acid, and that it is the same body, namely, true creasote, which has been described by Reichenbach and Ettling.

Another question is, whether this body is a completely pure chemical compound; whether it is to be regarded as a chemical individuum. That in creasote such a chemical individuum exists there can be no doubt, only it appears to be mixed therein with a small quantity of a body, differing in its carbon contents, but equal in its hydrogen contents. The peculiarities already pointed out respecting the boiling point of the pure product, renders this manifest above all things.

In conclusion, I will offer a practical remark. When it is desirable in commerce to distinguish whether a substance sold for creasote is carbolic or phenylic acid, or whether it is adulterated with this body, the boiling point perfectly affords the safest conclusion. But much simpler, and quite as certain, is to test the suspected fluid with chloride of iron, and ordinary acetic acid. In the presence of carbolic acid, chloride of iron causes always a blue violet coloration, and afterwards a whitish turbidity; and acetic acid completely dissolves carbolic acid, in a gentle heat. Creasote prepared from beech-wood tar is not changed by chloride of iron, and is only partly dissolved by ordinary acetic acid in the heat. To those accustomed to the odor of real creasote, the odor of the false will be a sufficient guide.

Whether in wood tar, and generally among the products of the dry distillation of wood, carbolic acid is contained, was by an extensive research of this nature principally to be learned. In tar water, obtained by the digestion of three pounds of beech-wood tar, with eighteen pounds of water, I could detect readily creasote, but not phenylic acid.—*Liebig's Annalen.*

# NEW TEST FOR QUININE.

BY A. VOGEL.

Some time since I made known a new reaction on sulphate of quinine, which consisted in this: that a solution of sulphate of quinine, mixed with chlorine water, assumed a dark red coloration upon the addition of a concentrated solution of ferrocyanide of potassium. Recently, Fresenius has asserted that this reaction is not established. This was to me surprising, as I have repeatedly exhibited this reaction in my lectures, and have had much practical experience with it without once miscarrying. Although, consequently convinced of the correctness of my observation, I have nevertheless, again undertaken the subject, to be able to learn the relations which have caused the failures in other hands. Believing that error lay in the quinine itself, I have examined several kinds of quinine derived from various sources, and obtained the reaction with all; the failure of the reaction must, therefore, be sought for in the method. By a series of researches it has been shown that, as was expected, the prevention of success is caused by the constitution of the reagents, the chlorine water, and the ferrocyanide of potassium. The chlorine water must be necessarily concentrated, freshly prepared, and free from muriatic acid. If the solution of ferrocyanide of potassium is not concentrated by solution in the heat, the red coloration appears later, but can be obtained directly, and also with a diluted solution of ferrocyanide of potassium, upon the addition of a few drops of ammonia; the failure also depends upon the quantities of the reagents. Only a proportionately small quantity of the chlorine water must be taken; on the contrary, a large excess of the solution of ferrocyanide of potassium, if it be desirable not to add a little ammonia. I have further remarked, that an aqueous solution of sulphate of quinine is to be preferred to a spirituous one, because the spirituous, when not sufficient chlorine water is present, precipitates the concentrated solution of ferrocyanide of potassium, and the establishment of red coloration is thereby rendered difficult. It needs be scarcely mentioned that the reagents must be applied in the prescribed order, as in any other way no reaction appears.

I now give the following method by which this reaction can be obtained, under all circumstances, by the most inexperienced. Sulphate of quinine is introduced into a test tube, and water poured on it, so that the greater part of the crystals remain undissolved. Some drops of this fluid, which is shaken to retain the sulphate of quinine in suspension, are poured into a watch glass, and so much chlorine water added, that a clear, somewhat yellowish, solution results. The quantity of chlorine water applied depends upon its concentration, and upon the quantity of quinine salt. When into this chlorinated quinine solution finely pulverized ferrocyanide of potassium is introduced, it acquires a bright rose-red color. The rose-red color passes over soon, and particularly rapidly, if still more of the pulverized ferrrocyanide be added, into a deep dark-red. By this method, the failure of this reaction is entirely removed, and the research may be in such way quite as easily and certainly conducted as the well-known reactions on strychnine with chromic acid, or with peroxide of lead and sulphuric acid.—*Annalen der Chemie.*

---

## ON THE PREPARATION OF CHROME YELLOW.

BY RIOT AND DELLISSE.

For some time, this pigment has been adulterated with as much as 50 per cent. of artificial sulphate of lead. This addition communicates very objectionable properties, for it is then difficult to use, and does not cover well; but it admits of a considerable reduction in the price of the yellow, the pure substance costing 350 francs for 100 kilogrammes, the impure substance but 35 francs for the same quantity. The latter, however, is practically the dearest, for it covers a less surface and the color is less durable.

It is evident that the substance which communicates the color to chrome yellow is the chromic acid, that is likewise what causes its high price; while the cheaper oxide of lead communicates the valuable property of covering well. We therefore proposed to ascertain whether the color of the chrome yellow would remain the same when the proportion of chromic acid, necessary to form chromate of lead, is diminished.

After a number of experiments, we have ascertained that the proportion of chromic acid may be reduced to nearly one half, and that twenty-five parts of neutral chromate of potash, instead of fifty-four parts for one hundred parts of chrome yellow, produced the same color.

It was then necessary to ascertain whether the difference between twenty-five and fifty-four could not be made up by another substance, for instance, oxide of lead or a lead of salt, so that the chrome yellow would be cheaper and at the same time cover well.

We, moreover, endeavored to obtain a bye-product, which in the ordinary way is lost. That method as is well known, consists in dissolving a certain quantity of acetate of lead in warm water, and decomposing it with a solution of neutral chromate of potash, by which means the acetate of potash is obtained in too diluted a state to repay the cost of evaporation.

The process which we adopt is the following: The acetate of lead is dissolved in warm water, the quantity of sulphuric acid necessary to convert the oxide of lead into sulphate is calculated and added; the clear liquid which remains after the precipitate has subsided contains the acetic acid, and may be drawn off and preserved for the preparation of acetate of lead. The sulphate of lead is then washed and treated with a hot solution of neutral chromate of potash, twenty-five parts being used for every seventy-five parts of sulphate of lead. The liquid then contains sulphate of potash, which may be made available, and the precipitate consists of chromate and sulphate of lead.

The product thus obtained covers as well as the pure chrome yellow, and has as good a color, while it is much cheaper.—*Armengaud's Génie Industriel*, April, 1853.

---

## NEW METHODS FOR MANUFACTURING PURE ACETIC ACID.

The decomposition of acetate of lime or lead by means of sulphuric acid has many inconveniences, and there is danger of the product being contaminated with sulphuric acid. Christl* was therefore induced to employ hydrochloric acid as a decomposing agent, and has found that when this acid is not used in excess, the distillate contains scarcely an appreciable trace of chlorine. A mixture of 100 lbs. of raw acetate of lime obtained from the distillation of wood, and containing 90 per cent. of neutral acetate, with 120 lbs. of hydrochloric acid (20° Baumé), is allowed to stand during a night, and then distilled in a copper vessel. The application of heat requires to be gradual, in order to prevent the somewhat thick liquor from running over. The product of acetic acid amounted to 100 lbs. of 8° Baumé; it had a faint yellow color and empyreumatic odour, which may be perfectly removed by treatment with wood-charcoal and subsequent rectification.

In order to obtain the acetate of lime sufficiently pure, Völckel † adopts the following process:—The raw pyroligneous acid is saturated with lime without previous distillation.

---

* Dingler's Polytech. Journal. † Ann. der Chem. und Pharm.

A part of the resinous substances dissolved in the acid are thus separated in combination with lime. The solution of impure acetate of lime is either allowed to stand until it becomes clear or filtered,* then evaporated in an iron pan to about one-half, and hydrochloric acid added until a drop of the cooled liquid distinctly reddens litmus-paper. The addition of acid serves to separate great part of the resin still held in solution, which collects together in the boiling liquid, and may be skimmed off; and likewise decomposes the compounds of lime with kreosote and some other imperfectly known volatile substances, which are driven off by further evaporation. As these volatile substances have little or no action upon litmus-paper, its being reddened by the liquor is a sign that not only are the lime compounds of these substances decomposed, but also a small quantity of acetate of lime. The quantity of acid necessary for this purpose varies, and depends upon the nature of the pyroligneous acid, which is again dependent upon the quantity of water in the wood from which it is obtained. 1.50 litres of wood-liquor require from 4 to 6 lbs. of hydrochloric acid.

The solution of acetate of lime is evaporated to dryness, and a tolerably strong heat applied at last, in order to remove all volatile substances. Both operations may be performed in the same iron pans, but when the quantity of salt is large, the latter may be more advantageously effected upon cast iron plates. The drying of the salt requires great care, for the empyreumatic substances adhere very strongly to the acetate of lime, as well as to the compound of resin and acetic acid mixed with it, and when not perfectly separated, pass over with the acetic acid in the subsequent distillation with an acid communicating to it a disagreeable odor. The drying must therefore be continued until upon cooling the acetate does not smell at all, or but very slightly. It then has a dirty brown color. The acetic acid is obtained by distillation with hydrochloric acid in a still

* A part is distilled off in a copper still in order to obtain wood-spirit.

with copper head and leaden condenser; when proper precautions are taken, the acetic acid does not contain a trace of either metal. The quantity of hydrochloric acid required cannot be exactly stated, because the acetate of lime is mixed with resin, and already formed chloride of calcium. In most instances, ninety or ninety-five parts by weight of acid, 1.16 spec. grav., are sufficient to decompose completely 100 parts of the salt, without introducing much hydrochloric acid into the distillate.

The distilled acetic acid possesses only a very faint empyreumatic odor, very different from that of the raw pyroligneous acid; it is perfectly colorless, and should only become slightly turbid on the addition of nitrate of silver. If the acid has a yellowish color, this is owing to resin having been spirted over in the distillation. It is therefore advisable to remove the resin which is separated on the addition of hydrochloric acid, and floats upon the surface of the liquid, either by skimming or filtration through a linen cloth. The distilled acid has a specific gravity ranging between 1.058 and 1.061, containing upwards of 40 per cent. of anhydrous acetic acid. It is rarely that acid of this strength is required; and as the distillation is easier when the mixture is less concentrated, water may be added before or towards the end of the distillation. Völckel recommends as convenient proportions—

100 parts acetate of lime,
90 to 95 hydrochloric acid,
25 parts water,

which yield from 95 to 100 parts of acetic acid of 1.105 spec. grav. 150 litres of raw pyroligneous acid yield about 50 lbs. of acetic acid of the above specific gravity.

The acid prepared in this way may be still further purified by adding a small quantity of carbonate of soda and redistilling; it is thus rendered quite free from chlorine, and any remaining trace of color is likewise removed. This slight empyreumatic smell may be removed by distilling the acid with about two or three per cent. of acid chromate of potash. Oxide of manganese is less efficacious as a purifying agent.

Although pure acetic acid may be procured by the distillation of vinegar, the whole of the acid cannot be obtained except by distilling to dryness, by which means the extractive substances are burnt, and the distillate rendered impure. In order to obviate this difficulty, Stein* proposes to add 30 lbs. of salt to every 100 lbs. of vinegar; the boiling point is thus raised, and the acid passes over completely.—*Chemical Gazette.*

---

## ON THE GENERAL DISTRIBUTION OF IODINE.

BY STEPHENSON MACADAM.

(*Communicated by the Author.*)

During the last twelve months I have been engaged in a series of experimental researches as to the general distribution of iodine and bromine.

My attention was first drawn to this subject by the announcement recently made by Chatin, that he had detected the presence of iodine in the atmosphere, in rain-water and in snow.

Believing that if iodine were present in the media referred to, its neighbor element (bromine) would be found there too, I was induced to undertake the investigation, partly with the hope of being able to corroborate the results communicated by Chatin in reference to iodine, but principally with a view to determine whether an appreciable quantity of bromine was present in the atmosphere.

Several minor experiments, in the course of which I subjected to examination quantities of air ranging from 150 to 4,000 cubic feet, having given a negative result, so far as the detection of iodine and bromine were concerned, I at length

* Polytech. Centralblatt, 1852, p. 395.

undertook an experiment, during which 100,000 cubic feet of air were transmitted through—

1st. A tube containing slips of starched paper;

2d. A gas-bottle containing iron-filings and water; and

3d. A similar bottle with solution of acetate of lead.

The starched papers and the liquid with iron-filings were intended to retain any *free* iodine, and the lead solution any soluble iodide. At the conclusion of the experiment, and when 625,000 gallons of air had been passed through the arrangement, it was found that the papers were not sensibly altered in tint, and that neither the water in which the iron-filings were suspended, nor the solution of acetate of lead contained the slightest trace of iodine.

I do not purpose to take up the time of the Society by minutely detailing the several steps of the process to which the liquids obtained at this and other parts of the inquiry were subjected; suffice it to say, that in every instance when the final testing of the solution was arrived at, I determined the presence or non-presence of iodine by aid of starch, nitrate of potassa, and hydrochloric acid.

Whilst these experiments on the atmosphere were proceeding, I was examining large quantities of rain-water which had fallen in different districts of Scotland.

In some instances, acetate of lead was simply added to the water, and the whole evaporated to dryness; in other cases, iron-filings were first added, and the liquid, after being agitated with an iron rod, was treated with acetate of lead, evaporated to dryness, and subsequently tested. In no instance, even when employing twelve gallons of water at one time, was there any indication of iodine.

Twelve gallons of water obtained from snow collected in the centre of Edinburgh, also twelve gallons from snow which had fallen in the country (at Pennecuick) ten miles south of that city, and twelve gallons from the neighborhood of Innerleithen, thirty miles south of Edinburgh, were severally treated with iron-filings and acetate of lead, and no iodine was found. The liquids ultimately obtained from the three quantities of snow-water, and which had been used in the starch-testing, were added together, neutralized with an alkali, evaporated to dryness, and carefully charred to decompose the starch; the liquid obtained from this, and which represented thirty-six gallons of snow-water, did not exhibit the slightest indication of the presence of iodine.

In these experiments, I was anxious to employ reagents which were perfectly free from iodine, and therefore refrained from using the fixed alkalies to any extent, although Chatin's papers lead me to believe that they were largely employed by him. The quantity of iodine in potashes seems to decrease by each refinement, but I have never yet encountered a sample of potash in which I did not find iodine when it was sought for. The purest is that obtained by calcining the bitartrate of potash. I have had occasion several times to use small quantities of the alkali thus obtained, and although the presence of iodine could not be detected in two ounces of a strong solution, yet in six ounces a trace was visible.

The negative results of these experiments lead me to believe that in the air, in the rain-water, and in the snow employed by me, there was not an appreciable quantity of iodine.

Before parting with this part of my subject, I may state that I am well aware that several communications have lately been laid before the Academy of Sciences which tend to verify the accuracy of Chatin's results; but one and all of them are objectionable, from the authors having employed potash and other materials, which, there is every reason to believe, would contain iodine originally.

Marchand employed nitrate of silver, hyposulphite of soda, and bicarbonate of potash; Grange, chloroform and caustic potash. Barral, in his late admirable researches on the atmosphere, failed to detect iodine in the rain-water which falls during January, February, March, April and May, but found a very small quantity in that of June. I have not seen a report of the process employed by him, but think it probable that he used the materials derived from some of the nitric acid experiments, and to which he had added caustic potash in order to fix the nitric acid.

So far as regards the process adopted by myself, it is worthy of remark, that Thénard, in commenting upon the researches of Chatin, recommends that the metals most susceptible of being iodized should be exposed for some time to the action of the air. Some months previous to this suggestion being read to the Academy of Sciences, I had used iron and lead in the search for iodine, and ten days prior to the date of Thénard's paper, a report of some of my experiments was published in the *Edinburgh Philosophical Journal*, in which the use of the metals was clearly stated.

Every trial for free iodine was accompanied by a search for bromine, but the result was, in every instance, a negative one, so far as the atmosphere, rain-water and snow are concerned.

Whilst differing from the views expressed by Chatin in reference to the atmospheric distribution of iodine, I very willingly agree with him in considering that this element will be found more generally distributed in the vegetable kingdom than it has formerly been supposed to be. In 45 plants, hitherto unknown to contain iodine, I have discovered that element. Amongst that number, there are representatives from different districts of Scotland, and also different altitudes, from the level of the sea to some 1,600 feet above it.

The determination of the presence of bromine in plants is somewhat more difficult, owing to the tests for that element being much less delicate in their action than the starch-test for iodine.

With the exception of the announcement of the presence of bromine in the ammoniacal liquids of the gas-works, in plants of the family of *Oscillariæ*, growing in thermal waters in the south of France, and a trace in carbonate of potash, I am not aware that the element in question has been shown to be a constituent of inland plants. In the greater number of plants tested by me, not a trace of bromine could be detected; but in potashes, in the ashes of the pear, the gooseberry, and apple-trees, I obtained very distinct evidence of the presence of this element. The tests I relied upon were the odor, the yellow color imparted to ether, and the production (to a greater or less extent) of the brown-red bromide of gold.

The failure which I encountered when testing for bromine in the majority of plants, I am inclined to ascribe to the small quantity of plant ashes which were at my disposal.

In conclusion, I would state that the presence of iodine and bromine in plants, more especially in the edible ones, implies that these substances are introduced into the system of even the highest animal; and though as yet unsuccessful, yet I trust that before long I shall be able to determine the presence of both these elements as normal constituents of the animal frame.—*Quarterly Journal of the Chemical Society.*

---

## ON IODINE REACTIONS.

BY A. OVERBECK.

Chatin and Gaultier de Claubry have, as a result of their recent investigations of the accuracy of the various methods for detecting and separating iodine, given the preference to the starch-test, and recommended for the liberation of the iodine, instead of chlorine or sulphuric acid, either nitric acid or a mixture of nitric and sulphuric acids.

The author states, that from comparative experiments he has found the following process more advantageous:

A little starch or sugar is treated with concentrated nitric acid in a test tube, and heated until a vigorous disengagement of gas commences. The gas which is then disengaged, without any further application of heat, is passed into the liquid to be examined, which has previously been mixed with starch paste. When only one millionth part of iodide of potassium is present, the blue color is immediately produced, and after continued application of the gas the iodide of starch separates in flocks.

By this method the author has detected iodine in the ashes of many plants: for instance, several ranunculaceæ, *ranunculus flammula*, *Ficaria ranunculoides*, &c.

He likewise represents it as possessing a degree of delicacy superior to any other test, and considers that it may be more advantageous, from the circumstance that the danger to be apprehended from the presence of chloride of iodine in the nitric acid* is even less immediate than in the method adopted by Chatin.—*Archiv. der Pharmacie*, February, 1853.

---

## THE SOLUBILITY OF BINIODIDE OF MERCURY IN COD-LIVER OIL.

I find by experiment that *cod-liver oil* possesses the property of dissolving *biniodide of mercury*, and as both are administered at the same time, the medical practitioner will find it convenient when these remedies are required to be given together, to dissolve the biniodide in the oil. Solution is readily effected at the ordinary temperature of the atmosphere to the extent of *half a grain* to the *fluid ounce*, by rubbing down the biniodide in a small portion of the oil, mixing it with the remainder in a bottle, and shaking for a few moments; at the temperature of 50° C. two grains are permanently dissolved by one fluid ounce of oil.

I also find that biniodide of mercury dissolves with the same facility in almond, olive, and castor oils, also in chloroform, pyroxilic spirit, and melted lard and spermaceti cerate.

J. B. BARNES.

1 *Trevor Terrace, Knightsbridge.*

—*Pharmaceutical Journal.*

---

* Böttgher has shown that all (?) strong nitric acid contains iodine in the state of chloride, and therefore considers that Chatin's experiments are not trustworthy.

## NOTES OF ALTERATIONS MADE IN SOME OF THE FORMULA OF U. S. P., 1851.

ACETA.—In these preparations the alcohol is omitted, probably as being unnecessary to their preservation.

ACID. ACETIC. DILUT.—The strength of this is increased from *one to ten* to *one to seven.*

ACID. NITRIC. DILUT.—The strength increased from *one to nine* to *one to six.*

AQUA CAMPHORÆ.—The carbonate of magnesia is increased from *one* to *four* drachms, and in the other waters from *half* to *one* drachm.

CERAT. CALAMIN.—The quantity of calamin and yellow wax are diminished *one-fourth.*

CERATUM CANTHARIDIS.—The proportion of wax, resin and lard are varied from equal parts to *seven* of the two former to *ten* of the latter. The proportion of cantharis the same. I have found the *consistence* of the older formula not all objectionable.

DECOCT. SARSA. CO.—Macerate the ingredients for twelve hours *before* boiling.

EMPLASTR. SAPONIS.—The proportion of soap is diminished one-third.

EXTRACT. CONII.—This is a new admission, and is directed to be evaporated either *in vacuo*, or by a *current of air* (dried?) *directed over the surface.*

EXTRACT. GENTIAN.—"Introduce into an apparatus for displacement" is exchanged for "transfer it to a percolator"—a tribute to elegance of phraseology scarcely to be expected; but when "met with," as it frequently is in the present edition, deserves to be made "a note of." I regret the same critical nicety did not cause the omission of the full length description of the process of percolation, which is appended in all its cumbrousness to the formula of the tinctures, wherever it is thought proper to be used. "Prepare by percolation" would have sufficed and been in better keeping.

EXTRACTA FLUIDA.—It may be said of the fluid extracts of cubebs and black pepper, that they are more properly ethereal oils than fluid extracts. This class of preparations is now first admitted.

TINCT. FERRI CHLORID.—Heat is now directed to be employed; most probably to effect more fully the solution of the subcarbonate of iron.

FERRI ET POTASS. TART—The hydrated oxyde of iron for this is directed to be obtained by the officinal method, instead of the previous complex, and I think not so perfect a manner.

LIQUOR IODID. FERRI.—Sugar is substituted for the honey.

FERRI PHOSPHAS.—In the test directions appended to this formula, the word *in*soluble is substituted for *soluble*—all the difference in the world.

HYDRARG. OXYD.-RUBR.—The quantity of nitric acid is increased from *fourteen* to *eighteen* fluid ounces.

INFUSA.—The duration of the maceration directed for some of these is reduced from *four* to *two* hours; as for instance, infus. buchu—a good general rule is to let them stand till cool.

MEL ROSÆ.—The proportion of rose leaves in this is increased, and the officinal directions rendered more definite.

OXYMEL SCILLÆ.—A pint and a half of honey is substituted for three pounds—a fair exchange.

PIL. CATHART. CO.—The extract of jalap is no longer directed "*in powder*," as formally.

PIL. RHEI CO.—The excipient "syrup of orange peel" is exchanged for "water." The syrup was useful in preventing the mass becoming too hard to admit of being rolled out when wanted for use, and was not objectionable in point of bulk.

POTASSÆ CARBONAS PURUS is now directed to be prepared by calcining bicarbonate of potass instead of by deflagration, as formerly—a very great and proper simplification.

POTASSII CYANURET.—Another simplification, which see!

SPIRITUS.—These preparations are for the most part *reformed*. The process of distillation is omitted, except in one or two instances. "Facilis descensus averni."

SYRUPUS ALLII.—This formula is much *redacted*. The garlic is to be *bruised*, *dilut. acetic acid* used instead of distilled vinegar, and sugar in coarse powder to be dissolved in the liquor by agitation, instead of by "proceeding in the manner directed for syrup."

SYRUP. IPECAC.—There is here an *alteration* without a *difference*, and there is still much room for improvement. This syrup can and should be much stronger.

SYRUP. KRAMERIÆ.—Another formula is added, in which rhatany root is directed instead of extract rhatany. The older formula is also retained secondarily.

SYRUPUS TOLUTAN. ET ZINGIB.—The tinctures of the substances are to be mixed with the sugar, heated to expel the alcohol, and syrupified. The former syrup is much better prepared by the *process* of the London Pharmacopœia.

TINCTURÆ.—There are now *two* officinal tinctures of aconite, viz.. "tinct. aconiti foliorum" instead of the "tinctura aconiti" of the older pharmacopœia, and "tinct. aconiti radicis," which last is *saturated*, and intended chiefly for external use. The distinction deserves to be borne in mind by physician and apothecary, and the old term, "tinctura aconiti," should never be used, but in every case the particular kind designated.

TINCT. CINCHONÆ.—*Yellow bark* is directed for this tincture, while *red bark* is directed for the compound tincture. Why this should be, I do not perceive. Red bark, I think, is best for both.

TINCT. JALAP.—The quantity of jalap is diminished from *eight* to *six* ounces. The previous formula corresponded nearly with the London and Dublin Pharmacopœias, now it does not correspond with any in the language.

TINCT. KINO.—This is a new admission, and is directed to be made by displacement. I fear that by this means it may be rendered more liable to deteriorate. It can be made equally well at least by maceration.

TINCT. SAPON. CAMPH.—A small quantity of water is now directed to be used in this, to prevent, I suppose, the congelation of a part of the soap, which is otherwise apt to take place.

UNG. AQUÆ ROSÆ.—The quantity of rose water is reduced one-half.

UNG. HYDRARG. NITRAT.—The nitric acid is increased from *eleven* to *fourteen* drachms.

UNG. IODINI.—A very small quantity (4 grs. to an oz.) of iodide of potassium is ordered in this, and water substituted for alcohol—quite an improvement.

UNG. STRAMONII.—Directed to be made from the extract instead of the fresh leaves.

VINA.—For these, white wine is specified as tho kind to be used.

ZINCI CARB. PUR.—The *precipitated* is substituted for the *prepared* carbonate, and the latter is exchanged, although ordered in a previous preparation (Turner's cerate). The former is made by decomposing sulphate of zinc with carbonate of soda.

On the whole, there is an improvement in this edition of the Pharmacopœia, quite up to the present *status*; and the chief drawback is to find the work in barbarous Anglo-Saxon instead of the language of science.

---

## EXTRACT OF CAPSICUM.

BY W. C. BAKES.

At the request of a physician of this city, I have been induced to prepare the above extract. Although the Pharmacopœia recognises the infusum capsici, and also the tinctura capsici, yet it is not always convenient to administer a medicine in the form of a liquid; therefore an extract was thought of as being, perhaps, the most convenient to the medical profession. After some experiments, I have found the following formula the most satisfactory:

Take of powdered capsicum, 8 ounces,
dilute alcohol, 1½ pint.

Moisten the capsicum with a sufficient quantity of the dilute alcohol, and set the mixture aside in a close vessel to macerate, for six days; then place it in a percolator, and pour dilute alcohol on it until four pints have been obtained, and evaporate by means of a water bath to the consistence of an extract. I have found eight ounces of the powder to yield two ounces of extract. It is very powerful; and when a small quantity is placed on the tongue, it produces an insupportable burning sensation immediately; and, if left too long, will act as an epispastic. It has been used with success combined with quinine, in cases of intermittent fever, occasioned by the too frequent use of ardent spirits. An ointment made in the following manner:

Take of extract capsicum, 1 drachm,
simple cerate, 1 ounce,

was found to act as a rubefacient in less than twenty minutes. It may be used with success where a simple rubefacient is required.—*Am. Jo. of Pharmacy.*

---

## OVERHEATED STEAM APPLIED TO THE CARBONIZING OF WOOD.

For several years past, overheated steam has been used in numerous industrial operations, and we may say generally that it may be employed in all processes in which a temperature between 100° and 500° C. is required. Among these processes are the extraction of wood-spirit, the continuous baking of bread, the preparation of sea-biscuit, the drying of wood, the preservation of meats, the extraction of volatile substances insoluble in water, the purification of fatty acids by MM. Leplay and Dubrunfaut, the extraction of the mercury from the residues of zinc amalgam, by M. Violette, and finally, the carbonizing of wood, by the same chemist. M. Violette is a member of the Commission on Powder and Saltpetre, and in this situation he has turned his attention to the ingredients of powder, the manufacture of which still admits of much improvement. The charcoal employed in this manufacture is of a quality intermediate between wood and ordinary charcoal (*charbon roux*), and is produced at 300° C.; at a higher temperature it becomes black charcoal, and at a lower the carbonization is incomplete.

By the old process of heating in closed cylinders, 10,000 kilogrammes of wood furnished 2,000 kil. of black charcoal, and 1,300 of red. The new process with steam yields a better article in larger quantity, for 10,000 kil. of wood give 4,000. The wood immersed in the vapor is readily carbonized, and as it is easy to regulate the temperature of the vapor, charcoal may be obtained of a constant and uniform character. It is some years since that overheated steam was first adopted in this process by M. Violette, and now the red charcoal, before employed only for the finest powder, is in general use for the cheaper kinds, so simple and certain is its preparation by means of steam.

M. Violette communicates to the Academy some new results. He shows that the change to charcoal takes place differently with different woods, and that the products of the same temperature differ in elementary constitution. Exposed to moist air, the charcoals absorb more water, the lower the temperature to which they were exposed, and the inverse is true of their power of conducting heat or electricity. Charcoal made at 1500° C. conducts much better than the charcoal of gas retorts, and serves perfectly for electric illumination. The density increases in the same proportion. When lighted, charcoals remain ignited for a time, which decreases as the temperature of carbonization increases. The charcoal made at 260° C. burns more easily and longer; that made between 1000° and 1500° C. will not ignite or burn.

The most inflammable of all charcoals is that of an agaricus. It takes fire spontaneously at 300° C. Other charcoals, prepared at the temperature 300° C., take fire in air spontaneously between 360° and 380°, according to the wood that has afforded them, the charcoals of the lighter woods burning the most readily.

When charcoals are mixed with sulphur, they inflame at a temperature much below that required when alone; the mixture of the two prepared between 150° and 400° C., is wholly consumed at 250° C. On the contrary, when the charcoal employed has been prepared at 1000° or 1500° C., only the sulphur burns.

To decompose saltpetre, the charcoal requires a higher temperature; a heat of 400° C, is needed for charcoals prepared between 150° and 432°, and a red heat for those made between 1000° and 1500°.

Sulphur decomposes saltpetre at a higher temperature than charcoal requires, viz., at 432°. The sulphur alone inflames in common air at 250° C., and not at 150°, as stated in treatises on chemistry.

The deflagration of powder takes place 250°, but its combustibility varies with the charge and the size of the grain. The powder in grain burns between 270° and 320°, while powder pulverized burns between 265° and 270°.

In view of these facts, M. Violette concludes that it is necessary to revise the charges employed, taking into consideration the actual composition of the charcoal. Trials made with this in view upon hunting powder, with charges calculated according to the actual composition of the charcoal, have given a range much beyond the standard rate obtained with the ordinary powder.—*J. Nickles, in Amer. Jour. of Science and Arts, Sept.* 1853.

## ON THE MANUFACTURE OF HUMULINE.

The hops used in the manufacture of humuline, or concentrated extract of hops, are first dried in a stove or oven, heated to 86° Fah., and when brittle, are rubbed through a sieve, the meshes of which are about one-tenth of an inch wide. The coarse powder thus obtained is next placed in a closed cylinder, and as much alcohol is poured on it as the powder will absorb, after which a further quantity is added until a layer af alcohol of the depth of 1½ inch covers the powder. The contents of the cylinder are then submitted to considerable pressure, and allowed to remain in this state for twenty-four hours, after which the alcoholic tincture is run off through a tap in the lower part of the cylinder into a tub or other suitable recipient. Water is then added to the hops in the cylinder until the liquor that passes out through the exit-tap is clear and colorless. This liquor is again added to the hops, and they are macerated in it for forty-eight hours, after which time the hops are again washed with fresh supplies of water, in order to remove all soluble extractive matter. By this process there are obtained an alcoholic tincture holding the essential oil of hops in solution, and an aqueous solution of the principles soluble in water.

To form the humuline, the following process is adopted:—The alcoholic tincture is placed in a suitable still heated by a water-bath, and the alcohol is distilled off, leaving as a residuum the essential oil and a brownish yellow resin, covered with a layer of yellowish liquor some inches in depth, composed of watery extract. This watery extract is then added to the aqueous solution before mentioned, and evaporated by steam heat to the consistence of a soft extract. To this extract the essential oil and resin are next added, and the product thus obtained is humuline.

Another extract is obtained from hops, by placing them either in a powdered or whole state in a closed cylinder, and submitting them to the action of steam. By the partial condensation of the steam a liquid extract of hops is obtained, the watery particles of which may be evaporated until it becomes of the same consistence as the humuline.—*Pharmaceut. Jo.*]

---

## SULPHATE OF QUININE.

A brief statement of a process which has been recently patented by Mr. Edward Herring, for the manufacture of sulphate of quinine, was communicated to the meeting.

The first part of the process consists in treating the bark with a boiling caustic alkali. The powdered bark is boiled with a solution of caustic soda or potash, and then pressed and washed with water until the whole of the coloring matter of the bark has been removed. After being thus treated, the bark, which has been deprived of its coloring matter, retains the greater part of the alkaloids in an uncombined state. The blood-red alkaline liquors resulting from the boiling and washing, which contain a small quantity of quinine, are retained for subsequent treatment. The bark is, in the next place, boiled with dilute sulphuric acid, so as to completely exhaust it of the alkaloids. The liquor is concentrated, filtered, and precipitated with solution of caustic soda or potash. The precipitated alkaloids are combined with sulphuric acid, and the sulphates of quinine, quinidine and cinchonine are separated from each other by repeated crystallization, and previously to the last crystallization are decolorized with pure animal charcoal.

The blood-red alkaline liquors, referred to above, are treated in the following manner:—Muriatic acid is added, so as to render them acid; they are then filtered, and precipitated with slaked lime. This precipitate is washed, pressed, dried and powdered. The alkaloids contained in this precipitate are dissolved out with benzole, and the solution in this menstruum is agitated with dilute sulphuric acid, by which the alkaloids are transferred to the latter, which is afterwards separated by decantation. This acid solution is precipitated with caustic soda or potash, and the alkaloids are treated as described in the former part of the process.

The sample of sulphate of quinine made by this process, which was on the table, was accompanied by a sample from each of the several manufacturers, both English and foreign. They comprised three English, three German, two French, three Italian and two American.—*Pharmaceut. Jo.*

---

## EXPLOSIVE COMPOUNDS.

BY MR. G. WINIWARTER.

No. 1.—Fulminating mercury, 300 parts; chlorate of potash, 288 parts; sulphate of antimony, 312 parts; charcoal and nitre (mixed in the proportion of 16 and 7), 60 parts; ferrocyanide of potassium, 23 parts; binoxide of lead, 6 parts; and etheroxylin, 900 parts.

No. 2.—Fulminating zinc, 75 parts; chlorate of potash, 4 parts; sulphate of antimony, 7 parts; binoxide of lead, 15 parts; ferrocyanide of potassium, 1 part; and etheroxylin, 224 parts.

No. 3.—Amorphous phosphorus, 75 parts; binoxide of lead, 64 parts; charcoal and nitre, 15 parts; and etheroxylin, 106 parts.

The etheroxylin is formed by dissolving 75 parts of gun cotton in 150 parts of sulphuric ether.

# EDITORIAL.

New York Journal of Pharmacy.—With the present number, the journal "published by authority of the College of Pharmacy of the city of New York" terminates. When it again appears—and if the contemplated arrangements are carried out, this will be after the regular monthly interval—the College will no longer be even nominally responsible for its contents or its pecuniary obligations. In looking back on its career, we think our readers will agree that the very moderate engagements entered into upon its commencement have been fulfilled. If, on the one hand, its columns have not received all the assistance which had been anticipated and even promised, on the other, it has met with support from quarters which had not been relied on. Its original articles have been extensively copied both at home and in England, and translations of many of them have appeared in the French and German journals. It has confined itself exclusively to matters of common interest, and its pages have never been used for the personal ends of any man or set of men.

For our successor, our "alter ego," we bespeak a candid and favorable reception; and we hope it may long continue to promote the true end of journalism—the fostering of scientific investigation and the spread of useful knowledge.

---

Citrine Ointment.—Every apothecary knows the difficulty of preparing the unguentum hydrargri nitratis so that it will retain its color and consistence for a length of time. An intelligent apothecary, Mr. R. A. Sands, informs us that he has for a long time prepared the ointment according to the formula of the Dublin College, substituting only a pound of butter, which has been carefully washed to remove the salt, for the olive oil directed in the formula. The acid nitrate of mercury requires to be gently heated before it is mixed with the fatty matter, when the quantity prepared at one time is not greater than that directed by the College. We have seen old ointment prepared in this manner which retained perfectly its soft consistence and fine yellow color.

---

Creasote.—We would call the attention of our readers to the paper of M. Gorup Besanez, republished in our present number. It will be seen that he takes a different view of the subject from that proposed by Mr. Edward Kent.* Both views have the support of eminent authority in their favor. It is important that this matter should be settled, and that if there be a difference in the therapetuic as well as in the chemical properties of carbolic acid, the creasote obtained from coal tar and that obtained from wood tar, and if the former be inferior, that we should have recourse to the old sources of supply. Most, if not all the creasote now sold is carbolic acid; and we have been struck with the fact that it has seemed less efficacious when used for arresting vomiting than that which was found in the city some twelve years ago.

---

* New York Journal of Pharmacy, Vol. II, No. 10, p. 289.

www.ingramcontent.com/pod-product-compliance
Lightning Source LLC
LaVergne TN
LVHW020116110826
845151LV00001B/175

* 9 7 8 1 4 2 5 5 4 2 9 2 4 *